STEDMAN'S
WordWatcher®
1995-1997

STEDMAN'S
WordWatcher®
1995-1997

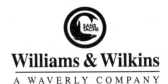

Williams & Wilkins

A WAVERLY COMPANY

BALTIMORE • PHILADELPHIA • LONDON • PARIS • BANGKOK
BUENOS AIRES • HONG KONG • MUNICH • SYDNEY • TOKYO • WROCLAW

Editor
Maureen Barlow Pugh
Williams & Wilkins, Baltimore, MD
Managing Editor
Darla Haberer, CMT
Indexer
Editorial Services
Proofreaders
Barbara Ferretti, Natalie Tyler, Martha Richards, RRA
Manager of Production and Inventory Operations
Martin T. Lannon
Williams & Wilkins, Baltimore, MD
Design
Parkton Art Studio, Inc.
Cover Design
MGP Direct, Inc.

Williams & Wilkins
A WAVERLY COMPANY
351 West Camden Street
Baltimore, MD 21201-2436

1-800-527-5597
410-528-4223 (Outside U.S. and Canada)
www.stedmans.com

STEDMANS

The Best Words in Medicine

NOTICE: DRUG ENTRIES in STEDMAN'S WordWatcher are intended to serve as quick reference to generic and brand names, usage, and dosages. Care has been taken to ensure accuracy; however, due to the nature of clinical trials, research protocols, and pending FDA approval, the editors, advisors, and Publisher cannot be responsible for the continued accuracy and changes in dosage, use, drug name, results of new developments, patient responses, side effects, etc. in new drugs. Further, usual dosage information is based on the stage of investigation and extent of usage of the drug in the general population. This information is not intended to serve as a basis for actual dosage amounts for prescribing purposes. Pharmaceutical company information is provided for further detailed product information.

98 99
1 2 3 4 5 6 7 8 9 10

TABLE OF CONTENTS

Preface

Stedman's WordWatcher has been a unique effort on the part of the Stedman's team. Always concerned with providing up-to-date and accurate medical language information to medical language specialists, we conceived of the idea of a periodical product that would fill the gap between word book and dictionary revisions. To that end, we published eight issues of *Stedman's WordWatcher* between 1995 and 1997.

Each *WordWatcher* issue contained new generic and recently approved brand name drugs and clinical trials; the newest surgical instruments, equipment, devices, and implants; breakthrough surgical operations with related anatomy and equipment; current laboratory tests; and emerging diagnostic procedures. Each issue was designed to be a professional medical language tool, providing precise, accurate, and case-correct information, with concise definitions, descriptions, and even recurring icons for faster lookup.

In *Stedman's WordWatcher 1995-1997*, we have combined all eight issues into one book, integrating all the entries in one easy-to-use A-Z list. Users can also find a term by looking in the cross-referenced A-Z, Specialty, and Topic Indices in the back of the book. This organization of the content makes *Stedman's WordWatcher 1995-1997* your single source for the newest terminology of cutting-edge advances in healthcare.

Like our other Stedman's reference products, *Stedman's WordWatcher* offers an authoritative assurance of quality and exactness to the wordsmiths of the healthcare professions — medical transcriptionists, medical editors and copy editors, health information management personnel, court reporters, and the many other users and producers of medical documentation.

We at Williams & Wilkins strive to provide you with the most up-to-date and accurate word references available. Your use of this book will prompt new editions, which will be published as often as warranted by changing terminology. We welcome your suggestions for improvements, changes, corrections, and additions — whatever will make this *Stedman's* product more useful to you. Please use the postpaid card at the back of this book and send your recommendations care of "Stedmans" at Williams & Wilkins.

Acknowledgments

We are grateful to the editorial advisors, who over the years spent countless hours poring over medical journals, literature, and the Internet, searching for new and exciting terms. A special thank you to Darla Haberer, CMT, who acted as Managing Editor in 1996 and 1997. Thanks also to Barb Ferretti, who played a vital role in many aspects of the publication process.

As with all our *Stedman's* word references, we have benefitted from the suggestions and expertise of our many contacts in the medical transcriptionist community. Thanks to all our reviewers and editors, AAMT meeting attendees, and others who have written in with requests and comments — keep talking, and we'll keep listening.

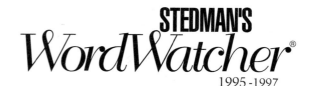

STEDMAN'S
WordWatcher®
1995 -1997

Editorial Advisory Board

abciximab

Brand name
ReoPro

Use
adjunctive agent to aspirin and heparin which may prevent early cardiac ischemic complications associated with percutaneous transluminal coronary angioplasty (PTCA) or directional coronary atherectomy in patients at high risk for abrupt closure of the treated coronary vessel

Usual dosage
intravenous: trial dosage of 0.25 mg/kg bolus followed by a 10 mcg/min infusion

Pharmaceutical company
Centocor Inc. Malvern, PA.

Source
University of Pittsburgh Drug Information and Pharmacoepidemiology Center. Pittsburgh, PA.

 abductory midfoot osteotomy

Description
technique for correction of metatarsus adductus, performed in the lesser tarsal region; enables transverse plane correction of adducted forefoot deformity; uses closing wedge technique to shorten the lateral column and opening wedge technique to lengthen the medial column

Anatomy
midfoot structures; extensor hallucis longus tendon; neurovascular bundle; capsuloperiosteal layer; extensor digitorum brevis muscle; intertarsal joints

Equipment
standard surgery equipment; 1/4-inch Key elevator; Kirschner wire guide; allogeneic or autogeneic bone graft; barbed bone staples; closed-suction drain system

Source
Adapted from Harley BD, Fritzhand AJ, Little JM, Little ER, Nunan PJ. Abductory midfoot osteotomy procedure for metatarsus adductus. The Journal of Foot and Ankle Surgery 1995; 34:153-162.

 Abelcet

Generic name
see amphotericin B lipid complex injection

ABO glycosyltransferase genotyping

Synonyms
none

Use
direct genotypic determination of patient or donor ABO red blood cell types

Method
allele-specific polymerase chain reaction (PCR)

Specimen
blood

Normal range
O1, O2, A1, A2, or B

Comments
particularly useful for prenatal diagnosis and forensic investigations

Source
Adapted from Gassner C, Schmarda A, Nussbaumer W, Schonitzer D. ABO glycosyltransferase genotyping by polymerase chain reaction using sequence-specific primers. Blood 1996;88:1852-1856.

 ## Above-Knee Suction Enhancement system

Description
fabric socks and sheaths with impregnated silicone bands (air seals) in the fabric to sustain suction; addresses residual-limb shrinkage and edema commonly experienced by lower-limb amputees; easy donning and doffing; loose suction sockets for less tissue compression; optimal fit by accommodating residual-limb volume changes

Source
Hypobaric Interfaces product information. Nashua, NH.

 ## acadesine

Brand name
Protara

Use
reduces ischemic damage in coronary artery bypass graft surgery

Usual dosage
intravenous: doses of 5-15 mg as a slow infusion have been used in clinical trials

Pharmaceutical company
Gensia Pharmaceuticals Inc. San Diego, CA.

Source
University of Pittsburgh Drug Information and Pharmacoepidemiology Center. Pittsburgh, PA.

acarbose

Brand name
Precose

Use
hypoglycemic agent investigated as a treatment for hyperlipoproteinemia, obesity, and dumping syndrome

Usual dosage
oral: 50 to 300 mg one to three times daily

Pharmaceutical company
Miles Inc. West Haven, CT.

Source
University of Pittsburgh Drug Information and Pharmacoepidemiology Center. Pittsburgh, PA.

 Accelerator II aspirator

Description
power aspiration unit that is very quiet and vibration free; dual-headed pumps are configured to pull independently against the patient, relieving back pressure and quickly reaching a sustaining, deep vacuum

Source
Byron Medical product information. (*Editor note:* advertising uses byron but company name correctly is Byron) Tucson, AZ.

 Accellon Combi biosampler

Description
cervical cytology collecting device that simplifies Pap smear process so that its fibers contact both exo- and endocervical mucosal surfaces, including critical transformation zone (T-zone); construction prevents intromission high in cervical canal

Source
Medscand Inc. product information. Hollywood, FL.

 Accents system

Description
motorized power unit with many needle styles for cosmetic enhancement and surgical micropigmentation procedures

Source
Newport Medical Products product information. San Luis Obispo, CA.

4

 Accolate

Generic Name
see zafirlukast

 ACCUJET dental needle

Description
disposable dental needle with a red dot to indicate the position of the bevel even when the tip is below the gum line; affords atraumatic anesthetic administration

Source
Astra USA Inc. product information. Westborough, MA.

 Accu-Measure personal body fat tester

Description
device designed to estimate total-body fat by measuring the amount of subcutaneous fat superior to the anterior iliac crest

Source
Accu-Measure Inc. product information. Parker, CO.

 AccuPressure heel cup

Description
reduces congestion of soft tissue to alleviate heel pain, plantar fasciitis, and bursitis; all-purpose boot with breathable, closed toe design provides year-round protection with high-top design and ankle strap to eliminate heel slippage

Source
Darco product information. Huntington, WV.

 Accuratome precurved papillotome

Description
surgical instrument with pre-curve enabling it to resist deformity induced by catheter memory and forces resulting from angulation of endoscope; piggyback needle-knife papillotome can be placed through wire-guided channel of the Accuratome

Source
Wiltek Medical Inc. product information. Winston-Salem, NC.

Accusite

Generic name
see fluorouracil/epinephrine

 Accusway balance measurement system

Description
computer-operated platform for measuring balance; software records center-of-pressure; summarizes data with sway-area, velocity, and frequency calculations

Source
Advanced Mechanical Technology Inc. product information. Watertown, MA.

 ACE Bone Screw Tack

Description
surgical tack made of titanium alloy with a low profile hexed head; shaft is designed with a retention collar and threaded upper shaft for rigid fixation, easy tightening and retrieval of laminar bone and membrane

Source
ACE Dental Implant System product information. Brockton, MA.

 acellular pertussis vaccine

Brand name
Acelluvax

Use
second generation genetically-detoxified pertussis vaccine used to immunize against *Bordetella pertussis* cough

Usual dosage
injectable: 5 µg per 0.5 ml to be given to infants along with diphtheria tetanus (DT) vaccine for 3 doses at age 6-12, 13-20, and 21-28 weeks of age, with 4 to 12 weeks between successive doses

Pharmaceutical company
Chiron Biocine. Emeryville, CA.

Source
Stadtlanders Managed Pharmacy Services. Pittsburgh, PA.

 Acelluvax

Generic name
see acellular pertussis vaccine

acemannan

Brand name
Carrisyn

Use
for the treatment of ulcerative colitis

Usual dosage
oral: 400 mg four times per day

Pharmaceutical company
Carrington Laboratories. Irving, TX.

Source
Stadtlanders Managed Pharmacy Services. Pittsburgh, PA.

 Ace/Normed osteodistractors

Description
bi-directional and multi-directional distractors for craniomaxillofacial callus distraction; allows for transverse movement for distraction in all planes

Source
Ace Surgical Supply Co. product information. Brockton, MA.

 acitretin

Brand Name
Soriatane

Use
retinoid used in the treatment of psoriasis, various nonpsoriatic dermatoses, and cutaneous lupus erythematosus

Usual Dosage
oral: initial doses of 25 mg or 50 mg once daily then adjusted upon efficacy and toxicity

Pharmaceutical company
Roche Laboratories. Nutley, NJ.

Source
University of Pittsburgh Drug Information and Pharmacoepidemiology Center. Pittsburgh, PA.

 Acorn II nebulizer

Description
provides effective delivery of aerosolized medication, i.e., Pulmozyme at nominal flow rates for better patient tolerance; hand-held or used for in-line ventilator treatments for cystic fibrosis

Source
Marquest Medical Products Inc. product information. Englewood, CO.

acquisition zoom magnification

Synonyms
none

Indications
for fluoroscopy and angiography in infants and children undergoing diagnostic cardiac catheterization; helps limit radiation exposure

Method
catheterization is performed; acquisition zoom technology allows use of lower dose 23-cm field of view; images digitally magnified during acquisition

Normal findings
not applicable

Comments
none

Source
Adapted from Ross RD, Joshi V, Carravallah DJ, Morrow WR. Reduced radiation during cardiac catheterization of infants using acquisition zoom technology. The American Journal of Cardiology 1997;79:691-693.

Acra-Cut blade

Description
reversible spiral craniotomy blade used during neurosurgical procedures

Source
Acra-Cut product information. Acton, MA.

acrivastine/pseudoephedrine

Brand name
Semprex-D

Use
antihistamine with decongestant used for allergic rhinitis and urticaria

Usual Dosage
oral: 8 mg acrivastine and 60 mg pseudoephedrine three times daily have been used

Pharmaceutical company
Burroughs Wellcome. Research Triangle Park, NC.

Source
University of Pittsburgh Drug Information and Pharmacoepidemiology Center. Pittsburgh, PA.

AcrySof intraocular lens

Description
acrylic, foldable, ultraviolet absorbing, and silicone-free intraocular lens

Source
Alcon Surgical Inc. product information. Fort Worth, TX.

Acthrel

Generic name
see corticorelin ovine triflutate

 Actifoam hemostat

Description
physiologically active, 100% collagen foam hemostat that potentiates a patient's natural clotting; easy to handle; readily adheres to tissue and easily removed; can be cut and/or sutured

Source
MedChem Products Inc. product information. Woburn, MA.

 Actifoam hemostat sponge

Description
collagen hemostatic sponge with foam agent that adheres to tissue easily; potentiates natural clotting

Source
MedChem Products Inc. product information. Woburn, MA.

 Action traction system

Description
indicated for muscle spasms, chronic low back pain, myofascial restrictions, some degenerative disk disease, bulging annulus, and contained herniated nucleus pulposus; combines traction and low-stress exercises

Source
Staodyn Inc. product information. Longmont, CO.

 Actiq

Generic name
see fentanyl citrate

 activated protein C resistance

Synonyms
APC; resistance activated protein C; RAPC

Use
identify etiology of recurrent thrombosis

Method
partial prothrombin time (PPT) performed with and without addition of activated protein C (APC); reference range is the ratio of the two

Specimen
blood
Normal range
APC ratio greater than 2
Comments
none
Source
Lexi-Comp Inc. database. Hudson, OH.

 Activa tremor control system

Description
electrode device implanted into the thalamus (deep in the brain) to reduce essential tremor in some patients with Parkinson disease; connected by lead wire under skin to pulse generator implanted in the chest; to turn stimulator off and on the patient touches a hand-held magnet over the pulse generator; generator battery life is three to five years
Source
Medtronic Corp. product information. Minneapolis, MN.

 Act joint support

Description
consists of knee, ankle and elbow performance supports; unlike neoprene, the Act products support the joints with a controlled compression that greatly improves proprioception
Source
Bauerfeind USA Inc. product information. Kennesaw, GA.

 Actonel

Generic name
see risedronate

 Acu-Ray x-ray unit

Description
XMA Acu-Ray portable x-ray unit provides shorter exposure time with up to 300 pre-programmed techniques
Source
X-Ray Marketing Associates Inc. product information. Romeoville, IL.

Acuson transducer

Description

transesophageal echocardiography (TEE) V5M transducer features variable speed rotation and 1-hand articulation with 3.5, 5, and 7 mHz frequencies

Source

Acuson Corp. product information. Mountain View, CA.

 ## AcuTrainer bladder retraining device

Description

hand-held electronic device assists patients with urge incontinence; records patient's activity and reminds them when to void with subtle beep or vibration

Source

UroSurge Inc. product information. Coralsville, IA.

 ## adapalene

Brand name

Differin

Use

treatment of acne vulgaris (facial acne)

Usual dosage

topical: 0.1% solution; to be applied topically once daily

Pharmaceutical company

Galderma. Fort Worth, TX.

Source

Stadtlanders Managed Pharmacy Services. Pittsburgh, PA.

 ## Adjusta-Wrist splint

Description

limits range of motion while keeping thumb and fingers free for functional tasks; used for arthritis, postoperative conditions, post-cast management, and adjunct to soft tissue contracture management

Source

Fred Sammons Inc. product information. Western Springs, IL.

"adoptable" baby cholangioscope

Description
small prototype Pentax cholangioscope that can be passed through a standard therapeutic duodenoscope; large-diameter duodenoscope ("mother and daughter scopes") no longer necessary for endoscopic retrograde cholangiopancreatography (ERCP)

Source
Pentax Precision Instrument Corp. product information. Orangeburg, NY.

 ## Advanced Surgical suture applier

Description
surgical device for laparoscopic procedures; consists of a pre-tied suture knot and removable introducer sheath; surgeon has ability to control suture tension independent of tying knot

Source
Advanced Surgical Inc. product information. Princeton, NJ.

 ## Advanced ultrasonography (AU3 and AU4) ultrasound units

Description
high-resolution imaging and ultra-sensitive Dopplers; AU3 color version for penile flow studies, impotency studies, prostatic exams, and cardiology; AU4 high-performance general imaging, i.e., radiology

Source
Biosound Inc. product information. Indianapolis, IN.

 ## Advent pachymeter

Description
instrument measures cornea with ultrasound; user maintains visualization through microscope and hears measurement values as taken; gives normal values for cornea or radial keratotomy procedures and lamellar values

Source
Mentor O & O Inc. product information. Santa Barbara, CA.

Aerosol Cloud Enhancer (ACE)

Description
metered-dose inhaler/spacer permits use in routine, oral inhalation as well as vent circuit, in conjunction with an endotracheal airway or resuscitation bag, and with an incentive spirometer; cone-shaped chamber maximized respirable volume while its clarity allows for easy confirmation of prescribed dose

Source
Diemolding Healthcare Division product information. Canastota, NY.

 AeroSonic personal ultrasonic nebulizer

Description
nebulizer unit that produces a therapeutic mist of highly concentrated, uniformly-sized particles that penetrate deeply into the lungs

Source
DeVilbiss Health Care Inc. product information. Somerset, PA.

 a-Fix cannula seal

Description
surgical device that securely maintains cannula position; unique "boot" allows full range of instrument maneuverability; seal placed around trocar and fixed to skin of patient with hypo-allergenic adhesive

Source
Advanced Surgical Inc. product information. Princeton, NJ.

 5-Agent Poet IQ monitor

Description
analyzes content of anesthetic gases being administered; automatically identifies presence and concentration of up to five different anesthetic agents given simultaneously; monitors oxygen and carbon dioxide on a breath-by-breath basis

Source
Criticare Systems Inc. product information. Milwaukee, WI.

 Aggrastat

Generic name
see tirofiban

Ahmed glaucoma valve implantation

Description
The Ahmed implant is an aqueous shunting device with valve designed to prevent postoperative hypotony; consists of elastomer membranes pretensioned to open and close in response to changes in intraocular pressure; venturi-shaped chamber uses Bernoulli principle to help drain aqueous humor from eye; a human donor scleral graft is placed over the tube and sutured to sclera; conjunctiva reapposed with absorbable sutures; intraocular pressure reasonably approximated by a gaussian distribution

Anatomy
anterior chamber; aqueous humor; choroid; conjunctiva; conjunctival space; corneal endothelial surface; corneoscleral limbus; fornix; iris plane; pars plana; recti muscles; suprachoroidal area; Tenon space

Equipment
standard ophthalmic surgery equipment; Ahmed glaucoma valve implant; 22- or 23-gauge needle; viscoelastic solutions

Source
Adapted from Coleman AL, Hill R, Wilson MR, Choplin N, Kotas-Newmann R, Tam M, Bacharach J, Panek C. Initial clinical experience with the Ahmed glaucoma valve implant. American Journal of Ophthalmology 1995;120:23-30.

 # AIDS vaccine glycoprotein 120 (gp 120)

Brand name
Remune

Use
gp 120-depleted inactivated HIV-1 vaccine for use in preventing HIV infection

Usual dosage
injectable: 100 µg doses every three months is currently studied in clinical trials

Pharmaceutical company
Genentech Inc. South San Francisco, CA.

Source
Stadtlanders Managed Pharmacy Services. Pittsburgh, PA.

 # AIDS vaccine (rgp 160)

Brand Name
VaxSyn

Use
recombinant HIV-1 envelope glycoprotein vaccine for use in preventing HIV infections

---

14

Usual Dosage
intramuscularly: dose varies in clinical trials; 160-640 µg at 0, 1, 6, and 12 months were used in some trials while 50 µg at 0, 1, 2, and 5 months or at 0, 1, 2, 3, and 4 months were used in others.

Pharmaceutical company
MicroGeneSys. Meriden, CT.

Source
University of Pittsburgh Drug Information and Pharmacoepidemiology Center. Pittsburgh, PA.

Aire-Cuf tracheostomy tube

Description
the traditional air-filled cuff design and all silicone construction decrease bacterial adhesions to tube; built-in swivel connector; low trauma tip

Source
Bivona Medical Technologies product information. Gary, IN.

Airlife cannula

Description
oxygen cannula available with flared or nonflared tips; angulated, flexible lip plate offers comfort at the tip of the nasal region

Source
Baxter Healthcare Corp. product information. Round Lake, IL.

Airlife MediSpacer

Description
provides a combination of dual valves and an efficient holding chamber that helps achieve accurate dosing; assists the patient in overcoming any coordination difficulties; allows the patient to tidal breathe through the device more easily; accurately and consistently dispenses medication in the holding chamber; aids in lung deposition

Source
Baxter Healthcare Corp. product information. Round Lake, IL.

AirLITE support pad

Description
sealed air support pad and durable contoured foam to enhance positioning, comfort, and support

Source
Crown Therapeutics Inc. product information. Belleville, IL.

air plethysmograph (APG)

Description
noninvasive diagnostic tool that quantifies the physiological components of chronic venous disease; measures true blood volume changes in milliliters and blood flow in milliliters per second; senses pressure changes in a large cuff that extends from knee to ankle

Source
ACI Medical product information. San Marcos, CA.

 Airprene hinged knee support

Description
"breathable" lining support gives more comfort than ordinary material; provides superior compression and muscle stability; hinged stainless steel side bars provide increased support

Source
Fred Sammons Inc. product information. Western Springs, IL.

 AkroTech mattress

Description
features kinetic rotation modalities for support and treatment of tissue trauma secondary to patient immobility

Source
Lumex product information. Bay Shore, NY.

 alar rim excision

Description
correction of thickened nasal rim; done in conjunction with standard rhinoplasty to correct internal nasal deformities

Anatomy
nose; nasal rim; nasal sill; nasal skin; alar base; alar cartilage; alar crease; alar groove; alar rim; vestibule; vestibular mucosa; vestibular skin; levator labii superioris; caput angular muscle; pars alaris musculi nasalis; depressor septi nasi; zygomaticus

Equipment
standard surgery equipment; intranasal packing; Telfa gauze; Aquaplast splint

Source
Adapted from Matarasso A. Alar rim excision: a method of thinning bulky nostrils. Plastic and Reconstructive Surgery 1996;97:828-834.

albendazole

Brand name
Albenza

Use
antihelminthic; for the treatment of malignant lesions (neurocysticercosis and hydatid diseases) caused by cyst-forming tapeworms, *Echinococcus multilocularis*

Usual dosage
oral: 400 mg twice a day

Pharmaceutical company
SmithKline Beecham. Philadelphia, PA.

Source
Stadtlanders Managed Pharmacy Services. Pittsburgh, PA.

 Albenza

Generic name
see albendazole

 albumin human 5% sonicated

Brand name
Albunex

Use
ultrasound microspheres/ultrasound contrast cardiac imaging agent for use with two-dimensional echocardiography

Usual dosage
intravenous: for left heart studies, the initial recommended dose is 0.08 ml/kg. A second dose of up to 0.22 ml/kg may be given; for right heart studies, the initial recommended dose is 2.0 ml; Albunex must be infused at a rate not to exceed 1 ml/sec; the total procedural dose should not exceed 0.30 ml/kg

Pharmaceutical company
Mallinckrodt Medical Inc. St. Louis, MO.

Source
University of Pittsburgh Drug Information and Pharmacoepidemiology Center. Pittsburgh, PA.

 albumin messenger ribonucleic acid (mRNA) detection

Synonyms
none

Indications
detection of albumin mRNA in hepatic and extrahepatic neoplasms

Method
localization of albumin mRNA using in situ hybridization (ISH); oligonucleotide probes for albumin and beta actin synthesized using automated synthesizer

Normal findings
staining for albumin mRNA regarded as positive if a distinct finely granular cytoplasmic staining was present, regardless of intensity

Comments
albumin is a ubiquitous protein that is synthesized only by hepatocytes

Source
Adapted from Krishna M, Lloyd RV, Batts KP. Detection of albumin messenger RNA in hepatic and extrahepatic neoplasms. American Journal of Surgical Pathology 1997;21:147-151.

 Albunex

Generic name
see albumin human 5% sonicated

 albuterol sulfate

Brand name
Epaq

Use
a non-chlorofluorocarbon formulation of albuterol for treatment of asthma

Usual dosage
inhalation: metered-dose inhaler; 1-2 inhalations (90-180 µg) every 4 to 6 hours in adults and children more than 4 years of age

Pharmaceutical company
3M Pharmaceuticals. St. Paul, MN.

Source
Stadtlanders Managed Pharmacy Services. Pittsburgh, PA.

 albuterol sulfate/ipratropium bromide

Brand name
Combivent

Use
for relief and prevention of bronchospasm in patients with reversible obstructive airway disease and for the prevention of exercise-induced bronchospasm

Usual dosage
inhalation: metered-dose inhaler containing albuterol sulfate 0.09 mg base
and ipratropium bromide 0.018 mg per inhalation; administered 1 to 2
inhalations every 4 to 6 hours as needed for bronchospasm; for prevention
of exercise-induced bronchospasm, use 2 inhalations 15 minutes prior to
exercise

Pharmaceutical company
Boehringer Ingelheim. Ridgefield, CT.

Source
Stadtlanders Managed Pharmacy Services. Pittsburgh, PA.

 ## Alcar

Generic name
see levacecarnine

 ## Aldara

Generic name
see imiquimod

 ## ALEC

Generic name
see dipalmitoylphosphatidylcholine

 ## alendronate sodium

Brand name
Fosamax

Use
oral: treatment and prevention of postmenopausal osteoporosis intravenous:
treatment for hypercalcemia and bone disease associated with metastatic
cancer and Paget disease

Usual dosage
oral: doses ranging from 5 to 40 mg daily have been used in clinical trials intravenous: infusion doses between 5 and 40 mg have been used in clinical trials

Pharmaceutical company
Merck & Co. Inc. West Point, PA.

Source
University of Pittsburgh Drug Information and Pharmacoepidemiology Center. Pittsburgh, PA.

ALEXlazr

Description
alternative to yttrium-aluminum-garnet (YAG) laser for tattoo removal

Source
Candela Corp. product information. Wayland, MA.

 Algisorb wound dressing

Description
sterile dressing for acute care setting; helps prevent maceration of tissue surrounding wound site

Source
Calgon Vestal Laboratories product information. St. Louis, MO.

 Alladin InfantFlow nasal continuous positive air pressure

Description
infant ventilatory support employs a patented fluid system that regulates pressure to the patient's demand, reducing work of breathing; eliminates the need to intubate and mechanically ventilate many term and pre-term infants

Source
Hamilton Medical product information. Reno, NV.

 Allegra

Generic name
see fexofenadine

 Allervax Cat

Generic name
see cat dander immunotherapeutic peptide

▶ *As of November 24, 1997, Immunologic Pharmaceutical Corporation reported that it is restructuring operations and that further clinical trials of its ALLERVAX® CAT and RAGWEED programs are on hold.*

 AlloDerm dermal graft

Description
acellular, human allograft implant facilitates effective soft tissue augmentation; eliminates donor site morbidity; provides unlimited tissue availability; can be folded or rolled to required thickness; eliminates painful donor site for patient

Source
LifeCell Corp. product information. The Woodlands, TX.

20

 allogeneic activated natural killer (NK) cell therapy

Synonyms
allogeneic NK cell treatment

Use
activation of donor marrow cell subpopulations to achieve graft-versus-tumor effect

Method
selection of donor lymphocyte subpopulations, activation of selected cells with interleukin-2, growth of the selected, activated population, and infusion of the cells into the transplant recipient

Specimen
donor lymphocytes

Normal range
not applicable

Comments
may be a more effective form of graft-versus-tumor effect than autologous natural killer cell activation

Source
Department of Laboratory Medicine and Pathology, University of Minnesota, Minneapolis, MN.

 allograft bone vise

Description
device designed to hold allograft bone for reaming, shaping, or cutting; two sets of vise jaws for reaming of femoral head

Source
Innomed Inc. product information. Savannah, GA.

 allograft reconstruction of fibular collateral ligament

Description
posterolateral complex reconstruction with allograft tissue to restore ruptured/insufficient fibular collateral ligament (FCL); extend lateral joint line incision distally and proximally to expose femur attachment; incise iliotibial band attachment along anterior border, preserving intramuscular septum attachment; expose knee and small area of FCL; secure circle allograft with sutures; incise behind FCL for inspection; soft tissue washer and interlocking suture fixation

Anatomy
knee; posterolateral ligament complex; fibula; peroneal nerve; fibular collateral ligament; fabellofibular ligament; arcuate ligament; popliteus tendon; muscle; biceps; Achilles tendon; femur; iliotibial band; vastus lateralis; tibia; fascia lata

Equipment
standard surgery equipment; surgical drill; curved curette; allograft material;
Ticron sutures

Source
Adapted from Noyes FR, Barber-Westin SD. Surgical reconstruction of severe chronic posterolateral complex
injuries of the knee using allograft tissues. American Journal of Sports Medicine 1995;23:2-12.

 Allotrap 2702

Generic name
see HLA-B2702 peptide

 All-Purpose Boot (A.P.B.) Hi

Description
all-purpose boot; high-top sneaker with closed toe for postoperative protection in all types of weather; adjustable straps at foot and ankle

Source
Darco International Inc. product information. Huntington, WV.

 Alond

Generic name
see zopolrestat

 Alpern cortex aspirator/hydrodissector

Description
ophthalmic surgical instrument; angled 45 degrees, 5 mm from end; both
right and left instruments

Source
Visitec Co. product information. Sarasota, FL.

 alpha$_2$ anti-plasmin antigen assay

Synonyms
alpha$_2$ anti-plasmin immunologic assay

Use
part of work-up of suspected dysantiplasminemia, a rare inherited cause of a
bleeding disorder

Method
Laurell rocket immunoelectrophoresis assay

Specimen
blood

Normal range
76% to 123% of result for normal pooled plasma

Comments
results of alpha$_2$ anti-plasmin antigen assay should be compared with results from functional assay

Source
University of Minnesota Department of Laboratory Medicine and Pathology. Minneapolis, MN.

 ## alpha$_2$ anti-plasmin chromogenic assay

Synonyms
alpha$_2$ anti-plasmin functional assay

Use
part of work-up of suspected dysantiplasminemia, a rare inherited cause of a bleeding disorder

Method
chromogenic (synthetic substrate) activity assay

Specimen
blood

Normal range
75% to 126% of result for normal pooled plasma

Comments
results of alpha$_2$ anti-plasmin functional assay should be compared with results from antigen assay

Source
University of Minnesota Department of Laboratory Medicine and Pathology. Minneapolis, MN.

 ## alpha$_2$ anti-plasmin crossed immunoelectrophoresis

Synonyms
antiplasmin CIEP

Use
alpha$_2$ crossed immunoelectrophoresis (CIEP) is the final step in work-up for suspected dysantiplasminemia, a rare inherited cause of a bleeding disorder

Method
two-dimensional (crossed) immunoelectrophoresis

Specimen
blood

Normal range
results given as interpretive report

Comments
blood specimen must be tested within 4 hours of collection

Source
University of Minnesota Department of Laboratory Medicine and Pathology. Minneapolis, MN.

Alphagan

Generic name
see brimonidine tartrate

alprostadil

Brand name
Muse

Use
another formulation of alprostadil; treatment of erectile dysfunction

Usual dosage
pelletized suppository: one pellet into urethra before intercourse available in 125, 250, 500, and 1,000 μg dosage strength with a urethral suppository applicator

Pharmaceutical company
Vivus Pharmaceuticals. Menlo Park, CA.

Source
Stadtlanders Managed Pharmacy Services. Pittsburgh, PA.

Alredase

Generic name
see tolrestat
► As of October 27, 1996, tolrestat drug has been withdrawn from the market by the manufacturer.

altitude simulation study

Synonyms
hypoxic response study

Indications
quantify decline of arterial oxygenation in persons with chronic obstructive pulmonary disease (COPD) or impaired gas exchange from other causes while breathing a gas mixture containing approximately 17% oxygen; simulate the conditions in domestic aircraft while flying

Method
supply patient with tubing and one-way breathing valve which carries 17.2% O_2 and balance N_2, which approximates the FiO_2 at 1650 meters; after patient breathes hypoxic mixture for 30 minutes, draw arterial blood gas

Normal findings
pO_2 less than 76 torr at sea level

Comments
useful guideline in determining whether supplemental oxygen might be required for air travel

Source
Lexi-Comp Inc. database. Hudson, OH.

Altona finger extension device

Description
extension apparatus that consists of metal traction bow, pulley assembly, five "S" hooks for connection to finger grips; for use when traction is needed

Source
Link America Inc. product information. Denville, NJ.

Alton Dean blood/fluid warmer

Description
portable unit attached to I.V. pole; individual holders simultaneously warm two different fluids (blood and/or irrigation fluids); adjustable flow rates; for surgical or trauma patients

Source
Alton Dean Medical Inc. product information. Woods Cross, UT.

altretamine

Brand name
Hexalen

Use
antineoplastic that has activity in ovarian carcinoma as a single agent or as combination therapy

Usual dosage
oral: 260 mg/m2/day in four divided doses, given after meals and at bedtime

Pharmaceutical company
Wyeth-Ayerst Laboratories. Wilmington, DE.

Source
University of Pittsburgh Drug Information and Pharmacoepidemiology Center. Pittsburgh, PA.

ALZET continuous infusion osmotic pump

Description
pump utilized for continuous infusion of medication via the intravenous route

Source
ALZA Corp. product information. Palo Alto, CA.

Amaryl

Generic name
see glimepiride

Ambicor penile prosthesis

Description
closed, fluid-filled, 2-piece penile prosthesis; 11, 13, and 15 mm diameters with lengths from 14 to 22 cm

Source
American Medical Systems Inc. product information. Minnetonka, MN.

 ## AmBisome

Generic name
see amphotericin B liposomal formulation

 ## Ambulatory infusion management (AIM) device

Description
ambulatory infusion management for multi-therapy delivery; a single-channel device for accurate medication delivery through multiple programming modes; 5 pumps in 1 for total parenteral nutrition, patient-controlled analgesia, variable time (circadian rhythm), or continuous therapy

Source
Abbott Laboratories product information. North Chicago, IL.

 ## Amerge

Generic name
see naratriptan

 ## Amfit orthotics

Description
custom orthoses that are functional and accommodative; assist in treatment of structural and functional abnormalities such as pes cavus symptoms, gait abnormalities, hip, low back and knee pain, shin splints, athletic overuse foot syndromes, excessive pronation, heel pain, metatarsalgia, various arthritides, diabetic foot, and limb-length discrepancies

Source
Amfit Inc. product information. Santa Clara, CA.

amifostine

Brand name
Ethyol

Use
selective tissue protectant to protect from hematologic toxicity and nephro-toxicity associated with chemotherapy and radiation therapy in patients with cancer

Usual dosage
intravenous: 740 to 910 mg/m² as a 15-minute infusion

Pharmaceutical company
U.S. Bioscience. West Conshohocken, PA.

Source
University of Pittsburgh Drug Information and Pharmacoepidemiology Center. Pittsburgh, PA.

 amikacin LF

Brand name
MiKasome

Use
liposomal formulation: treatment of drug resistant tuberculosis, *Pseudomonas aeruginosa* infections in immunocompromised patients, and *Mycobacterium avium* infections associated with AIDS

Usual dosage
intravenous: 10 mg/kg was investigated in clinical trials

Pharmaceutical company
AmpliMed Corp. Tucson, AZ.

Source
Stadtlanders Managed Pharmacy Services. Pittsburgh, PA.

 Amino acid cervical cream

Generic name
see methionine/cystine cream

 amiprilose

Brand name
Therafectin

Use
treatment of rheumatoid arthritis

Usual dosage
oral: 6 gm/day was used in early clinical trials
Pharmaceutical company
Boston Life Sciences Inc. Boston, MA.
Source
Stadtlanders Managed Pharmacy Services. Pittsburgh, PA.

 amlexanox

Brand name
Aphthasol
Use
treatment of aphthous ulcers
Usual dosage
topical: 5% oral paste applied to ulcer 4 times a day, after meals and at bed-time
Pharmaceutical company
Block Drug. Jersey City, NJ.
Source
Stadtlanders Managed Pharmacy Services. Pittsburgh, PA.

 amlodipine/benazepril

Generic Name
Lotrel
Use
calcium channel blocker and angiotensin converting enzyme inhibitor used for the treatment of hypertension
Usual Dosage
oral: one capsule daily. Available strengths include: 5/10 mg, 5/20 mg, and 2.5/10 µg of amlodipine/benazepril respectively
Pharmaceutical company
Ciba-Geigy. Summit, NJ.
Source
University of Pittsburgh Drug Information and Pharmacoepidemiology Center. Pittsburgh, PA.

 Ammonilect

Generic name
see sodium benzoate/sodium phenylacetate

AMO-PhacoFlex Lens and Inserter

Description
foldable intraocular lenses have ultraviolet absorbing benzotriazole blockers
to protect from potential harmful effects of ultraviolet after cataract surgery;
also AMO-PhacoFlex Inserter for maintaining small phaco incision and stability of sulcus or in-the-bag fixation

Source
Allergan Inc. product information. Irvine, CA.

AMO-Prestige Phaco System

Description
applied stable eye technology for control of fluidic condition in the anterior
chamber during surgery; senses changes and adjusts the fluidics to preserve
equilibrium to maintain chamber depth and control capsule flutter for techniques such as phaco chop

Source
Allergan Inc. product information. Irvine, CA.

Amphotec

Generic name
see amphotericin B colloidal dispersion (ABCD)
► Marketed outside of the U.S. as Amphocil.

amphotericin B colloidal dispersion (ABCD)

Brand name
Amphotec

Use
has been studied for treatment of fungal infection (aspergillosis) in patients
who are intolerant of or refractory to conventional amphotericin B therapy

Usual dosage
injectable: 1-7 mg/kg/day has been used in clinical trials in the treatment of
fungal infections (coccidioidomycosis, candidiasis, and aspergillosis)

Pharmaceutical company
SEQUUS Pharmaceuticals Inc. Menlo Park, CA.

Source
University of Pittsburgh Drug Information and Pharmacoepidemiology Center. Pittsburgh, PA.

amphotericin B lipid complex injection

Brand name
Abelcet

Use
treatment of fungal infection (aspergillosis) in patients who are intolerant of or refractory to conventional amphotericin B therapy

Usual dosage
injectable: 5.0 mg/kg as a single IV infusion dose; administered at a rate of 2.5 mg/kg/hr

Pharmaceutical company
Liposome Co. Princeton, NJ.

Source
University of Pittsburgh Drug Information and Pharmacoepidemiology Center. Pittsburgh, PA.

 amphotericin B liposomal formulation

Brand name
AmBisome

Use
liposomal formulation of amphotericin B used in the treatment of severe and life-threatening systemic fungal infections; may be less nephrotoxic compared to original formulation

Usual dosage
intravenous: doses from 2.5 to 5 mg/kg/day for up to 6 weeks have been used in clinical trials

Pharmaceutical company
Fujisawa USA Inc. Deerfield, IL.

Source
University of Pittsburgh Drug Information and Pharmacoepidemiology Center. Pittsburgh, PA.

 amrinone stimulation test

Synonyms
Inocor stimulation test

Indications
severe baseline left ventricular dysfunction patient

Method
intravenous infusion stimulation with amrinone

Normal findings
none

Comments
augmentation of myocardial contraction by amrinone in patients with chronic coronary artery disease and severe baseline left ventricular dysfunction; predicts improvement in left ventricular ejection fraction after coronary artery bypass graft surgery

Source
Adapted from Perez-Balino N, Masoli O, Meretta A, et al. Amrinone stimulation test: ability to predict improvement in left ventricular ejection fraction after coronary artery bypass surgery in patients with poor baseline left ventricular function. Journal of the American College of Cardiology 1996;28:1488-1492.

 anakinra

Brand name
Antril

Use
anti-inflammatory; for the treatment of rheumatoid arthritis

Usual dosage
subcutaneous: doses of 30 mg, 75 mg, or 150 mg a day was investigated in clinical trials

Pharmaceutical company
Amgen Inc. Thousand Oaks, CA.

Source
Stadtlanders Managed Pharmacy Services. Pittsburgh, PA.

 anal sonography with an intraluminal probe

Synonyms
none

Indications
defecatory problems, especially fecal incontinence

Method
ultrasound of the anal canal utilizing a rectal transducer

Normal findings
not applicable

Comments
sonography has a sensitivity and specificity of almost 100% in the detection of anal sphincter defects and of more than 90% in the location and assessment of the extent of the lesion

Source
Adapted from Enek P, von Giesen HJ, Schafer A et al. Comparison of anal sonography with conventional needle electromyography in the evaluation of anal sphincter defects. The American Journal of Gastroenterology 1996;91:2539-2543.

anaritide acetate (atrial natriuretic peptide)

Brand name
Auriculin

Use
cardiac hormone used to regulate fluid balance in renal and cardiac diseases

Usual dosage
intravenous: 0.02 mcg/kg/min x 24 hr

Pharmaceutical company
Scios Nova Inc. Mountain View, CA.

Source
University of Pittsburgh Drug Information and Pharmacoepidemiology Center. Pittsburgh, PA.

 ## anastrazole

Brand Name
Arimidex

Use
aromanase inhibitor for the treatment of postmenopausal women with advanced breast cancer who develop progressive disease while receiving tamoxifen

Usual Dosage
oral: 1 mg daily

Pharmaceutical company
Zeneca Pharmaceutical. Wilmington, DE.

Source
Samford University Global Drug Information Service. Birmingham, AL.

 ## Anchor soft tissue biopsy device

Description
has a sharp-cutting surgical needle on pistol-grip handle; permits excellent control during soft tissue biopsy procedures

Source
Anchor Products Co. product information. Addison, IL.

 ## ancrod

Brand name
Arvin

Use
anticoagulant derived from venom of the Malayan pit viper for use in patients with stroke

32

Usual dosage
intravenous or subcutaneous (intravenous route preferred): initial doses of 1 to 2 units/kg intravenous infusion over 6 to 24 hr followed by maintenance doses based on fibrinogen plasma levels (usually 1 to 2 units/kg/day)

Pharmaceutical company
Knoll Pharmaceuticals. Whippany, NJ.

Source
University of Pittsburgh Drug Information and Pharmacoepidemiology Center. Pittsburgh, PA.

 Androderm

Generic name
see testosterone transdermal patch

 AndroTest-SL

Generic name
see testosterone

 Angiopeptin

Generic name
see lanreotide

 Ank-L-Aid brace

Description
provides structural protection and stability to help rehabilitate injured or weakened ankles secondary to chronic conditions

Source
Ank-L-Aid Braces product information. Armore, PA.

 ankle rehab pump

Description
strengthens and rehabilitates motions most affected by ankle injuries; uses hydraulics for isokinetic resistance through a full adjustable range of inversion and eversion to strengthen muscles and tendons around the ankle to regain function and stability

Source
Ortho Dynamics product information. Albany, NY.

AnkleTough ankle rehabilitation system

Description
a system that consists of resistive tension straps and exercises designed to round out the rehab program; aids in the rehab of ankle injuries, such as sprains

Source
DM Systems Inc. product information. Evanston, IL.

 ## ANNE anesthesia infuser

Description
anesthesia infusion system; calculates weight-dependent dose and delivers drugs either as a bolus or as continuous infusion

Source
Abbott Laboratories product information. North Chicago, IL.

 ## anoscope with slot

Description
disposable surgical instrument for visualization of and access to anal tissue; wide distal slot allows for visualization of a selective segment and access for hemorrhoid treatment as well as other therapeutic treatments

Source
Circon Corp. product information. Santa Barbara, CA.

 ## Anspach 65K instrument system

Description
for working with biometals, bioplastics, and bones; used for removal of broken stems/acetabular cups, spinal procedures, microsurgery, hip revision, cranial procedures, shoulder surgery, craniofacial/maxillofacial procedures

Source
Anspach product information. Lake Park, FL.

 ## Antense anti-tension device

Description
electromyogram biofeedback monitoring device; good indicator of relaxation techniques

Source
BioSig Instruments Inc. product information. Champlain, NY.

anterior active mask rhinomanometry

Synonyms

Indications

nasal obstruction

Method

one nostril is occluded with a pressure transducer, which reflects transnasal pressure through the opposite, nonoccluded nostril; airflow is measured by a face mask connected to a pneumotachograph

Normal findings

greater than 0.01

Comments

able to assess nasal valvular function while previous rhinomanometry could only assess the degree of obstruction produced by the septum and turbinates

Source

Adapted from Constantian MB, Clardy RB. The relative importance of septal and nasal valvular surgery in correcting airway obstruction in primary and secondary rhinoplasty. Plastic and Reconstructive Surgery 1996;98:38-54.

anterior cervical approach to cervicothoracic junction

Description

a number of approaches to the upper thoracic vertebrae have been proposed combining thoracotomy, sternotomy or clavicle resection with anterior dissection into the superior mediastinum; an anterior cervical approach for patients with disease limited to one vertebral level is presented, in which midline ventral decompression is the goal; the angle of the approach to the cervicothoracic junction is dictated by the manubrium

Anatomy

aortic arch; apical lung pleura; carotid sheath; cervical fascia; carotid and subclavian arteries; esophagus; innominate vessels; inferior thyroidal artery; inferior laryngeal nerve; jugulosubclavian junction; larynx; ligamentum arteriosum; longus colli muscles; manubrium sterni; mediastinum; omohyoid muscles; platysma muscle; sternal notch; sternocleidomastoid muscle; sternothyroid and sternohyoid muscles; subclavian artery; superior vena cava; trachea; tracheoesophageal groove; thyroid gland; uncovertebral joints; vertebral bodies

Equipment

cervical periosteal elevators; hand-held retractors; high-speed drill; long-bladed, self-retaining retractor system (Farley retractor); methyl methacrylate construct; Steinmann pin

Source

Adapted from Gieger M, Roth PA, Wu JK. The anterior cervical approach to the cervicothoracic junction. Neurosurgery Journal 1995;37:704-709.

anti-CD34 antibody-binding flow cytometric assay

Synonyms
flow cytometry-based assay for anti-CD34 antibody binding

Use
evaluation of binding of various anti-CD34 antibodies

Method
recognition of epitope tag in flow cytometry

Specimen
purified antibody

Normal range
not applicable

Comments
allows comparison of various antibodies specific for CD34, the molecule currently most commonly used in stem cell selection for bone marrow transplantation

Source
Adapted from Benedict CA, MacKrell AJ, Anderson WF. Determination of the binding affinity of an anti-CD34 single-chain antibody using a novel, flow cytometry based assay. Journal of Immunologic Methods 1997;201:223-231.

anti-D enzyme-linked immunosorbent assay (ELISA)

Synonyms
anti-D ELISA

Use
for measurement of anti-D antibody in plasma samples and immunoglobulin preparations

Method
microtiter plate enzyme immunoassay using papainized red blood cells

Specimen
plasma

Normal range
variable; determined by nature of source material and purpose for measurement

Comments
precise and more readily performed than conventional hemagglutination method

Source
Adapted from Hirvonen M, Tervonen S, Pirkola A, Sievers G. An enzyme-linked immunosorbent assay for the quantitative determination of anti-D in plasma samples and immunoglobulin preparations. Vox Sanguinis 1995;69:341-346.

anti-liver microsomal antibody detection

Synonyms
none

Use
identify antibody described mainly in patients with various hepatic disorders; other conditions in which the microsomal antibodies have been described include acute hepatitis (viral or drug hypersensitivity), hepatocellular carcinoma, and "subclinical hepatitis"

Method
indirect fluorescent antibody (IFA)

Specimen
blood

Normal range
no antibody detected

Comments
although seen in less than 1% of patients with liver disease, it has been described in persons with active chronic hepatitis

Source
Lexi-Comp Inc. database. Hudson, OH.

 antinuclear antibody screening by enzyme immunoassay (EIA)

Synonyms
EIA detection of ANAs (antinuclear antibodies)

Use
screening test for diagnosis of numerous rheumatic and connective tissue diseases

Method
single and multi-antigen enzyme immunoassay

Specimen
serum

Normal range
titer of 1:160 or lower

Comments
positive specimens should be confirmed with conventional indirect fluorescent antibody (IFA)

Source
Adapted from Jaskowski TD, Schroder C, Martins TB, Mouritsen CL, Litwin CM, Hill HR. Screening for antinuclear antibodies by enzyme immunoassay. American Journal of Clinical Pathology 1996;105:468-473.

antithymocyte immunoglobulin

Brand name
Thymoglobulin

Use
a pasteurized, rabbit antithymocyte polyclonal antibody preparation for the treatment of acute organ rejection

Usual dosage
intravenous: clinical trials have used 1.5 mg/kg/day for 7 to 14 days

Pharmaceutical company
SangStat Medical Corp. Menlo Park, CA.

Source
Stadtlanders Managed Pharmacy Services. Pittsburgh, PA.

 ## Antizol

Generic name
see fomepizole

 ## Antocin

Generic name
see atosiban

 ## Antril

Generic name
see anakinra

 ## Anzemet

Generic name
see dolastron mesylate

 ## Apdyne phenol applicator kit

Description
phenol kit enables surgeon to perform myringotomy faster than with ion-tophoresis; eliminates pain of a Xylocaine injection

Source
Apdyne Medical Co. product information. Minneapolis, MN.

Aphthasol

Generic name
see amlexanox

 Apollo hot/cold Paks

Description
slip-on hot/cold packs confirm to body curves for maximum effectiveness
(Editor note: Paks is the correct spelling in the name of this product.)
Source
The Saunders Group product information. Chaska, MN.

 Apollo³ papillotome

Description
precurved triple-lumen wire-guided papillotome for biliary endoscopy
Source
Bard International Products Division product information. Billerica, MA.

 APOPPS, transtibial

Description
adjustable postoperative protective prosthetic socket (APOPPS) for transtibial amputations; accommodates compression and swelling of wound area; helps build tolerance for permanent socket
Source
Flo-Tech Orthotic and Prosthetic Systems product information. Geneva, NY.

 A-Port, A²-Port

Description
implantable ports for vascular access
Source
Arrow International product information. Reading, PA.

 Applied Medical mini ureteroscope

Description
triangular-shaped tip ureteroscope that allows easy entry into the ureteral orifice, often without pre-stenting or dilation; two channels provide improved working efficiencies
Source
Applied Medical Urology Division product information. Laguna Hills, CA.

applied stapling technique in radical retropubic prostatectomy

Description
use of the endoscopic gastrointestinal anastomosis (GIA) stapler as the sole source of ligation for division and hemostasis of the dorsal vein complex

Anatomy
pelvic area; urethra; bladder; ureters; prostate; symphysis pubis; pubovesical fascia; puboprostatic ligament; dorsal vein complex; endopelvic fascia

Equipment
standard surgical; GIA stapling device

Source
Adapted from Gould DL, Borer J. Applied stapling technique in radical retropubic prostatectomy: efficient, effective and efficacious. Journal of Urology 1996;155:1008-1010.

 aptiganel hydrochloride

Brand name
Cerestat

Use
treatment of inadequate blood flow to the brain, including stroke and traumatic brain injury

Usual dosage
intravenous: doses up to 100 µg/kg were used in clinical trials

Pharmaceutical company
Boehringer Ingelheim Pharmaceuticals Inc. Ridgefield, CT.

Source
Stadtlanders Managed Pharmacy Services. Pittsburgh, PA.

 Aqua-Cel heating pad system

Description
full-length back applications; non-electric, non-chemical portable pad is heated in a microwave oven; heat transfer is immediate and the pad remains hot for over 1 hour

Source
Aqua-Cel Corp. product information. Santa Ana, CA.

 Aquacel Hydrofiber wound dressing

Description
fibrous dressing for management of moderately to heavily draining wounds

Source
ConvaTec product information. Princeton, NJ.

AquaMED

Description
water jet hydrotherapy device

Source
JTL Enterprises product information. Clearwater, FL.

 AquaSens

Description
fluid monitoring system that consolidates fluid supply and collection into one portable unit

Source
Aquintel product information. Mountain View, CA.

 AquaShield orthopaedic cast cover

Description
one-piece completely waterproof reusable cast cover; works under water; SkidSafe sole; pediatric sizes available

Source
Orthomed Products Inc. product information. Grass Valley, CA.

 Aqua Spray

Description
nail debridement system that utilizes a fine alcohol/water mist to lubricate and prevent nail dust from becoming airborne during nail debridement

Source
Boyd Industries Inc. product information. Largo, FL.

 Aquatrend water workout station

Description
stainless-steel station in which a person can do a series of exercises or rehabilitation protocols on a regular basis while remaining partially submerged in water; includes an underwater treadmill, stepper, bicycle, and Roman chair

Source
Aquatic Trends Inc. product information. North Palm Beach, FL.

arch bar cutter

Description
cutting instrument that allows the oral surgeon to cut the arch bar in the patient's mouth, thus eliminating errors caused by cutting the bar too short or too long; holds the cut end of the bar preventing it from dropping into the patient's mouth

Source
IKON Instruments Inc. product information. Huntington Beach, CA.

 argatroban

Brand name
Novastan

Use
direct antithrombin agent used as an adjunctive to thrombolysis in acute myocardial infarction

Usual dosage
intravenous: 41-200 µg/kg/min infusion

Pharmaceutical company
Texas Biotechnology. Houston, TX.

Source
Stadtlanders Managed Pharmacy Services. Pittsburgh, PA.

 argyrophilic inclusion positive erythrocyte count

Synonyms
AE count; RE system testing

Use
evaluation of splenic reticuloendothelial (RE) function in patients with suspected hyposplenia or asplenia

Method
light microscopic examination of silver-stained and eosin-stained blood smear

Specimen
EDTA (ethylenediaminetetraacetic acid)-anticoagulated blood

Normal range
<3 % of the erythrocytes examined

Comments
simplest and most rapid test of splenic reticuloendothelial function; similar to pocked erythrocyte count, but a different technique

Source
Adapted from Tham KT, Teague MW, Howard CA, Chen SY. A simple splenic reticuloendothelial function test. American Journal of Clinical Pathology 1996;105:548-552.

argyrophilic nucleolar organizer regions (AgNORs) staining

Synonyms
none

Indications
AgNORs represent a tissue marker of cell proliferative activity; study done for assessment of prognostic value of AgNORs expression in oral squamous cell carcinoma (SCC)

Method
AgNORs area/nucleus studded in paraffin sections; staining done by using modified one-step silver colloid method; various solutions of different concentrations applied to paraffin-embedded blocks

Normal findings
time free of disease was considered a dependent variable of a binary indicator of AgNORs expression

Comments
AgNORs area evaluation increased the capability of predicting patients who have a high risk of recurrence of cancer

Source
Adapted from Teixeira G, Antonangelo L, Kowalski L et al. Argyrophilic nucleolar organizer regions staining is useful in predicting recurrence-free interval in oral tongue and floor of mouth squamous cell carcinoma. American Journal of Surgery 1996;172:684-687.

 Aricept

Generic name
see donepezil

 Arimidex

Generic Name
see anastrazole

 Arkin-Z

Generic name
see vesnarinone

 ArrowFlex intra-aortic balloon catheter

Description
catheter which flexes at any point and in any direction without kinking or collapsing; made of Cardiothane 51 bioelastomer

Source
Arrow International Inc. product information. Reading, PA.

Arrow FlexTip Plus catheter

Description
epidural catheter with unique wire reinforcement, virtually kink-free; soft tip designed to deflect when it comes in contact with the dura or veins in spinal column

Source
Arrow International Inc. product information. Reading, PA.

 ## Arrowsmith corneal marker

Description
corneal incision marker

Source
Accurate Surgical & Scientific Instrument Corp. product information. Westbury, NY.

 ## Arrow TwistLock catheter hub

Description
locking catheter device that holds catheter securely in place without restricting flow of vital infusates by twisting center section; twist other way, and catheter again slides easily

Source
Arrow International Inc. product information. Reading, PA.

 ## ArtAssist arterial assist device

Description
patented technology dramatically increases blood flow to chronic wounds; noninvasive; applies a unique regimen of external compression to the foot, ankle, and calf to patient in a comfortable sitting position

Source
ACI Medical product information. San Marcos, CA.

 ## artemether

Brand name
Paluther

Use
treatment of severe malaria caused by *Plasmodium falciparum*

Usual dosage
intramuscular: 4 mg/kg stat, then 2 mg/kg every 8 hours

Pharmaceutical company
Rhone-Poulenc Rorer Pharmaceuticals Inc. Collegeville, PA.

Source
Stadtlanders Managed Pharmacy Services. Pittsburgh, PA.

ArthroGuide carbon dioxide (CO_2) laser delivery system

Description
laser instrument adaptable to gas or saline insufflation; provides easier access to confined articular spaces, superior contouring of cartilage surfaces, and hemostasis in partial synovectomies

Source
Heraeus Surgical Inc. product information. Milpitas, CA.

 ## Arthroplasty Products Consultants (APC) foot and leg holder

Description
orthotic device designed for immobilization of foot during foot and ankle surgery; can also be used for tibial rodding

Source
Innomed Inc. product information. Savannah, GA.

 ## Arthrotec

Generic name
see diclofenac sodium and misoprostol

 ## Arvin

Generic name
see ancrod

 ## Asherman chest seal

Description
AE-1700 Asherman chest seal; sterile dressing for open chest wounds or other injuries that could compromise the pleural space of the chest cavity; designed for first responders to manage an open pneumothorax totally eliminating outside air intake through the wound hole into the pleural space; can be used to prevent tension pneumothorax and/or re-inflate a collapsed lung without using invasive procedures; also ideal for use with needle thoracentesis

Source
Armstrong Medical Industries Inc. product information. Lincolnshire, IL and San Diego, CA.

Aslan endoscopic scissors

Description
endoscopic scissors that reduce cutting effort and have an in-line actuator that doubles as the handle

Source
Aslan Medical Technologies product information. Kalamazoo, MI.

 ## Aspen ultrasound system

Description
ultrasound imaging platform with digital system architecture providing full digital control of the ultrasound echos from the transducer to the captured digital exam, advancing image quality with higher level of performance in 2D imaging using Convergent Color Doppler blood flow dynamics

Source
Acuson Corp. product information. Mountain View, CA.

 ## Aspisafe nasogastric tube

Description
disposable, traction-elastic tube counteracts gastroesophageal reflux aspiration or regurgitation; inflated gastric balloon placed under tension at the cardia; prevents reflux during induction of anesthesia

Source:
Braun product information. Melsungen, Germany.

 ## Assess esophageal testing kit

Description
device for performing precise pH and manometry tests; evaluates esophageal acid exposure, esophageal body pressures, effectiveness of peristaltic action, sphincter length and tone, and sphincter asymmetry

Source
Medtronic Synectics Medical product information. Shoreview, MN.

 ## Assistant Free retractor

Description
knee retractor system holds instrument utilizing Velcro straps; helps eliminate obstruction of surgeon's operative area, and frees assisting personnel

Source
Innomed Inc. product information. Savannah, GA.

Astelin

Generic name
see azelastine

 Aston cartilage reduction system

Description
nasal scissors, rasps, and supercut blades; designed by Sherrell J. Aston, MD, for accurate reduction of cartilaginous dorsum and lowering of upper lateral cartilages

Source
Snowden-Pencer product information. Tucker, GA.

 Atad cervical ripening device

Description
double-balloon device for cervical ripening and labor induction; uterine and cervicovaginal balloons inflated with normal saline; uterine balloon covers internal cervical os; cervicovaginal balloon located at external os

Source
Emerand Ltd. product information. Rehovot, Israel.

 Athena High Frequency (HF) mammography system

Description
screening and diagnostic imaging instrument; provides constant optical density of entire range of breast densities and sizes; effective for modified views of augmented breasts; diagnostic detail provides for early detection of cancer

Source
Fischer Imaging Corp. product information. Denver, CO.

 Athymil

Generic Name
see mianserin

 atorvastatin

Brand name
Lipitor

Use
cholesterol lowering agent; used to reduce elevated low density lipoprotein cholesterol (LDL) and triglycerides

Usual dosage
oral: 10 mg/day, may titrate up to a maximum dose of 80 mg/day
Pharmaceutical company
Parke-Davis Division of Warner Lambert Co. Morris Plains, NJ.
Source
Stadtlanders Managed Pharmacy Services. Pittsburgh, PA.

 ## atosiban

Brand name
Antocin
Use
oxytocin antagonist; treatment of acute premature/preterm labor in pregnant women
Usual dosage
injection: 2-6.5 mg bolus dose follow by 100-300 m µg/minute to control premature contractions
Pharmaceutical company
Ortho-McNeil Pharmaceuticals. Raritan, NJ.
Source
Stadtlanders Managed Pharmacy Services. Pittsburgh, PA.

 ## atovaquone

Brand Name
Mepron
Use
second-line treatment and prophylaxis of AIDS-related *Pneumocystis carinii* pneumonia
Usual Dosage
oral suspension: 750 mg/5ml twice a day with food
Pharmaceutical company
Burroughs Wellcome. Research Triangle Park, NC.
Source
University of Pittsburgh Drug Information and Pharmacoepidemiology Center. Pittsburgh, PA.

 ## atovaquone/proguanil

Brand name
Malarone
Use
antiparasitic and antimalarial agent; for the treatment of multi-drug resistant *Plasmodium falciparum*

Usual dosage
oral: 1000 mg of atovaquone plus 400 mg of proguanil once daily for 3 days
Pharmaceutical company
Glaxo Wellcome Inc. Research Triangle Park, NC.
Source
Stadtlanders Managed Pharmacy Services. Pittsburgh, PA.

 ## ATO walker

Description
solid, stable walking/standing frame reduces stress on the lower extremities; provides split-sectioned padding support for the upper extremities and torso
Source
Smith & Nephew Rolyan Inc. product information. Germantown, WI.

 ## Auriculin

Generic name
see anaritide acetate (atrial natriuretic peptide)

 ## Austin chevron osteotomy fixation

Description
V-shaped transverse osteotomy of the head of the first metatarsal for hallux valgus surgery with application of bioabsorbable 3.3-mm diameter poly-L-lactic acid screw
Anatomy
metatarsophalangeal joint; extensor hallucis longus tendon; metatarsal head; medial eminence; articular cartilage
Equipment
K-wire; specially shaped 3.3-mm diameter tap, 3.3-mm diameter poly-L-lactic acid (PLLA) cortical screw with fully threaded stem; dynamometric screwdriver; 3.6-mm drill bit
Source
Adapted from Barca F, Busa R. Austin-chevron osteotomy fixed with bioabsorbable poly-L-lactic acid single screw. The Journal of Foot & Ankle Surgery 1997;36:15-20.

 ## Auto-Kerato-Refractometer

Description
Topcon KR-7000 combines auto-refractometer and keratometer in a single diagnostic instrument; minimal 2.5-mm pupil diameter
Source
Topcon America Corporation product information. Paramus, NJ.

autologous activated natural killer (NK) cell therapy for malignancy

Synonyms
activated NK therapy

Use
treatment of advanced malignancy

Method
interleukin-2 activation of autologous NK cells followed by reinfusion

Specimen
peripheral blood lymphocytes

Normal range
not applicable

Comments
currently in multiple clinical trials

Source
Adapted from Benyunes MC, Higuchi C, York A, et al. Immunotherapy with interleukin-2 with or without lymphokine-activated killer cells after autologous bone marrow transplantation for malignant lymphoma: a feasibility trial. Bone Marrow Transplantation 1995;16:283-288.

autologous peripheral blood stem cell collection

Synonyms
autologous stem cell collection; peripheral stem cell collection; progenitor cell collection

Use
collect enough peripheral stem cells to repopulate patient's bone marrow after heavy chemotherapy and/or irradiation sufficient to obliterate marrow function and then, it is hoped, to destroy remaining malignant cells

Method
patient undergoes course of chemotherapy and may receive hematopoietic growth factor (e.g. GM-CSF, G-CSF) stimulation; stem cell protocol leukapheresis

Specimen
blood

Normal range
absence of malignant cells

Comments
indicated for patients with malignant disease not responding to conventional therapy

Source
Lexi-Comp Inc. database. Hudson, OH.

automated colorimetric HIV-1 drug susceptibility testing

Synonyms
automated rapid HIV-1 drug susceptibility testing
Use
determination of drug susceptibilities in strains of HIV-1
Method
automated colorimetric tetrazolium dye MT-2 cell viability measurement
Specimen
isolated HIV-1 strain
Normal range
not applicable
Comments
may replace current expensive and time consuming methods of viral
susceptibility testing
Source
Adapted from Jellinger RM, Shafer RW, Merigan TC. A novel approach to assessing the drug susceptibility and
replication of human immunodeficiency virus type 1 isolates. Journal of Infectious Diseases 1997;175:561-566.

 automated Pap smear screening

Synonyms
AutoPap 300 QC Automatic Pap Screener System, PAPNET
Use
quality control re-evaluation of Pap smear slides previously classified as normal
Method
computerized image-analysis microscopy
Specimen
Pap smear
Normal range
No evidence of dysplasia
Comments
recently granted FDA pre-market approval
Source
University of Minnesota Department of Laboratory Medicine and Pathology. Minneapolis, MN.

 autonomous erythroid growth flow cytometric assay

Synonyms
flow cytometric assay for erythroid precursors capable of autonomous growth
Use
diagnosis of polycythemia vera

Method
two-stage peripheral blood mononuclear cell culture to maximize growth of erythropoietin-independent erythroid cells, detected and enumerated by immunofluorescence flow cytometry

Specimen
peripheral blood mononuclear cells

Normal range
investigational, may be in the range of <5% autonomously growing erythroid colonies

Comments
flow cytometric read-out should make this assay superior to current autonomous erythroid development in vitro assays requiring erythroid colony scoring

Source
Adapted from Manor D, Rachmilewitz EA, Fibach E. Improved method for diagnosis of polycythemia vera based on flow cytometric analysis of autonomous growth of erythroid precursors in liquid culture. American Journal of Hematology 1997;54: 47-52.

 AutoSet portable system

Description
computer controlled nasal continuous positive airway pressure (CPAP) system for management of obstructive sleep apnea in adults; automatic titration of CPAP; measures and stores patient data on apnea, snoring, oxygen saturation, mask pressure and other respiratory disturbances; can print out results

Source
ResMed product information. San Diego, CA.

 Avan

Generic Name
see idebenone

 Avapro

Generic name
see irbesartan

 Avonex

Generic Name
see interferon beta-1a

azapropazone

Brand Name
Rheumox

Use
nonsteroidal anti-inflammatory drug with analgesic, anti-inflammatory, and antipyretic and uricosuric properties

Usual Dosage
oral: 600 mg twice daily

Pharmaceutical company
Robins/Wyeth-Ayerst Labs. Philadelphia, PA.

Source
University of Pittsburgh Drug Information and Pharmacoepidemiology Center. Pittsburgh, PA.

 ## azelaic acid

Brand name
Azelex

Use
topical treatment of mild-to-moderate inflammatory acne vulgaris

Usual dosage
topical 20% cream supplied in 30 gm tubes; apply twice daily

Pharmaceutical company
Allergan Pharmaceuticals. Irvine, CA.

Source
University of Pittsburgh Drug Information and Pharmacoepidemiology Center. Pittsburgh, PA.

 ## azelastine

Brand Name
Astelin

Use
anti-inflammatory agent used in the treatment and prophylaxis of seasonal and perennial allergic rhinitis

Usual Dosage
intranasal: 0.14 mg per nostril twice daily

Pharmaceutical company
Carter-Wallace. Cranbury, NJ.

Source
University of Pittsburgh Drug Information and Pharmacoepidemiology Center. Pittsburgh, PA.

Azelex

Generic name
see azelaic acid

 Backbar device

Description
barbell-shaped, hand-held device that uses the principles of self-administered symmetrical acupressure to relieve back pain; adjustable for any size individual
Source
The Outlook Design Co. product information. Andover, MA.

 Back Bull lumbar support system

Description
patented lumbar support that is a specialized miniature version of a standard lumbar support cushion
Source
Posture Dynamics Inc. product information. Brick, NJ.

 BackCycler continuous passive motion device

Description
microprocessor-controlled pneumatic cushion combining spinal mobilization and lordotic support; gently moves spine back and forth, shifting patterns of stress on the vertebrae, muscles, and ligaments; increases fluid and nutrient movement in and out of the intervertebral disks; designed for use in car seats and at home
Source
Ergomedics Inc. product information. Winooski, VT.

 Back-Huggar lumbar support

Description
ergonomically contoured lumbar support in standard, bucket seat, extra-wide, and secretary chairs
Source
Bodyline Comfort Systems product information. Jacksonville, FL.

Backjoy seat

Description
device to relieve and prevent back pain
Source
Sunsource International Inc. product information. Maui, HI.

back range of motion device

Description
measures back range of motion (BROM) including rotation and lateral flexion; positioned against the sacrum
Source
Performance Attainment Assoc. product information. St. Paul, MN.

BackThing lumbar support

Description
neoprene lumbar wrap for flexible joint and tissue support
Source
SportsTech/R.U. product information. Victor, ID.

Bactalert platelet concentrate microbial testing

Synonyms
Bactalert platelet testing
Use
monitoring of microbial contamination of platelet concentrates
Method
semi-automated microbial culture carbon dioxide detection
Specimen
platelet concentrate
Normal range
no evidence of contamination
Comments
automated microbial testing permits monitoring of platelet concentrates, the blood product at greatest risk for microbial contamination
Source
Adapted from Smith N, Fincham A, Bissell L et al. Bacterial surveillance of platelet concentrates using the Bactalert system. Transfusion Science 1996;12:5.

Baerveldt implant

Description
glaucoma shunt for intraocular pressure control; 200, 350, and 500 mm² (surface area) affords intraocular pressure control with few medications; superior temporal quadrant placement; models include BG103-250, BG101-350, BG103-425

Source
Iovision product information. Irvine, CA.

 ## Bag Bath

Description
ideal bathing alternative; heat one unopened package in a microwave oven for approximately 30 seconds or until warm to the touch, use one cloth for each of the areas of the body in a sequence that matches your bathing protocol

Source
Incline Technologies Inc. product information. Incline Village, NV.

 ## BagEasy disposable manual resuscitator

Description
bag oxygen resuscitator with built-in PEEP (peak end-expiratory pressure or positive end-expiratory pressure); oxygen reservoir is up front where it can be seen; 360 degree swivel and flexible front end with conformable CircleSeal mask that conforms to the contour of the patient's face and retains the shape for an easy seal; adult, child, and infant sizes

Source
Respironics Inc. product information. Murrysville, PA.

 ## balsalazide disodium

Brand name
Colazide

Use
to maintain remission in ulcerative colitis

Usual dosage
oral: 2.25 grams three times a day was used in clinical trials

Pharmaceutical company
Astra-Salix. Westboro, MA.

Source
Stadtlanders Managed Pharmacy Services. Pittsburgh, PA.

Bard BladderScan

Description
bladder volume instrument; portable ultrasound scanner for noninvasive bladder measurement; minimizes risks of urinary tract infection; eliminates catheter insertion trauma

Source
CR Bard Patient Care product information. Murray Hill, NJ.

 Bard bladder tumor-associated analytes (BTA) test

Synonyms
BTA test

Use
test aids in detection of bladder cancer more accurately

Method
diagnostic strip

Specimen
single voided urine sample

Normal range
not applicable

Comments
results available in three minutes

Source
Bard Urological Division product information. Covington, GA.

 Bard Touchless Clean-Cath Ultra

Description
vinyl intermittent catheterization products; each catheter is enclosed in a see-through pouch; insertion of catheter into urethra is performed by advancing the catheter within the pouch; user's hands never come in contact with the catheter; available with a 14 French (14-Fr) 6 inch long catheter for females or 14 French (14-Fr) 16 inch long unisex catheter

Source
Bard Inc. product information. Murray Hill, NJ.

 Barrett hydrodelineation cannula

Description
cannula (25 gauge) for cataract procedures; beveled up to provide easy insertion and injection of fluid for hydrodelineation of the lens nucleus

Source
Storz Ophthalmics product information. St. Louis, MO.

Bartonella henselae detection

Synonyms
Rochalimaea henselae detection

Use
identification of *Bartonella henselae* in patients suspected of infection

Method
BacT/Alert blood culture system with immunofluorescent confirmation

Specimen
blood

Normal range
no evidence of growth

Comments
Bartonella henselae is only presumptively identifiable by standard detection methods

Source
American Journal of Clinical Pathology 1995;104:530-536.

 basal cell-specific anti-cytokeratin antibody

Use
diagnosis of prostate cancer

Method
immunostaining for basal cell-specific cytokeratin

Specimen
prostate epithelium

Normal range
not applicable; cancer graded with Gleason system; if patient is cancer free, no antibody detected

Comments
useful tool in confirming, establishing, or changing diagnosis on questionable foci in surgical pathology; most useful in workup of foci of atypical glands on needle biopsy and in differentiating low-grade adenocarcinoma from adenosis on transurethral resection of prostate (TURP)

Source
Adapted from Wojno K, Epstein J. The utility of basal cell-specific anti-cytokeratin antibody (34BE12) in the diagnosis of prostate cancer: a review of 228 cases. American Journal of Surgical Pathology 1995;19:251-259.

basiliximab

Brand name
Simulect

Use
immunosuppressive agent used in combination with cyclosporine for the prevention of acute kidney rejection

Usual dosage
intravenous: 20-60 mg/day

Pharmaceutical company
Novartis. East Hanover, NJ.

Source
Stadtlanders Managed Pharmacy Services. Pittsburgh, PA.

 Baycol

Generic name
see cerivastatin sodium

 Baypress

Generic name
see nitrendipine

 Bazooka support surface

Description
specialty bed with dynamic air flotation, compression therapy and pressure relief that compensates for patient weight and movement to enhance capillary blood flow and assist in reduction of tissue edema

Source
Universal Hospital Services Inc. product information. Bloomington, MN.

 bead-mediated platelet-specific antibody assay

Synonyms
bead-mediated platelet assay

Use
detection and differentiation of platelet-bound antibodies

Method
isolation of human platelet glycoproteins using flow cytometric standardization beads following incubation of typed platelets with human sera

Specimen
serum

Normal range
no evidence of platelet-specific antibody

Comments
rapid, sensitive assay may replace or augment monoclonal antibody-specific immobilization of platelet antigen assay and modified antigen-capture enzyme-linked immunosorbent assay

Source
Adapted from Helmberg W, Folsch B, Wagner T, Lanzer G. Detection and differentiation of platelet-specific antibodies by flow cytometry: the bead-mediated platelet assay. Transfusion 1997;37:502-506.

 becaplermin

Brand name
Regranex

Use
recombinant human platelet derived growth factor used topically in wound healing

Usual dosage
topical: once daily application of 100 or 300 µg/ml has been used in the clinical trial for the treatment of deep pressure ulcers

Pharmaceutical company
Chiron Therapeutics. Emeryville, CA.

Source
University of Pittsburgh Drug Information and Pharmacoepidemiology Center. Pittsburgh, PA.

 Becker orthopaedic spinal system (B.O.S.S.) orthotic device

Description
incorporates features orthotists deem essential: locking lever, adjustable sides, serrated discs, and flexible back

Source
Becker Orthopaedic product information. Troy, MI.

 Bedfont carbon monoxide monitor

Description
micro and mini Smokerlyzers; carbon monoxide and carboxyhemoglobin monitors; noninvasive method of verifying if patient is smoking while on nicotine patches

Source
Bedfont Innovative Associates product information. Medford, NJ.

 Benefix

Generic name
see factor IX

BengalScreen

Synonyms
none

Use
rapid immunodiagnostic test for direct detection of *Vibrio cholerae* O139 (Bengal strain)

Method
monoclonal antibody-based coagglutination reaction

Specimen
water or stool

Normal range
no evidence of agglutination

Comments
highly portable and requires less than 5 minutes to complete

Source
Adapted from Hasan JA, Huq A, Nair GB, Garg S, Mukhopadhyay AK, Loomis L, Bernstein D, Colwell RR. Development and testing of monoclonal antibody-based rapid immunodiagnostic test kits for direct detection of *Vibrio cholerae* O139 synonym Bengal. Journal of Clinical Microbiology 1995;33:2935-2939.

 bentoquatam

Brand name
IvyBlock

Use
helps protect against poison ivy, poison oak, and sumac when applied before contact occurs

Usual dosage
topical: applied as a 5% lotion 15 minutes prior to possible contact with poisonous plant

Pharmaceutical company
EnviroDerm. Louisville, KY.

Source
Stadtlanders Managed Pharmacy Services. Pittsburgh, PA.

 Bergland-Warshawski phaco/cortex kit

Description
ophthalmic adapter kit allowing removal of cortex at the 12 o'clock position through a microvitreoretinal puncture at the 2 o'clock position

Source
Eagle Laboratories product information. Rancho Cucamonga, CA.

Bertin hip retractor

Description
self-retaining hip fracture surgical instrument, which allows surgeon to achieve excellent exposure; allows access to lateral side of femur for surgical instrumentation and implant insertions

Source
Innomed Inc. product information. Savannah, GA.

 Beta-Cap closure system for catheters

Description
Beta-Cap adapter, clamp, and cap system components; when filled with povidone-iodine provides infection barrier for peritoneal catheters; useful for patients on intermittent or continuous ambulatory peritoneal dialysis

Source
Quinton Instrument Co. product information. Seattle, WA.

 Betafectin

Generic name
see zymosan

 betaine anhydrous

Brand name
Cystadane

Use
treatment of homocystinuria; a rare genetic disorder caused by various inborn errors of methionine metabolism

Usual dosage
oral solution: 100 mg/kg/day and then increase weekly by 100 mg/kg increments for children less than 3 years old; for ages 3 years to an adult: 3 gm twice a day, up to 20 gm per day

Pharmaceutical company
Orphan Medical Inc. Minnetonka, MN.

Source
Stadtlanders Managed Pharmacy Services. Pittsburgh, PA.

bicalutamide

Brand Name
Casodex

Use
treatment of prostate cancer in combination with luteinizing hormone-releasing hormone agonist

Usual Dosage
oral: 50 mg once daily

Pharmaceutical company
Zeneca. Wilmington, DE.

Source
University of Pittsburgh Drug Information and Pharmacoepidemiology Center. Pittsburgh, PA.

 bifurcated vein graft (autologous pedal) for vascular reconstruction

Description
autologous vein grafts are the material of choice for small- to medium-size artery reconstruction; a composite vein graft to recreate an arterial bifurcation is occasionally required; reconstruction of arterial bifurcations is sometimes complicated by inability to mobilize arterial branches; use of autogenous material is preferred over prosthetic material for small caliber reconstructions

Anatomy
(harvested area) dorsum of foot; greater saphenous vein; medial malleolus; valves (reconstruction areas) arterial branches; common carotid artery; hepatic artery; renal artery; superior mesenteric artery; tibioperoneal trunk; valves

Equipment
standard surgery equipment; intraluminal shunt; Mill valvulotome; valvulotomy scissors

Source
Adapted from Carpenter JP, Weinmann EE. Autologous bifurcated vein graft for vascular reconstructions. Journal of American College of Surgeons 1995;181:83-84.

 bilateral retroperitoneal renal allografts

Description
shortage of donor organs has resulted in innovative techniques for transplantation of marginal organs; this technique uses the placement of both donor kidneys into a single recipient, while each donor kidney would be unsuitable when considered as a single allograft; use of both kidneys theoretically provides sufficient nephron mass for effective glomerular filtration; placement of both organs through a standard lower abdominal midline incision is the adopted technique

Anatomy

dome of bladder; external iliac artery and vein; iliac fossa; inferior epigastric vessels; iliopsoas and quadratus lumborum muscles; infraumbilical area; kidney; linea alba; peritoneal envelope; parietal peritoneum; preperitoneal fat; rectal fasciae

Equipment

standard urologic surgical equipment

Source

Adapted from Kuo PC, delaTorre A, Johnson LB, Schweitzer EJ, Bartlett ST. Bilateral retroperitoneal renal allografts: technique for placement though midline incision. Journal of American College of Surgeons 1997;183:529-530.

 ## bilobed digital neurovascular island flap

Description

reconstructive treatment of complete degloving digital injury in a one-stage procedure including microneurorrhaphy

Anatomy

phalanx; nail bed; neurovascular bundle; profundus flexor tendon; ulnar nerve and superficial sensory branch ulnar nerve; palmar digital artery

Equipment

standard surgical equipment

Source

Adapted from Tsai C, Lin S, Lai C, Chou C. Reconstruction of the totally degloved little finger with a bilobed digital neurovascular island flap. Annals of Plastic Surgery 1995;35:529-533.

 ## Bio-Eye ocular implant

Description

natural hydroxyapatite implant; integrated with rectus muscles and orbital tissues, can be coupled directly to artificial eye; provides motility, fibrovascular ingrowth, and resistance to migration and extrusion

Source

Integrated Orbital Implants Inc. product information. San Diego, CA.

 ## Biogel Reveal glove

Description

two-layer latex glove with a light-colored outer layer and a dark-green inner layer; puncture of outer layer in presence of fluid produces color change to dark green

Source

Regent Hospital Products product information. Greenville, SC.

64

Biogel sensor surgical glove

Description

provide sensitivity for delicate procedures; although more than 20% thinner than the Biogel glove, they puncture in use considerably less often than standard gloves

Source

Regent Hospital Products Ltd. product information. Greenville, SC.

BioGlide catheter

Description

hydrophilic surface modification enhances lubricity, allowing easier insertion; when hydrated prior to insertion a portion of the solution is absorbed, giving hydrophilic qualities to the surface

Source

Medtronic PS Medical product information. Goleta, CA.

BioGran resorbable synthetic bone graft

Description

resorbable synthetic bone; FDA market clearance for periodontal defects, extraction sites, and ridge augmentations

Source

Orthovita product information. Malvern, PA.

Bio-Guard spectrum catheter

Description

antimicrobial bonded central venous catheter that provides prophylaxis against catheter infections; cross-resistance with vancomycin or ß-lactam antibiotics not exhibited

Source

Cook Surgical product information. Bloomington, IN.

BioKnit garment electrodes

Description

conductive garment made of dust-free monofilament light-weight nylon for those who suffer from pain, swelling, and repetitive strains

Source

BioMedical Life Systems Inc. product information. Vista, CA.

Biologically Quiet reconstruction screw

Description
biodegradable screw for bone-tendon grafting; completely absorbed and replaced by new cancellous bone after six months; eliminates need for surgery to remove hardware

Source
Instrument Makar Inc. product information. Okemos, MI.

 Biologics Airlift bed

Description
dynamic pressure relief air fluid bed for management of decubitus ulcers; designed to eliminate risk of dehydration and shear/friction related skin injuries; provides inflatable air chamber when repositioning is necessary

Source
Red Line Medical product information. Golden Valley, MN.

 BioLon

Generic name
see sodium hyaluronate

 biomechanical evaluation of foot function during stance phase of gait

Synonyms
(related terms) kinematics; kinetics

Indications
measurement of foot function in patients with pathological conditions (rheumatoid arthritis; pronated foot) and those without foot pathology

Method
biomechanical tools include electrogoniometers and imaging techniques, 3D computerized movement analysis (Vicon), and force platform mounted flush with the floor

Normal findings
adequate assessment and measurements of rocker function of foot as compared to a normal subject: measurement of heel rocker as foot is lowered to floor, ankle rocker as tibia advances over fixed foot, and forefoot rocker as heel rises for push-off; movements occur in sagittal plane

Comments
technique demonstrated ability to differentiate normal from pathological function

Source
Adapted from Siegel KL, Kepple TM, O'Connell PG, et al. A technique to evaluate foot function during the stance phase of gait. Foot and Ankle International Journal 1995;16:764-770.

Bio-Medicus arterial catheter

Description
large-bore catheter 15 to 21F with Luerlock side-port for rapid infusion of volume before and after initiation of bypass; inserted via Seldinger technique
Source
Bio-Medicus product information. Eden Prairie, MN.

 BioMend

Description
periodontal material used to cover defect sites; made of bovine Achilles tendon
Source
Calcitek product information. Carlsbad, CA.

 Bio-Oss bone filler

Description
bovine-derived natural bone matrix from which protein has been removed; bone filler used in oral and maxillofacial surgery; eliminates rejection or immunological reaction; osteoconductive; reproduces the pore system of natural bone
Source
Osteohealth Co. product information. Shirley, NY.

 Biopatch antimicrobial dressing

Description
nontoxic, nonirritating antimicrobial dressing with center-hole for placement around orthopaedic pins; inhibits growth of bacteria; reduces risk of infection
Source
Johnson & Johnson Medical Inc. product information. Piscataway, NJ.

 Biopharm leeches

Description
leeches, "the biting edge of science," are generally used on any skin flap or other tissue suffering from impaired venous circulation (venous congestion); called leeching or hirudinization
Source
Biopharm Leeches Ltd. product information. Charleston, SC.

Bioplant hard tissue replacement (HTR) synthetic bone

Description
microporous bone substitute used in post-extraction implant procedures

Source
Septodont Inc. product information. New Castle, DE.

 Bioplate screw fixation system

Description
self-tapping, fluted titanium alloy screws utilize a press-fit center-drive system for craniomaxillofacial surgical procedures (Editor note: these screw sizes do show the 0 before the 1.5 which is a deviation from normal use when the 0 is dropped and only 1.5 mm is used, i.e., 01.0 mm to 01.5 mm)

Source
Bioplate Inc. product information. Los Angeles, CA.

 biopsy urease test (BUT)

Synonyms
rapid urease test (RUT)

Use
diagnose *Helicobacter pylori* among patients undergoing endoscopy

Method
gastric antral mucosal biopsy specimen

Specimen
gastric mucosal biopsy

Normal range
absence of *Helicobacter pylori*; no color change in the pH indicator

Comments
results are available within 24 hours; there are three rapid urease tests including CLOtest, Hpfast and Pyloritek (Editor note: CLOtest got its name from "*Campylobacter*-like organism" test. At the time CLOtest was patented in 1985, *H. pylori* was called a *Campylobacter*, which means "curved bacteria". Now there are enough of these bacteria to warrant their own genus called *Helicobacter*, which means "spiral or helical bacteria".)

Source
Adapted from Editorials. The new urea membrane tests: BUT, RUT, or what? Gastrointestinal Endoscopy 1996;44(5):519-521, 626-627.

68

Bio-R-Sorb resorbable poly-L-lactic acid mini-staples

Description
bioresorbable high molecular weight poly-L-lactic acid staples that are slow-ly and gradually reabsorbed over a period of 24-36 months

Source
Adapted from Barca F, Busa R. Resorbable poly-L-lactic acid mini-staples for the fixation of Akin osteotomies. The Journal of Foot and Ankle Surgery 1997;36:106-111.

BioSkin support

Description
nonbinding compression support with anatomical design that fits like skin; made of patented material designed to replace neoprene compression devices; provides support for protection of extremities

Source
Cropper Medical product information. Ashland, OR.

Biosyn suture

Description
synthetic absorbable Glycomer monofilament sutures for general surgery

Source
United States Surgical Corp. product information. Norwalk, CT.

Biothotic orthotic mold

Description
high-tech mold for precise control of foot function; easily posted and adjust-ed functional and accommodative orthotics; resin sets in 3 minutes, provid-ing permanent support; orthotic can be posted with wedges and is available in various degrees

Source
Orthofeet Inc. product information. Northvale, NJ.

Bio-Tropin

Generic name
see somatropin

Bisolvon

Generic name
see bromhexine

Bivona-Colorado voice prosthesis

Description
accessories and puncture kits for attachment to dummy prosthesis for sizing post total laryngectomy

Source
Bivona Medical Technologies product information. Gary, IN.

BladderManager ultrasound scanner

Description
portable ultrasound scanner used to measure amount of urine in the bladder; designed for patients with spinal cord injuries, multiple sclerosis, or spina bifida

Source
Diagnostic Ultrasound product information. Redmond, WA.

bladder wall pedicle wraparound sling

Description
modification of current bladder neck reconstruction developed to provide tapering, circumferential compression, and suspension of the bladder neck; involves wrapping a pedicle and suspending it to the symphysis pubis; results are encouraging in female patients; applicability to male patients is more limited

Anatomy
anterior bladder wall; anterior rectus fascia; bladder neck; Cooper ligament; detrusor muscle; dome of bladder; internal sphincter; mucosa; prostate; prostatic urethra; rectus abdominis fascia; seminal vesicles; symphysis pubis; ureter; urethra; urinary sphincter; vagina

Equipment
standard urologic surgery equipment; coudé-tip catheter; electrocautery; right-angle clamp; suprapubic tube; umbilical tape; urethral catheter

Source
Adapted from Kurzrock EA, Lowe P, Hardy BE. Bladder wall pedicle wraparound sling for neurogenic urinary incontinence in children. Journal of Urology 1996;155:305-308.

Blake silicone drain

Description
fluted, 4-flow channel drain provides greater tissue contact area to maximize fluid entry; no holes for tissue to occlude or invaginate into making removal less painful; increased tensile strength for use in virtually all surgical procedures when closed wound drainage is indicated

Source
Johnson & Johnson Medical Inc. product information. Arlington, TX.

70

 blepharoplasty, modified Loeb and de la Plaza techniques

Description

two different techniques were described: Loeb "sliding pad" technique modified by carrying it out with a transconjunctival approach; the de la Plaza technique consisting of placing the fat from the palpebral bags back into the orbital cavity, and its retention by suturing the capsulopalpebral fascia to the periosteum of the orbital rim; lifting of the upper two-thirds of the face often needs to be done with eyelid surgery, which has a favorable effect on the tissues of the orbita and periorbita

Anatomy

canthal ligament; capsulopalpebral fascia; facial mimic muscles; Horner muscle; orbicularis oculi muscle; palpebral raphe; septum orbitale; tetrastructure of superficial fascial system

Equipment

standard blepharoplasty surgical equipment; de la Plaza retractor

Source

Adapted from de la Plaza R, de la Cruz L. A new concept in blepharoplasty. Aesthetic Plastic Surgery 1996;20:221-232.

 blocking or stimulating thyroid stimulating hormone (TSH) receptor antibody

Synonyms

Use

advanced workup of suspected thyroid dysfunction

Method

immunoassay using peptide-specific monoclonal antibodies

Specimen

blood

Normal range

negative

Comments

discrepant thyroid function testing results may require differentiation of blocking and stimulating TSH receptor antibodies

Source

Adapted from Reinhardt MJ, Moser E. An update on diagnostic methods in the investigation of diseases of the thyroid. European Journal of Nuclear Medicine 1996;23:587-594.

 blood ethyl benzene detection

Synonyms

Use

monitor exposure to ethyl benzene

Method
gas chromatography

Specimen
blood

Normal range
none detected; limit of detection: 0.05 mg/L

Comments
none

Source
Lexi-Comp Inc. database. Hudson, OH.

 Blumenthal anterior chamber maintainer

Description
ophthalmic instrument that maintains the chamber without use of viscoelastics; provides a continuous high flow of fluid to the anterior chamber

Source
Visitec product information. Sarasota, FL.

 BMSI 5000

Description
instrument for long-term electroencephalography (EEG) epilepsy monitoring system; other potential applications include cerebral function monitoring in neonates, long-term EEG monitoring of intensive care patients, and correlated sleep and epilepsy studies

Source
Nicolet Biomedical Inc. product information. Madison, WI.

 Body Armor walker cast

Description
hard polyurethane shell acts like a cast; protects lower leg and ankle; provides compression to decrease edema; adjustable straps and cut-out vents; open-toe shoe

Source
Darco International product information. Huntington, WV.

 Bondek suture

Description
multifilament, synthetic, absorbable suture; coated with Polyglyd for ease in gliding through tissue

Source
Snowden Pencer DSP product information. Fall River, MA.

72

 bone augmentation for atrophic jaw

Description
thin, collapsed alveolar ridge split and filled in with bone chips; if implant is fixed in base of atrophic alveolar ridge and supported by palatal bone wall, buccally exposed implant threats are covered with autogenous bone grafts; simultaneous insertion of implants along with free bone grafts allows early functional loading and stimulates bone remodeling; implant-supported prostheses are used for oral rehabilitation

Anatomy
maxilla; alveolar ridge

Equipment
standard surgical equipment

Source
Adapted from Weingart D, Schilli W, Assael L. Bone augmentation procedures in atrophic jaws. Implant Dentistry 1996;5:56.

 bone culture

Use
determine precise bacterial etiology of osteomyelitis

Method
microbiologic culture for aerobic bacteria and Haemophilus

Specimen
bone biopsy

Normal range
no growth detected

Comments
aspirated specimens may be used in suspected acute infections

Source
University of Minnesota Department of Laboratory Medicine and Pathology. Minneapolis, MN.

 BoneSource hydroxyapatite cement

Description
cement used for filling cranial defects and restoring contours; easily sculptured, moldable and sets with little or no heat release

Source
Howmedica Leibinger Inc. product information. Dallas, TX.

Bot-B

Generic name
see botulinum toxin type B

 botulinum toxin type B

Brand name
Bot-B

Use
botulinum toxin type B used in the treatment of cervical dystonia

Usual dosage
injectable: doses of 100 MU to 1,910 MU administered as single injection at two neck muscles in an early pilot study

Pharmaceutical company
Athena Neurosciences. San Francisco, CA.

Source
Stadtlanders Managed Pharmacy Services. Pittsburgh, PA.

 brachioradialis transfer for wrist extension

Description
brachioradialis tendon transferred to the extensor carpi radialis longus and brevis tendons to restore active extension of the wrist; used with patients who have traumatic tetraplegia; provides extension of the wrist that is strong enough for useful function of the hand; uses a side-weave technique

Anatomy
brachioradialis tendon; extensor carpi radialis tendon; brevis tendons; radius; radial sensory nerve

Equipment
standard orthopaedic equipment

Source
Adapted from Johnson DL, Gellman H, Waters RL, Tognella M. Brachioradialis transfer for wrist extension in tetraplegic patients who have fifth-cervical-level neurological function. The Journal of Bone and Joint Surgery 1996;78:1063-1067.

 branched DNA signal amplification assay for hepatitis B

Synonyms
HBV bDNA signal amplification

Use
measurement of patient's hepatitis B viral load

Method
chemiluminescent DNA capture and amplification assay
Specimen
serum
Normal range
hepatitis B DNA not detected
Comments
quantitation of hepatitis B viral DNA in human serum investigational, but has been used to measure hepatitis B viral DNA in serum
Source
American Journal of Clinical Pathology 1995;104:537-546.

Branemark System for craniofacial rehabilitation

Description
implants that establish a bone-anchored foundation aesthetically designed prosthesis; for patients in need of head and neck cancer reconstruction, or with congenital and trauma-related facial defects
Source
Nobelpharma product information. Westmont, IL.

Bravavir

Generic Name
see sorivudine

breast cancer scintigraphy

Synonyms
scintimammography; breast tumor scintigraphy; breast imaging
Indications
effective test for evaluating palpable breast masses
Method
inject thallium-201 or technetium-99m sestamibi (Cardiolite); image breast area with gamma camera
Normal findings
no accumulation of radioactivity on the scintigram strongly indicates a benign lesion
Comments
none
Source
Lexi-Comp Inc. database. Hudson, OH. Nuclear Medicine Consultant. Stedman's Medical Dictionary, 26th edition.

Breast Implant Protector (B.I.P.)

Description
protective shield for use in breast augmentation, reconstruction, and expansion surgeries; easily inserted between implant and subcutaneous tissues; protects implant from nicks and punctures; when closure is completed protector is removed; provides ease for surgeons in closing subcutaneous tissues over the implant

Source
Adept-Med International product information. El Dorado Hills, CA.

breast tissue telomerase activity

Synonyms
none

Use
diagnosis of suspected malignant breast lesions

Method
direct measurement of cellular telomerase enzyme activity

Specimen
breast biopsies and fine-needle aspirates

Normal range
investigational

Comments
may permit identification of cells that have lost normal growth regulation, a critical step in malignant transformation

Source
Adapted from Sugino T et al. Telomerase activity in human breast cancer and benign breast lesions: diagnostic applications in clinical specimens, including fine-needle aspirates. International Journal of Cancer 1996;69:301-306.

Breast Vest EXU-DRY one-piece wound dressing

Description
wound dressing that covers the chest wall and hard-to-dress axilla; excellent for moist skin desquamation that may develop in post mastectomy patients

Source
Kaysons International Inc. product information. Tarrytown, NY.

breathing pacemaker

Description
device with external transmitter and antennas that transmit energy to bilaterally implanted receivers that convert radio signals to stimulating pulses delivered to phrenic nerves by electrodes; for ventilation-dependent patients

Source
Avery Laboratories Inc. product information. Long Island, NY.

 breath test detects *Helicobacter pylori*

Synonyms
none

Indications
dyspepsia

Method
an oral dose of urea given; if *H. pylori* is present in gastric mucosa the urea breaks down to ammonia and carbon dioxide (CO_2) which are detectable in the breath indicating *H. pylori* infection

Normal findings
negative

Comments
diagnosis and treatment of most cases of dyspepsia, gastritis, and peptic ulcer disease can be simplified by breathtaking technology; most patients complaining of dyspepsia could have infection treated by general internist

Source
Adapted from Phillips M. Breathtaking technology for the detection of *Helicobacter pylori*. American Journal of Gastroenterology 1995;90:2089-2090.

 brimonidine tartrate

Brand name
Alphagan

Use
for lowering intraocular pressure in patients with open-angle glaucoma or ocular hypertension

Usual dosage
ophthalmic: one drop in the affected eye(s) three times daily; approximately eight hours apart

Pharmaceutical company
Allergan. Irvine, CA.

Source
Stadtlanders Managed Pharmacy Services. Pittsburgh, PA.

Brisman-Nova carotid endarterectomy shunt

Description
internal shunt consisting of balloon, inflation arm, and cone-shaped bulb; inflation balloon provides atraumatic method for preventing backflow around internal shunt

Source
Heyer-Schulte NeuroCare product information. Pleasant Prairie, WI.

 brofaromine

Brand Name
Consonar

Use
selective reversible monamine oxidase inhibitor type-A used in the treatment of depression and panic disorders

Usual Dosage
oral: in clinical trials doses were initiated at 25-50 mg/day in two divided doses and then titrated up to 150 mg/day as tolerated

Pharmaceutical company
Ciba-Geigy Pharmaceuticals. Summit, NJ.

Source
University of Pittsburgh Drug Information and Pharmacoepidemiology Center. Pittsburgh, PA.

 bromfenac

Brand name
Duract

Use
non-narcotic and nonsteroidal anti-inflammatory agent used to treat mild to moderate pain and inflammation

Usual dosage
oral: clinical trials included administration of single daily doses ranging from 25-100 mg

Pharmaceutical company
Wyeth-Ayerst Laboratories. Philadelphia, PA.

Source
Stadtlanders Managed Pharmacy Services. Pittsburgh, PA.

bromhexine

Brand name
Bisolvon

Use
expectorant/mucolytic agent for use in Sjogren syndrome and mild or moderate chronic bronchitis

Usual dosage
oral: 8 to 16 mg three times daily or 30 mg twice daily

Pharmaceutical company
Boehringer Ingelheim. Ridgefield, CT.

Source
University of Pittsburgh Drug Information and Pharmacoepidemiology Center. Pittsburgh, PA.

 bromocriptine

Brand name
Ergoset

Use
used as monotherapy or in combination with oral sulfonylureas to control blood glucose levels in Type II diabetes

Usual dosage
oral: 1.6 to 2.4 mg a day

Pharmaceutical company
Ergoscience Corp. Boston, MA.

Source
Stadtlanders Managed Pharmacy Services. Pittsburgh, PA.

 bropirimine

Brand name
Remisar

Use
treatment of carcinoma in situ bladder cancer and/or superficial bladder cancer

Usual dosage
oral: 250 mg tablets; phase I and II trials have used the total daily dose ranging from 1.5 g to 4.5 g/day. The daily dose is to be administered every 2 hours in 3 divided doses every day for 3 consecutive days and to repeat every 12 weeks

Pharmaceutical company
Pharmacia and Upjohn. Kalamazoo, MI.

Source
Stadtlanders Managed Pharmacy Services. Pittsburgh, PA.

buccal mucosa harvest for urethral reconstruction

Description
urethral substitution in complex hypospadias repairs and traumatic urethral repairs

Anatomy
mouth area; cheek; buccal mucosa; penis; urethra; glans, corona

Equipment
standard surgical equipment; Steinhauser mucosa stretcher

Source
Adapted from Morey AF, McAninch JW. Technique of harvesting mucosa for urethral reconstruction. Journal of Urology 1996;155:166-167.

 buccinator myomucosal flap

Description
floor-of-mouth reconstruction is treatment of choice following ablative tumor surgery; intraoral and extraoral approaches are two techniques of harvesting the flap; reconstructs defects of the floor of the mouth using free-tissue transfer

Anatomy
buccinator muscle; buccal fat pad; carotid artery; gingivobuccal sulcus; mandible, maxilla; oral commissure; orbicularis oris muscle; parotid duct; pterygomandibular raphe; pterygoid plexus; parotideomasseteric fascia; periodontal gingiva; periosteum

Equipment
standard surgery equipment; loupe magnification; methylene blue; Doppler; Silastic tubing; Xeroform bolster dressing

Source
Adapted from Stofman GM, Carstens MH, Berman PD, Arena S, Sotereanos GC. Reconstruction of the floor of the mouth by means of an anteriorly based buccinator myomucosal island flap. The Laryngoscope 1995;105:90-96.

 budesonide

Brand name
Rhinocort

Use
glucocorticoid to treat the symptoms of seasonal allergic rhinitis

Usual dosage
intranasal: 2 sprays in each nostril in the morning and evening

Pharmaceutical company
Astra USA Inc. Westborough, MA.

Source
University of Pittsburgh Drug Information and Pharmacoepidemiology Center. Pittsburgh, PA.

Buedding squeegee cortex extractor and polisher

Description
ophthalmic instrument; irrigating cortex extractor with silicone sleeve for the 12 o'clock position; 23 mm long

Source
Eagle Laboratories product information. Rancho Cucamonga, CA.

 ## Buphenyl

Generic name
see sodium phenylbutyrate

 ## bupropion hydrochloride

Brand name
Zyban

Use
nicotine-free smoking cessation agent that works in the brain to decrease cravings and withdrawal symptoms

Usual dosage
oral: 150 mg twice a day for 7-12 weeks

Pharmaceutical company
GlaxoWellcome Inc. Research Triangle Park, NC.

Source
Stadtlanders Managed Pharmacy Services. Pittsburgh, PA.

 ## Buratto ophthalmic forceps

Description
acrylic intraocular lens (IOL) folding forceps; provide even and equal folding of the IOL while preventing the lens from reverse folding

Source
American Surgical Instruments Corp. product information. Westmont, IL.

 ## buried K-wire fixation in digital fusion

Description
Kirschner wire (K-wire) placement in digital fusion is mostly in callous bone; motion between the pin-skin and pin-bone interface is easily accomplished; buried K-wire has reduced the concern of pin-tract infection while providing adequate fixation; bending the K-wire within the digit directly after implantation potentially can improve the cosmesis and functional result of the fused digit

Anatomy
cancellous bone; distal aspect of toe; distal phalanx; distal phalangeal tuft; digit; metatarsophalangeal joint space; middle phalanx; opposing articular surfaces; proximal phalangeal base; proximal interphalangeal joint

Equipment
standard orthopaedic surgery equipment; Kirschner wire; pins

Source
Adapted from Creighton RE, Blustein SM. Buried Kirschner wire in digital fusion. Journal of Foot and Ankle Surgery 1995;34:567-570.

 ## buried penis, surgical correction

Description
the congenital anomaly of buried penis is due to a deficiency of penile shaft skin, and abnormal attachments of the tunica dartos to Buck fascia; the otherwise normal penis is entrapped in the subcutaneous tissue of the prepubic area; a new technique for correction consists of resection of abnormal dartos attachments, unfurling of prepuce, and correction of deficient shaft skin by reapproximating the preputial skin flaps to obtain adequate penile skin coverage

Anatomy
Buck fascia; coronal sulcus; dorsal neurovascular bundle; glans penis; mons pubis; penile shaft; penis; phallus; prepuce; prepubic region; preputial skin; scrotum; tunica dartos

Equipment
standard genitourinary surgery equipment; compression dressing; drip catheter; 5-0 polydioxanone sutures; 6-0 polyglactin sutures

Source
Adapted from Boemers TML, De Jong T. The surgical correction of buried penis: a new technique. The Journal of Urology 1995;154:550-552.

 ## Busenkell posterior hip retractor

Description
orthopaedic surgical instrument used to impact into bone posteriorly; retractor is slipped along the posterior border of ischium; point of instrument is impacted into ischium with mallet

Source
Innomed Inc. product information. Savannah, GA.

 ## BuSpar patch

Generic name
see buspirone transdermal patch

buspirone transdermal patch

Brand name
BuSpar patch

Use
another dosage form of buspirone; used for the treatment of anxiety, depression, smoking cessation, and attention-deficit disorder (ADD)

Usual dosage
topical: 5-10 mg patches; 1-3 patches daily

Pharmaceutical company
Bristol-Myers Squibb Co. Princeton, NJ.

Source
Stadtlanders Managed Pharmacy Services. Pittsburgh, PA.

 butenafine hydrochloride

Brand name
Mentax

Use
antifungal for interdigital tinea pedis (athlete's foot fungal infection)

Usual dosage
topical: 1% cream; apply to affected area between toes 3 to 4 times per day

Pharmaceutical company
Schering/Penederm. Kenilworth, NJ.

Source
Stadtlanders Managed Pharmacy Services. Pittsburgh, PA.

 butoconazole nitrate

Brand name
Femstat One

Use
controlled release form of lotion; a single dose treatment of vaginal yeast infections

Usual dosage
intravaginal: one vaginal suppository containing 2% butoconazole for one-time treatment

Pharmaceutical company
Roche Laboratories. Nutley, NJ.

Source
Stadtlanders Managed Pharmacy Services. Pittsburgh, PA.

bypass coaptation for cervical nerve root avulsion

Description
restores neurological function in patients with various cervical nerve root avulsions

Anatomy
cervical spine; cervical nerve root; sternocleidomastoid; jugular vein; primary rami; brachial plexus; supraclavicular and infraclavicular regions; shoulder

Equipment
standard neurosurgical equipment

Source
Adapted from Yamada S, Lonser RR, Iacono RP, Morenski JD, Bailey L. Bypass coaptation procedures for cervical nerve root avulsion. Neurosurgery 1996;38:1145-1152.

 ## Byrne expulsive hemorrhage lens

Description
ophthalmic lens designed to help stop effusion of ocular material in event of hemorrhage during anterior segment surgery; radial slot allows suturing to close incision while pressure is applied to globe

Source
Ocular Instruments Inc. product information. Bellevue, WA.

 ## cabergoline

Brand name
Dostinex

Use
long-acting dopamine-agonist for the treatment of hyperprolactinemic disorders

Usual dosage
oral: 0.5-1 mg twice a week

Pharmaceutical company
Pharmacia & Upjohn Co. Kalamazoo, MI.

Source
Stadtlanders Managed Pharmacy Services. Pittsburgh, PA.

 ## calbindin-D$_{28K}$ detection

Synonyms
none

Use
evaluation of suspected medulloblastomas and neuroblastic tumors

Method
immunohistochemical staining

Specimen
tissue biopsy

Normal range
undetermined

Comments
investigational

Source
Archives of Pathology and Lab Medicine 1995;119:734-743.

 calcipotriene

Brand name
Dovonex

Use
synthetic vitamin D_3 derivative indicated for the treatment of moderate plaque psoriasis

Usual dosage
topical: 50 mcg/g ointment, applied as a thin layer twice daily

Pharmaceutical company
Bristol-Myers Squibb Co. Princeton, NJ.

Source
University of Pittsburgh Drug Information and Pharmacoepidemiology Center. Pittsburgh, PA.

 calcitonin (salmon)

Brand name
Miacalcin Nasal Spray

Use
treatment of osteoporosis in estrogen-insensitive women who are >5 years postmenopausal

Usual dosage
nasal spray: one spray (200 IU) in one nostril per day, alternating nostrils every other day

Pharmaceutical company
Sandoz Pharmaceutical Co. East Hanover, NJ.

Source
University of Pittsburgh Drug Information and Pharmacoepidemiology Center. Pittsburgh, PA.

 Calcort

Generic name
see deflazacort

calretinin immunohistochemistry

Synonyms
calretinin marker analysis for mesothelioma

Use
diagnosis of malignant mesothelioma

Method
immunohistochemistry with anti-calretinin polyclonal antisera

Specimen
tissue biopsy or serous effusion specimens

Normal range
nonreactive

Comments
a uniquely sensitive and specific immunocytochemical marker for malignant mesothelioma; expected soon to become a standard marker for diagnosis of this disease

Source
Adapted from Doglioni C, Dei Tos AP, Laurino L, et al. Calretinin: a novel immunocytochemical marker for mesothelioma. American Journal of Surgical Pathology 1996;20:1037-1046.

 # Calypte HIV-1 urine EIA (enzyme immunoassay)

Synonym
none

Use
testing safer, easier and more accessible compared with standard blood test; detects antibodies to HIV present in simple plastic cup specimens of urine using an enzyme-linked immunosorbent assay (ELISA) method to detect the presence of antibodies to HIV-1; previous HIV tests use either blood or oral fluid samples; any initially reactive sample will be retested twice; for confirmation of a positive urine test, the patient must be tested with a more accurate blood test (Editor note: Also marketed under Sentinel HIV-1 urine EIA manufactured by Seradyn Inc. of Berkeley, CA)

Method
urinalysis

Specimen
urine

Normal range
none

Source
Adapted from Altman LK. The Houston Chronicle, August 7, 1996:12A and Internet www.fda.gov.

Camber Axis Hinge (CAH)

Description
another option available for thermoformable orthoses; range of motion or fixed ankle position can be set by inserting the color-coded keys that are included with each kit

Source
Becker Orthopedic product information. Troy, MI.

 Camptosar

Generic name
see irinotecan hydrochloride

 Campylobacter **resistotyping**

Synonyms
none

Use
identification of enteric *Campylobacter* subtypes

Method
bioassay for microbial resistance patterns to multiple pharmacologic agents

Specimen
Campylobacter isolate

Normal range
not applicable

Comments
a simple, accurate, reproducible and inexpensive method for identification of microbial subtypes; may replace pyrolysis mass spectrometry

Source
Adapted from Ribeiro CD, Thomas MT, Kembrey D, Magee JT, North Z. Resistotyping of Campylobacters: fulfilling a need. Epidemiology & Infection 1996;116:169-175.

 Cannula cushion

Description
cushion for prevention of skin irritation and breakdown behind the ears and on cheeks with the use of an oxygen nasal cannula; made from unique pink polyurethane foam; viscoelastic properties provide excellent cushioning; designed so that the spiral cut allows the two layers of foam to overlap and cling to each other; disposable; can be used anywhere tubing comes in contact with skin

Source
Wear Care Products LLC product information. McDonough, GA.

capecitabine

Brand name
Xeloda

Use
pro-drug of 5-fluorouracil used in the treatment of patients with advanced colorectal cancer

Usual dosage
oral: dosage range from 502-2510 mg/m^2/day were used in clinical trials

Pharmaceutical company
Roche Laboratories. Nutley, NJ.

Source
Stadtlanders Managed Pharmacy Services. Pittsburgh, PA.

 Capener finger splint

Description
spring coil extension assist splint (also called "Wynn Parry" splint); uses coil springs placed lateral to and in line with proximal interphalangeal (PIP) joint; indicated for PIP flexion tightness

Source
DeRoyal/LMB product information. San Luis Obispo, CA.

 Capnocheck capnometer

Description
hand-held capnometer to spot-check readings of end-tidal carbon dioxide (ETCO$_2$); also provides intubation verification and respiratory rate measurements from neonate to adult patients

Source
BCI International product information. Waukesha, WI.

 Capnostat Mainstream carbon dioxide module

Description
gas analyzer that functions with Tram monitoring instrument; audible and visual alarms for inspired carbon dioxide (CO$_2$), expired CO$_2$, respiratory rate, and no breath detected; measures and displays CO$_2$ concentrations and respiratory rates

Source
Marquette Electronics Inc. product information. Milwaukee, WI.

Capture-S syphilis test

Synonyms
nontreponemal, qualitative syphilis screening test

Use
blood donor syphilis screening by serological detection of reagin antibodies

Method
solid-phase adherence assay using anti-IgM-coated indicator erythrocytes

Specimen
serum or plasma

Normal range
seronegative

Comments
similar in sensitivity and specificity to the standard RPR card test, but more readily accommodates high-volume testing and automation

Source
Adapted from Stone DL, Moheng MC, Rolih S, Sinor LT. Capture-S, a nontreponemal solid-phase erythrocyte adherence assay for serological detection of syphilis. Journal of Clinical Microbiology 1997;35:217-222.

 ## Carabelt lower back support

Description
belt that supports lower back with a bi-density pad; reduces pressure on vertebrae and muscles; vertical spinal groove gives firm support without spinal loading or restricting movement

Source
Bollinger Healthcare product information. Irving, TX.

 ## carbamazepine

Brand name
Carbatrol

Use
sustained-released formulation of carbamazepine to control seizures in epileptic patients

Usual dosage
oral: 300-600 mg as a single daily dose was studied in clinical trials

Pharmaceutical company
Athena Neurosciences Inc. South San Francisco, CA.

Source
Stadtlanders Managed Pharmacy Services. Pittsburgh, PA.

Carbatrol

Generic name
see carbamazepine

 Carbicarb

Generic name
see sodium bicarbonate/sodium carbonate

 CarboMedics "top-hat" supra-annular valve

Description
cardiac implantable valve designed for supra-annular placement; potential of
up to 60% increase in valve flow area; for double/multiple valve procedures
Source
CarboMedics Inc. product information. Austin, TX.

 Carbon Copy 2 Light prosthesis

Description
lightweight prosthetic foot with modular heel inserts allowing modification
of heel durometer controlling heel compression and optimizing gait; recessed
keel attachment point allows the prosthesis to be used with ankle units;
prosthesis is thinner from ankle to toe for less resistance during heel-off and
toe-off and aids in more normal gait, and is thicker at midfoot for greater
resistance during higher levels of activity
Source
Ohio Willow Wood Co. product information. Mount Sterling, OH.

 Carbon Monotube external fixation system

Description
fixation system for long bone fractures; black radiolucent tube with multi-
planar clamps at either end to hold bone pins; clamps move along tube and
also rotate right-left and tilt up-down for adjustment
Source
Howmedica Inc. product information. Rutherford, NJ.

Carden bronchoscopy tube

Description
diagnostic or therapeutic flexible bronchoscope; wide at upper distal portion and narrower at proximal portion for access through and below the vocal cords; reduces the resistance to flow of gas through the tube when the fiberoptic bronchoscope is in place; Carden jetting device and swivel connectors facilitate time saving jet ventilation during microlaryngeal surgery or rigid bronchoscopy procedures

Source
Bivona Medical Technologies product information. Gary, IN.

Cardiac T rapid assay

Synonyms
cardiac troponin T; serum troponin T

Indications
rapid identification of patients with myocardial damage, microinfarcts, acute MI

Method
one-step disposable test for cardiac troponin T; results in 1 to 20 minutes; uses less than 1 cc of whole blood; reported more sensitive than troponin I testing; troponin C not currently being tested for this indication

Normal findings
negative test result

Comments
can be performed at bedside; easy to read visual positive or negative indicator

Source
Boehringer Mannheim Corp. product information. Indianapolis, IN.

cardiac troponin I assay

Synonyms
cTn-I assay

Use
detection of myocardial injury, particularly infarction

Method
rapid immunoassay

Specimen
serum

Normal range
not yet established

Comments
likely to become widely used due to high degree of cardiospecificity

Source
Adapted from Keffer JH. Myocardial markers of injury. American Journal of Clinical Pathology 1996;105:305-320.

 ## Cardifix EZ cardiac pacing lead

Description
pacing lead with shielded corkscrew utilizing soluble protective cover of polyethylene glycol (PEG); after introduction this tip dissolves in 2-4 minutes, exposing corkscrew for easy fixation in either atrium or ventricle

Source
Intermedics Inc. product information. Angleton, TX.

 ## Cardionyl suture

Description
polyamide monofilament sutures; an alternative to polypropylene; supple, yet strong

Source
Promedica Distribution product information. Newport Beach, CA.

 ## Cardiovit AT-10 monitor

Description
portable system combination ECG monitor and spirometer monitor with built-in battery and printer

Source
Schiller America Inc. product information. Tustin, CA.

 ## carmustine

Brand name
Gliadel

Use
nitrosurea derivative alkylating agent used alone or in combination in the treatment of various neoplastic conditions such as Hodgkin disease, brain tumors, multiple myeloma, and non-Hodgkin lymphoma

Usual dosage
intravenous: as a single agent, 150 to 200 mg/m2 every six weeks given as a single dose or divided into two daily doses

Pharmaceutical company
Scios Nova Inc. Mountain View, CA.

Source
University of Pittsburgh Drug Information and Pharmacoepidemiology Center. Pittsburgh, PA.

Carpentier-Edwards Physio annuloplasty ring

Description
heart valve ring that preserves the natural 3:4 leaflet relationship of a normal mitral valve

Source
Baxter Healthcare Corp. product information. Irvine, CA.

 carposcope

Description
fiberoptic light retractor that allows easy and safe release of the carpal tunnel through a short transverse incision under direct visualization of the transverse carpal ligament

Source
ESI product information. Rochester, NY.

 Carrisyn

Generic name
see acemannan

 Carter Tubal Assistant

Description
surgical instrument that isolates and captures fallopian tube through a small abdominal incision, cutting down surgical time during tubal ligation

Source
CooperSurgical product information. Shelton, CT.

 carvedilol

Brand name
Coreg, Kredex

Use
beta blocker used for the treatment of hypertension

Usual dosage
oral: starting dose is 6.25 mg twice daily for 7-14 days then increase to 12.5 mg twice daily for 7-14 days if needed; maximum dose should not exceed 25 mg twice daily (50 mg/day)

Pharmaceutical company
SmithKline Beecham. Philadelphia, PA.

Source
University of Pittsburgh Drug Information and Pharmacoepidemiology Center. Pittsburgh, PA.

Casodex

Generic Name
see bicalutamide

 Catatrol

Generic Name
see viloxazine

 cat dander immunotherapeutic peptide

Brand name
Allervax Cat

Use
prevention of hypersensitivity symptoms in people with allergic reaction to cat dander

Usual dosage
injectable: 750 μg twice weekly for 2 weeks was used in clinical studies

Pharmaceutical company
Marion Merrell Dow. Kansas City, MO.

Source
Stadtlanders Managed Pharmacy Services. Pittsburgh, PA.

 Cath Caddie

Description
abdominal binder specifically made for Hickman catheters and PEG tubes; provides easy access for treatments and feedings; contains and controls catheter coil for greater patient comfort; helps prevent accidental removal of catheter

Source
Mark-Clark product information. Topeka, KS.

 cathepsin D tissue detection

Synonyms
tissue cathepsin D detection

Use
assess high levels of cathepsin D, an estrogen-induced lysosomal protease; may have clinical significance in predicting decreased shorter metastasis-free survival and decreased overall survival in women with node-negative breast cancer

Method
enzyme immunoassay (EIA)

Specimen
solid tumor; frozen (free of excess fat and blood), confirmed as cancer by histologic examination

Normal range
investigational use

Comments
performance characteristics have not been established

Source
Lexi-Comp Inc. database. Hudson, OH.

 Cath-Secure tape

Description
hypoallergenic tape featuring hook-and-loop tab that holds various tubing in place; allows changing of tube without changing of tape; used for jejunostomy, gastrostomy, peritoneal dialysis tubing, central line ports, suprapubic catheter tubing, and wound drainage tubing

Source
MC Johnson Co. product information. Naples, FL.

 cautery-assisted uvulopalatoplasty

Description
snoring and mild obstructive sleep apnea syndrome (OSAS) are treated surgically with uvulopalatoplasty; the tongue is retracted using a Harrington (sweetheart) retractor; Yankauer sucker placed inside corner of mouth for smoke evacuation; electrocautery dispersive pad placed on patient's flank; uvula grasped with straight Allis clamp; approximately three-fourths of uvula is removed; uvular base marked with cautery before making lateral cuts; subsequent stages performed no less than four weeks apart; procedure performed in similar manner; uvula is further shortened only if found redundant

Anatomy
flank; palatal musculature; pharyngeal wall; soft palate; tongue; uvula; uvular artery; velopharyngeal (pertaining to the velum palatinum and posterior nasopharyngeal wall)

Equipment
Allis clamp; electrocautery; electrocautery dispersive pad; Harrington retractor; Yankauer sucker

Source
Adapted from Zinder DJ, Postma GN. Outpatient cautery-assisted uvulopalatoplasty. Laryngoscope 1995;105:1256-1257.

Cavernotome C&R

Description
instrument for implantation of penile prosthesis

Source
Southwest Instrument Co. product information. Van Buren, AR.

 ## CCOmbo catheter

Description
gives continuous cardiac output monitoring and accurate venous oxygen saturation; latest member of the Swan-Ganz catheter family

Source
Baxter Healthcare Corp. product information. Irvine, CA.

 ## CD4 analysis

Synonyms
CD4 FACS, CD4 flow cytometry

Use
prognostic factor in acute leukemias

Method
two-color flow cytometry

Specimen
bone marrow

Normal range
investigational

Comments
likely to be used in conjunction with CD13 and CD33 analysis, to assess likelihood of non-lymphoid differentiation

Source
American Journal of Clinical Pathology 1995;104:204-211.

 ## CD44, marker for early tumor detection

Synonyms
none

Indications
testicular biopsy sent for routine pathology

Method
employment of specific antiseminoma monoclonal antibody to specimen

Normal findings
negative pathologic findings

Comments
CD44 binds selectively to seminoma cells that are in earliest stages of malignant transformation and metastasis; can identify neoplasm positively in biopsies of most patients before tumor becomes clinically apparent

Source
Adapted from Hadziselimovic F, Herzog B, Emmons LR. The expression of CD44 adhesion molecules on seminoma cells: a new marker for early detection of the tumor. Cancer 1996;77(3):429-430.

 CD34-positive selection

Synonyms
stem cell positive selection

Use
enrichment of CD34-positive cells, the presumed stem and progenitor population, prior to transplantation or gene therapy Method immunologic isolation of cells expressing the CD34 surface antigen

Specimen
bone marrow; peripheral blood stem cell cytapheresis product; umbilical cord blood

Normal range
investigational use

Comments
methods currently in use include immunoaffinity and immunomagnetic separation

Source
University of Minnesota Department of Laboratory Medicine and Pathology. Minneapolis, MN.

 CD34 progenitor cell quantitation

Synonyms
precursor cell quantitation; stem cell enumeration

Use
determine appropriate interval for harvesting peripheral blood stem cells following growth factor mobilization; quantify CD34 cells following bone marrow purging and processing procedures; enumerate total number of stem cells in cord blood

Method
direct fluorescent antibody (DFA) using monoclonal antibodies and flow cytometry

Specimen
blood; leukapheresis product; bone marrow; cord blood

Normal range
investigational use

Comments
performance characteristics have not been established

Source
Lexi-Comp Inc. database. Hudson, OH.

 ## CD34 progenitor subset analysis

Synonyms
stem cell subset analysis; flow cytometry subset analysis

Use
determine specific progenitor cell subpopulations in bone marrow, peripheral blood stem cell cytapheresis products, and umbilical cord blood

Method
direct and indirect fluorescent antibody staining using lineage-specific monoclonal antibodies and flow cytometry

Specimen
bone marrow; peripheral blood stem cell cytapheresis product; umbilical cord blood

Normal range
investigational use

Comments
performance characteristics and appropriate interpretation of results have not been established

Source
University of Minnesota Department of Laboratory Medicine and Pathology. Minneapolis, MN.

 ## Cedax

Generic Name
see ceftibutin

 ## cefazolin assay

Synonyms
cefazolin clearance

Use
determines the serum level of cefazolin, which is used as an antibiotic prophylaxis

Method
levels in serum determined with a Quanta-4000 capillary electrophoresis system equipped with a 254-nanometer ultraviolet detector

Specimen
serum

Normal range
none

Comments
minimum inhibitory concentration of cefazolin is 0.5 microgram per milliliter for the usual infecting organisms

Source
Adapted from Meter JJ, Polly DW, Brueckner RP, Tenuta JJ, Asplund L. Effect of intraoperative blood loss on the serum level of cefazolin in patients with total hip arthroplasty. The Journal of Bone and Joint Surgery 1996;78-A:1201-1205.

 cefdinir

Brand name
Omnicef

Use
oral cephalosporin with advantage of increased gram-positive activity effective in the treatment of otitis media, skin and soft tissue infections

Usual dosage
oral: 300 mg twice daily

Pharmaceutical company
Warner-Lambert/Parke-Davis. Morris Plains, NJ.

Source
Stadtlanders Managed Pharmacy Services. Pittsburgh, PA.

 cefepime

Brand name
Maxipime

Use
fourth generation cephalosporin antibiotic used to treat serious hospital-acquired bacterial infections, as well as other infections caused by aerobic gram-negative bacteria

Usual dosage
intravenous: 1 to 2 g every 8 to 12 hours

Pharmaceutical company
Bristol-Meyers Squibb Co. Princeton, NJ.

Source
University of Pittsburgh Drug Information and Pharmacoepidemiology Center. Pittsburgh, PA.

 cefodizime

Brand Name
Kenicef

Use
third generation cephalosporin antibiotic used in the treatment of various infectious diseases

Usual Dosage
IM or IV: normal dose 1-4 g daily in 1 or 2 divided doses for 5-14 days; gonorrhea and uncomplicated urinary tract infections single dose therapy of 0.5-2 g; children 60 mg/kg/day in 3 or 4 divided doses for 7-14 days

Pharmaceutical company
Fujisawa USA Inc. North Deerfield, IL.

Source
University of Pittsburgh Drug Information and Pharmacoepidemiology Center. Pittsburgh, PA.

 cefpirome

Brand name
Cefrom

Use
classified as third or fourth generation cephalosporin with an improved gram-positive spectrum of activity; effective against gram-negative and gram-positive bacteria in respiratory, enteric, skin and soft tissue, and urinary tract infections

Usual dosage
injectible: 1 to 2 gm every 12 hours intravenously

Pharmaceutical company
Hoechst-Roussel. Somerville, NJ.

Source
Stadtlanders Managed Pharmacy Services. Pittsburgh, PA.

 Cefrom

Generic name
see cefpirome

 ceftibuten

Brand Name
Cedax

Use
third generation cephalosporin antibiotic used in the treatment of urinary tract infections and various other infectious disorders

Usual Dosage
oral: adults 400 mg once daily; children 9 mg/kg/day

Pharmaceutical company
Schering. Kenilworth, NJ.

Source
University of Pittsburgh Drug Information and Pharmacoepidemiology Center. Pittsburgh, PA.

celiprolol

Brand Name
Selecor

Use
cardioselective beta-adrenergic blocking agent used for the treatment of hypertension and angina pectoris

Usual Dosage
oral: trial doses from 200 mg-600 mg once daily

Pharmaceutical company
Rhone-Poulenc Rorer Pharmaceuticals Inc. Collegeville, PA.

Source
University of Pittsburgh Drug Information and Pharmacoepidemiology Center. Pittsburgh, PA.

 CellCept

Generic name
see mycophenolate mofetil

 Cell-DYN 3500 hematology analysis

Synonyms
Abbott CD 3500

Use
a method to determine complete blood count profile and differential leukocyte count

Method
impedance measurement and multiple angle polarized light scatter separation

Specimen
EDTA (ethylenediaminetetraacetic acid)-anticoagulated blood

Normal range
not applicable; individual reference ranges exist for all 15 blood cell parameters

Comments
recently developed automated instrument for new way to determine standard blood cell parameters; new methods infrequently introduced

Source
Vives-Corrons J-L, Besson I, Jou JM, Gutierrez G. Evaluation of the Abbott Cell-DYN 3500 hematology analyzer in a university hospital. American Journal of Clinical Pathology 1996;105:553-559.

cell flow cytometry crossmatch

Synonyms
FCXM

Use
measurement of maternal anti-paternal leukocyte antibody levels in women with history of recurrent spontaneous abortions

Method
flow cytometric detection of circulating HLA antibodies

Specimen
maternal blood

Normal range
no evidence of anti-paternal leukocyte antibodies

Comments
the method of choice when determining the need for alloimmunotherapy and to monitor the effectiveness of treatment

Source
Adapted from Matzner W, Chong P, Xu G, Ching W. A comparison of flow cytometry and microcytotoxicity for the evaluation of alloimmune therapy in patients with recurrent spontaneous abortions. American Journal of Reproductive Immunology 1995;33:10-13.

 Celsite brachial port

Description
subcutaneous implantable titanium port for inserting drugs; silicone septum allows up to 1,500 leak-tight punctures with 22-gauge Huber needle

Source
Braun Medical Inc. Cardiovascular Division product information. New Orleans, LA.

 Cencit imaging system

Description
optical surface scanner produces highly repeatable images for measuring landmark dimensions; three-dimensional surface landmarks coordinate to reconstruct surfaces and volumes

Source
Cencit Inc. product information. St. Louis, MO.

 CenTNF

Generic name
see humanized monoclonal antibody (MAb)-cA2

CeraOne abutment implant

Description
gold cylinder endosseous dental implant luted to a metal abutment; for fabrication of cemented single tooth implant-supported restorations

Source
Nobel-pharma USA product information. Westmont, IL.

cerebellar aggregation cultures for teratogenicity testing

Synonyms
cerebellar aggregation cultures

Use
prediction of drug teratogenic potency

Method
effects on aggregation and fiber formation of cerebellar neurons measured, following treatment with test drug, in primary cultures of dissociated cerebella from 6-day-old mice

Specimen
pharmacologic agent

Normal range
cerebellar neural development unaffected

Comments
potential screening test for drug teratogenic potential

Source
Adapted from Maar TE, Ellerbeck U, Bock E, Nau H, Schousboe A, Berezin V. Prediction of teratogenic potency of valproate analogues using cerebellar aggregation cultures. Toxicology 1997;116:159-168.

cerebrospinal fluid (CSF) cytomegalovirus (CMV) polymerase chain reaction (PCR)

Synonyms
CSF CMV PCR

Use
detection of CMV in cerebrospinal fluid of immunocompromised patients

Method
PCR assay with CMV nucleic acid-specific primers

Specimen
cerebrospinal fluid

Normal range
undetectable

Comments
may be particularly valuable in evaluation of new-onset neurologic symptoms in immunocompromised patients

Source
Adapted from Vogel JU, Cinatl J, Lux A, Weber B, Driesel AJ, Doerr HW. New PCR assay for rapid and quantitative detection of human cytomegalovirus in cerebrospinal fluid. Journal of Clinical Microbiology 1996;34:482-483.

 Cerebyx

Generic name
see fosphenytoin

 Cerestat

Generic name
see aptiganel hydrochloride

 Cerezyme

Generic Name
see imiglucerase

 cerivastatin sodium

Brand name
Baycol

Use
used in the treatment of hypercholesterolemia

Usual dosage
oral: 0.3 mg daily in the evening

Pharmaceutical company
Bayer Pharmaceuticals. West Haven, CT.

Source
Stadtlanders Managed Pharmacy Services. Pittsburgh, PA.

 cervical esophagogastrostomy, stapled anastomotic technique

Description
anastomotic leakage can occur after operation for carcinoma of the esophagus; various stapling techniques have been used to decrease the incidence; a modification of cervical esophagogastrostomy using a P-CEEA (Premium circular end-to-end anastomosis) stapler is reported; a rubber tube is used with the stapler enabling modification of the technique for performing safe surgery in the small field of the neck region; the technique can be done without resection of the manubrium, or the head of the left clavicle

Anatomy

antrum; apical point of fundus; cervical esophagus; clavicle; clavicular head; esophagus; fourth and fifth branches of right gastric artery; manubrium; stomach; xiphoid process

Equipment

standard surgery equipment; Auto Suture GIA 80 stapler; P-CEEA 25 mm stapler; Penrose drain; Maloney bougie; hydrostatic balloon; 7- or 8-cm rubber tube; trocar

Source

Adapted from Mafune K, Tanaka Y. Stapled anastomotic technique for cervical esophagogastrostomy. Journal of American College of Surgeons 1995;181:85-87.

 ## cervical range of motion device

Description

measures cervical range of motion (CROM); flexion and extension; positioned on the bridge of the nose and over the ears

Source

Performance Attainment Assoc. product information. St. Paul, MN.

 ## cervical-vaginal telecytology

Synonyms

Use

offsite diagnosis and automated screening of cervical-vaginal specimens

Method

cytologic examination by video microscopy

Specimen

cervical-vaginal smear

Normal range

benign

Comments

video microscopy has not yet achieved the diagnostic accuracy of light microscopy

Source

Adapted from Raab SS, Zaleski MS, Thomas PA, Niemann TH, Isacson C, Jensen CS. Telecytology: diagnostic accuracy in cervical-vaginal smears. American Journal of Clinical Pathology 1996;105:599-603.

 ## Cervidil

Generic Name

see dinoprostone

Cer-View vaginal retractor

Description
surgical instrument that has been contoured and shaped to fit into a standard speculum and expand beyond the width of the blades; retracts sidewalls of vaginal vault for better view of cervix

Source
EURO-MED division of Cooper Surgical product information. Shelton, CT.

CerviSoft cytology collection

Description
cervical cell collection device that is more comfortable for the patient, made of nonabrasive foam bonded to a 7-inch plastic shaft

Source
Hardwood Products Co. product information. Guilford, ME.

Cervitrak device

Description
cervical traction for home use; indicated for nerve root compression and myofascial restrictions, nuclear prolapse, and whiplash; prevents and reduces adhesion formation; reduces pain, muscle guarding, and spasms

Source
Staodyn Inc. product information. Longmont, CO.

cetirizine

Brand name
Reactine; Zyrtec

Use
antihistamine for treatment of seasonal allergic rhinitis, chronic urticaria, or allergen-induced asthma

Usual dosage
oral: 5 to 10 mg once or twice daily

Pharmaceutical company
Pfizer Laboratories Inc. New York, NY.

Source
University of Pittsburgh Drug Information and Pharmacoepidemiology Center. Pittsburgh, PA.

CE-3000 video technology

Description
provides real-time video surgery during endoscopic plastic and reconstructive surgeries

Source
DigiVision product information. San Diego, CA.

Chagas antibody EIA

Synonyms
Trypanosoma cruzi (*T. cruzi*) ELISA

Use
screening potential blood donors at risk for transmitting *T. cruzi*, the causative agent of Chagas disease

Method
limited-sensitivity ELISA specific for *T. cruzi* antibodies

Specimen
blood

Normal range
nonreactive

Comments
an extremely specific test, possibly suitable for screening at-risk donors

Source
Adapted from Mercer SD, Rawlinson PSM. An evaluation of two ELISA methods for the detection of *Trypanosoma cruzi* antibodies in volunteer blood donors. Transfusion Science 1996;12:5.

Chagatest ELISA

Synonyms
Trypanosoma cruzi ELISA

Use
screening potential blood donors at risk for transmitting *T. cruzi*

Method
T. cruzi antibody-specific ELISA

Specimen
blood

Normal range
nonreactive

Comments
test has comparatively poor specificity, but is widely marketed

Source
Adapted from Mercer SD, Rawlinson PSM. An evaluation of two ELISA methods for the detection of *Trypanosoma cruzi* antibodies in volunteer blood donors. Transfusion Science 1996;12:5.

chemiluminescent in situ hybridization for detection of CMV (cytomegalovirus) DNA

Synonyms
CMV detection by chemiluminescent in situ hybridization

Use
diagnosis of viral infection

Method
in situ hybridization using chemiluminescent substrate

Specimen
biopsy or other tissue specimens

Normal range
CMV DNA (deoxyribonucleic acid) not detected

Comments
investigational, but likely to become clinically important

Source
Adapted from Musiano M, Roda A, Zerbini M, et al. Chemiluminescent in situ hybridization for the detection of cytomegalovirus DNA. American Journal of Pathology 1996;148:1105-1112.

 chemiluminescent microtiter protein kinase activity assay

Synonyms
microtiter protein kinase assay

Use
identification of protein kinase inhibitor compounds

Method
chemiluminescent protein kinase assay, with monoclonal antibodies used to detect phosphorylation of biotinylated substrate peptides immobilized in streptavidin-coated microtiter wells

Specimen
pharmacologic agent

Normal range
not applicable

Comments
rapid, sensitive, and readily automated assay; likely will be used in academic and industrial laboratories to identify new classes of protein kinase inhibitors

Source
Adapted from Lehel C, Daniel-Issakani S, Brasseur M, Strulovici B. A chemiluminescent microtiter plate assay for sensitive detection of protein kinase activity. Analytical Biochemistry 1997;244:340-346.

 ChinUpps cervicofacial support

Description
one-piece, one-step application face and neck support; comfortable fit leaves ears unobstructed; made of fabric that maintains elasticity

Source
Tulip Co. product information. San Diego, CA.

Chiroslide

Description
hand-held device to measure leg length difference

Source
Chiroslide product information. Congers, NY.

Chirotech x-ray system

Description
x-ray equipment designed specifically for the chiropractic profession; radiation can be reduced by use of Lo-Dose collimation system; utilizes a rare earth x-ray beam filter that vastly reduces absorbed dose for spinal radiography

Source
Summit Industries Inc. product information. Chicago, IL.

CholestaGel

Generic name
see colesevelam

chondrocutaneous flap for ear reconstruction

Description
moderate-sized cancers of upper third of ear excised, including cartilage; unsupported soft tissue of upper ear reconstructed by rotating position of composite flap of skin and cartilage from middle third of ear; thick split-skin grafts from postauricular area used to cover flap donor site

Anatomy
ear; cartilage; superior helix; postauricular area; antihelix; concha

Equipment
standard plastic surgery equipment

Source
Adapted from Cocke WM. Radial composite chondrocutaneous flap for ear reconstruction. The American Surgeon 1995;61:347-349.

Cho-Pat strap

Description
Achilles tendon strap for Achilles tendonitis; original knee strap for kneecap tendonitis; patellar stabilizer strap for quadriceps tendonitis; tennis elbow splint for forearm tendonitis; upper arm strap for bicipital and tricipital tendonitis; shin splint sleeve; ankle support for sprains

Source
Cho-Pat Inc. product information. Hainesport, NJ.

chorionic villus deoxyribonucleic acid (DNA) analysis for triosephosphate isomerase (TPI) gene mutation

Synonyms
TPI deficiency mutation analysis

Use
prenatal diagnosis of triosephosphate isomerase deficiency

Method
TPI gene-specific polymerase chain reaction amplification of chorionic villus DNA

Specimen
chorionic villus sample

Normal range
no evidence of mutation

Comments
first example of prenatal molecular diagnosis of a human glycolytic enzyme disorder

Source
Adapted from Arya R, Lalloz MRA, Nicolaides KH, Bellingham AJ, Layton DM. Prenatal diagnosis of triosephosphate isomerase deficiency. Blood 1996;87:4507-4509.

 Christoudias approximator

Description
multifunctional laparoscopy tool eliminates the need for two instruments; dual jaw arrangement, cleaning port, dual push-button controls

Source
Marlow Surgical Technologies Inc. product information. Willoughby, OH.

 cidofovir

Brand name
Vistide

Use
antiviral for the treatment of acquired immunodeficiency syndrome (AIDS)-related cytomegalovirus retinitis

Usual dosage
intravenous: 5 mg/kg weekly for 2 weeks then bi-weekly thereafter is currently being investigated

Pharmaceutical company
Gilead Sciences Inc. Foster City, CA.

Source
University of Pittsburgh Drug Information and Pharmacoepidemiology Center. Pittsburgh, PA.

cidofovir (gel)

Brand name
Forvade

Use
HIV/AIDS-related CMV retinitis

Usual dosage
ophthalmic: new topical formulation of cidofovir is available in 0.3% and 1% solution, applied once a day to eye(s) for 5 days

Pharmaceutical company
Gillead Sciences. Foster City, CA.

Source
Stadtlanders Managed Pharmacy Services. Pittsburgh, PA.

 cifenline

Brand name
Cipralan

Use
class I, antiarrhythmic agent used to treat chronic ventricular arrhythmias

Usual dosage
oral: clinical trials have used titration of doses in step-wise fashion. Early clinical trials used doses starting from 130 mg to 160 mg every 12 hours, then slowly titrating down to 80 mg and 100 mg as arrhythmias are controlled

Pharmaceutical company
Roche/Glaxo. Nutley, NJ.

Source
Stadtlanders Managed Pharmacy Services. Pittsburgh, PA.

 cilazapril

Brand name
Inhibace

Use
angiotensin-converting enzyme inhibitor studied for the treatment of hypertension and congestive heart failure (CHF)

Usual dosage
oral: 0.5 to 10 mg daily

Pharmaceutical company
Roche Laboratories. Nutley, NJ.

Source
University of Pittsburgh Drug Information and Pharmacoepidemiology Center. Pittsburgh, PA.

Cimochowski cardiac cannula

Description
three-tier balloon retrograde cardioplegia surgical instrument used for maximum occlusion of the coronary sinus; conforms anatomically to the native coronary sinus; need for pursestring suture at ostium eliminated

Source
Research Medical Inc. product information. Midvale, UT.

 ## Cipralan

Generic name
see cifenline

 ## Cipramil

Generic name
see citalopram

 ## Circline magnifier

Description
all-purpose illuminated magnifier allowing patients with deteriorating eyesight to pursue activities; available on casters or pedestal base

Source
Dazor Manufacturing Corp. product information. St. Louis, MO.

 ## CircPlus bandage/wrap system

Description
bandage/wrap system providing adjustable, nonelastic compression for easy maintenance and treatment of edema and stasis ulcers

Source
CircAid Medical Products product information. San Diego, CA.

 ## Circulaire aerosol drug delivery system

Description
aerosol device allows a shorter, more focused therapy while delivering maximum dosage to lungs; defined as microscopic aerosol therapy (MAT)

Source
WestMed product information. Tucson, AZ.

Circul'Air shoe process system

Description
a system whereby air is propelled from the rear to the front of the shoe; has a reverse air-lock ball that keeps air from flowing back to the heel; also has numerous air holes to ensure an even distribution of fresh air; each pressure of the heel activates the system

Source
Lemaitre Securite French Co. product information. Chicago, IL.

 ## Cirrus foot prosthesis

Description
high-strength composite prosthetic foot allows customization of the patient's gait through substitution of toe and/or heel springs; independent toe springs provide stability as each maintains contact with the ground surface while the leg achieves angles up to 32 degrees without a separate articulating ankle; features a true heel spring allowing uniform roll-through from heel to toe, removing the hesitation characteristic of many amputee patients; comes with a custom-made anatomical foot-shell and Spectra sock to provide durability and aesthetic appeal

Source
Second Nature product information. Salt Lake City, UT.

 ## cisatracurium

Brand Name
Nimbex

Use
adjunct to general anesthesia to facilitate endotracheal intubation and to relax skeletal muscle during surgery or mechanical ventilation

Usual Dosage
intravenous: bolus dose of 0.15 to 0.2 µg/kg for intubation and a maintenance dose of 0.5 to 10.2 µg/kg/min (mean dose of 3 µg/kg/min) has been used in clinical trials

Pharmaceutical company
Burroughs Wellcome. Research Triangle Park, NC.

Source
University of Pittsburgh Drug Information and Pharmacoepidemiology Center. Pittsburgh, PA.

citalopram

Brand name
Cipramil

Use
selective serotonin reuptake inhibitor (SSRI) for use in depression

Usual dosage
oral: 40 mg daily was used in clinical trials

Pharmaceutical company
Forest Pharmaceuticals Inc. St. Louis, MO.

Source
Stadtlanders Managed Pharmacy Services. Pittsburgh, PA.

 ## citicoline sodium

Brand name
Sintoclar

Use
used in clinical trials to treat memory disorders caused by ischemic stroke or head trauma

Usual dosage
oral: 500 or 2,000 mg daily currently under investigation
injectible: intravenous or intramuscular injection in doses up to 1000 mg per day has been used in the clinical trial

Pharmaceutical company
Interneuron. Lexington, MA.

Source
Stadtlanders Managed Pharmacy Services. Pittsburgh, PA.

 ## CKS

Description
Continuum knee system (CKS) offers implants and single interchangable instrumentation system for both primary and revision arthroplasty knee surgery; unique selection of patented wedge-lock spacers and stem extensions for tibia and femur

Source
Techmedica product information. Camarillo, CA.

ClearCut 2 instrument

Description
single surgical handpiece instrument for cutting, coagulation, light, and smoke evacuation; delivers bright light directly to operative site; evacuates smoke plume generated during electrosurgery

Source
Medtronic Surgical Products product information. Grand Rapids, MI.

 ClearView uterine manipulator

Description
disposable uterine sound and cervical dilator; natural curved design to follow cervical canal; marked for accurate sounding (4 to 10 cm)

Source
Clinical Innovations product information. Murray, UT.

 Climara

Generic name
see estradiol (patch)

 clopidogrel

Brand name
Plavix

Use
an antiplatelet agent for the prevention of acute thromboembolic artery occlusions in cardiovascular and cerebrovascular diseases, such as myocardial infarction and stroke

Usual dosage
oral: daily doses of 25, 50, or 75 mg were used in the clinical trials

Pharmaceutical company
Bristol-Meyers Squibb Co. Princeton, NJ.

Source
Stadtlanders Managed Pharmacy Services. Pittsburgh, PA.

 CM-Band 505N brace

Description
lightweight, flexible wrist/thumb brace for the treatment of carpometacarpal (CM) joint arthrosis, rheumatism, tenosynovitis, etc.

Source
Nakamura Brace Co. Ltd. product information. Oda, Japan.

CMS AccuProbe 450 system

Description
cryoprobe unit quickly freezes and ablates large quantities of targeted internal tissue; ultrasonic guide for placement and control of tissue destruction

Source
Cryomedical Sciences Inc. product information. Rockville, MD.

 ## Coach incentive spirometer

Description
"coaches" patients into correctly performing and monitoring their own postoperative breathing exercises; goal indicator lets patients adjust the Coach to their prescribed daily volume levels; inspiratory flow guide helps patients maintain slow, deep inspirations; 1-way valve ensures patients inhale rather than exhale into the Coach; dual-sided calibrations make volume reading easy; capacities of 2, 2.5, and 4 liters

Source
DHD product information. Syracuse, NY.

 ## cocaethylene (CE) assay

Synonyms
none

Use
forensic and clinical evaluation of suspected concurrent cocaine and ethanol abuse

Method
gas chromatography/mass spectrometry

Specimen
blood

Normal range
investigational

Comments
metabolite resulting from simultaneous cocaine and ethanol abuse

Source
American Journal of Clinical Pathology 1995;104:187-192.

 ## Colace Microenema

Generic name
see docusate sodium

Colazide

Generic name
see balsalazide disodium

Cold-Eeze

Generic name
see zinc lozenges

Coleman microinfiltration system

Description
instrumentation for removal of aspirant from a donor site as well as preparation and precise microinfiltration at the recipient site; Coleman aspiration cannulae allow passage of aspirant optimally sized for each infiltration procedure

Source
Byron Medical product information. Tucson, AZ.

colesevelam

Brand name
CholestaGel

Use
a nonabsorbable cholesterol reducing agent for the treatment of hypercholesterolemia

Usual dosage
oral: 2.4 and 7.2 grams daily being studied in clinical trials

Pharmaceutical company
GelTex Pharmaceuticals Inc. Waltham, MA.

Source
Stadtlanders Managed Pharmacy Services. Pittsburgh, PA.

Cole uncuffed endotracheal tube

Description
pediatric siliconized tube, 15 cm long with 15-mm connector; minimizes airway resistance

Source
Rusch Inc. product information. Duluth, GA.

CollaCote, CollaPlug, CollaTape wound dressing

Description
absorbable collagen wound dressings for dental surgery; CollaCote designed
for small shallow oral wounds such as palatal donor or recipient sites, under
and over mucosal flaps, and around interosseous defects; CollaPlug has a bul-
let-shape for treating deep wounds such as biopsy and extraction sites; Col-
laTape offers broadest range of use including closure of grafted sites

Source
Calcitek Inc. product information. Carlsbad, CA.

collagen injection for intrinsic sphincteric deficiency

Description
collagen injections have appeared to be effective in treatment for male urinary incontinence due to intrinsic sphincteric deficiency; injections were
performed transurethrally through a blunt end sheath; general or local anesthesia was administered; collagen injected submucosally proximal to the
external sphincter on both sides until urethral mucosa coaptation was
achieved; the end point for treatment was either cure or administration of
five injections

Anatomy
bladder; detrusor muscle; external sphincter; intrinsic sphincter; lumen;
prostate; submucosa; sacral roots; urethra; urethral wall; urethral mucosa

Equipment
standard urologic endoscopic surgery equipment; 21 French (21-F) blunt end
sheath with 25-degree lens; side channel for insertion of 22-gauge metal needle; phosphate-buffered physiological saline solution; collagen

Source
Adapted from Aboseif SR, O'Connell HE, McGuire EJ. Collagen injection for intrinsic sphincteric deficiency in
men. Journal of Urology 1996;155:10-13.

collimated beam handpiece (CBH-1) for laser surgery

Description
LaserSonics handpiece designed specifically for aesthetic carbon dioxide
(CO_2) laser surgery; produces a collimated beam of 3 mm in diameter, which
guarantees the same spot size at any distance

Source
Heraeus Surgical Inc. product information. Milpitas, CA.

Collins SurveyTach with MicroTach assembly

Description
pneumotachometer system for screening spirometry, bedside spirometry, or
bronchoprovocation studies

Source
Collins/Cybermedic product information. Braintree, MA.

Colloral

Generic name
see type II collagen

ColoCARE Self-Test for fecal occult blood testing

Synonyms
none

Indications
rule out colorectal neoplasia

Method
ColoCARE Self-Test pad placed in toilet bowl after bowel movement; if
occult blood is present, positive result is indicated by appearance of blue
color in test area of pad

Normal findings
no color

Comments
patients may prefer simplicity and convenience of ColoCARE; test is not
sensitive for detection of colorectal neoplasia; patients may not feel comfortable interpreting the results without medical personnel; more sensitive
screening self-test is needed

Source
Adapted from Foliente RL, Wise GR, Collen MJ, et al. ColoCARE self-test versus Hemoccult II Sensa for fecal
occult blood testing. American Journal of Gastroenterology 1995;90:2160-2163.

Colorado microdissection needle

Description
precise ultrasharp tip for electrosurgery and tissue dissection to allow for
minimal scarring and faster healing

Source
Colorado Biomedical Inc. product information. Evergreen, CO.

Color Bar Schirmer strips

Description
a blue dye imprinted on millimeter-scaled strips that travel the tear flow and leave a soft blue vignette that is easy to read; strips are printed R (right) and/or L (left) on the bottom for appropriate use

Source
Eagle Vision product information. Memphis, TN.

 colorectal/ovarian carcinoma localization scintigraphy

Synonyms
OncoScint CR/OV; monoclonal antibody B72.3 scan

Indications
determine location and extent of extrahepatic metastasis in patients with known colorectal or ovarian cancer

Method
inject indium-111-conjugated labeled monoclonal antibody B72.3 and image patient using a gamma camera; evaluate for abnormal localization of radioactivity indicating tumor presence

Normal findings
no accumulation of radioactivity in unexpected areas under study

Comments
relatively low sensitivity and specificity limits utility

Source
Lexi-Comp Inc. database. Hudson, OH.
Nuclear Medicine Consultant. Stedman's Medical Dictionary, 26th edition.

 colorimetric *Candida albicans* susceptibility testing assay

Synonyms
C. albicans susceptibility

Use
determination of *Candida albicans* antibiotic susceptibility patterns

Method
Alamar Blue-based colorimetric assay

Specimen
Candida albicans culture specimen

Normal range
susceptible

Comments
assay sometimes involves a microdilution modification

Source
Adapted from Tiballi RN, He X, Zarins LT, Revankar SG, Kauffman CA. Use of a colorimetric system for yeast susceptibility testing. Journal of Clinical Microbiology 1995;33:915-917.

color kinesis (CK) echocardiography

Synonyms
none

Indications
assessing regional wall motion in patients with severe left ventricular dysfunction

Method
echocardiographic imaging performed; overall, time, and lateral gain compensations optimized and endocardial border identified using acoustic quantification edge-display method; when the color kinesis display is operated and the endocardial boundary moves inward during systole, a single color hue is added to mark endocardial pixels that change from blood to tissue; a different color is added for each frame; when endocardial wall segments are dyskinetic, endocardial pixels change from tissue to blood and a red color is displayed

Normal findings
not applicable

Comments
dyskinetic segments are characterized by significantly more red, dyskinetic motion than the other wall grades

Source
Adapted from Vandenberg BF, Oren RM, Lewis J, Aeschilman S, Burns TL, Kerber RE. Evaluation of color kinesis, a new echocardiogram method for analyzing regional wall motion in patients with dilated left ventricles. The American Journal of Cardiology 1997;79:645-650.

 color power angiography

Synonyms
none

Indications
imaging of vascular anatomic structures

Method
imaging of total volume of red blood cells; Cineloop lets film be rewound to take second look; persistence function stabilizes image by averaging several frames to minimize motion

Normal findings
normal blood flow through structure

Comments
superior to color Doppler; uses technology of color Doppler with just a software upgrade

Source
Adapted from Maltz G. Color power angiography improves fetal imaging. Ob.Gyn. News 1996;31:18.

Color Screening Inventory

Synonyms
none

Indications
detection of individuals with deficient color perception

Method
10-item color screening, with quadratic regression analysis for conversion to standard 100 hue test scores

Normal findings
normal color perception

Comments
rapid and simple means of testing color discrimination

Source
Adapted from Coren S, Hakstian AR. Testing color discrimination without the use of special stimuli or technical equipment. Perceptual and Motor Skills 1995;81:931-938.

 # Columbus McKinnon assist for lifting or transfer

Description
Columbus McKinnon (CM) device is a freestanding motorized device that assists in lifting and transferring patients who lack mobility; no discomfort or strain for patient or care giver

Source
Columbus McKinnon Corp. product information. Amherst, NY.

 # Columbus McKinnon Hugger device

Description
accessory device to Columbus McKinnon (CM) assist offers secure yet gentle upper body support; enables many persons to make independent transfers at home

Source
Columbus McKinnon Corp. product information. Amherst, NY.

 # CombiDERM Absorbent Cover Dressing (ACD)

Description
a nonadherent, super absorbent, waterproof pad that keeps excess exudate away from the wound, yet keeps the healing environment moist

Source
Bristol-Myers Squibb Co. product information. Princeton, NJ.

Combi Multi-Traction System

Description
table system series for traction therapy; designed as an all-in-one system for total control over treatment; includes cervical, lumbar, static, intermittent, and intersegmental traction capabilities; spinal profile system measures in/out 10 times per second to adjust each prescribed parameter; traction combinations include heat and soft tissue massage

Source
Williams Healthcare Systems product information. Elgin, IL.

 combined pelvic osteotomy for bladder exstrophy

Description
combined vertical and horizontal pelvic osteotomy (bilateral innominate and posterior vertical iliac osteotomy); approach for primary and secondary repair of primary bladder and cloacal exstrophy

Anatomy
pubic diastasis; tensor sartorius; iliac crest; pectineal tubercle; sacroiliac joints; ureters; sciatic notch

Equipment
standard surgical equipment; external fixator and pins for osteotomies

Source
Adapted from Gearhart J, Forschner D, Jeffa R, Ben-Chaim J, Sponseller P. A combined vertical and horizontal pelvic osteotomy approach for primary and secondary repair of bladder exstrophy. The Journal of Urology 1996;5(2):689-693.

 combined resection arthroplasty and arthrodesis

Description
surgical correction of severe rheumatoid forefoot deformities; manual correction of joint deformities preoperatively; circumferential dissection at base of phalanx; toe distraction; plate and capsule dissection; saw resection of surfaces for coaptation; medial-to-lateral arc resection of lesser joints and joint heads; pin placement protrudes from toes and is brought out from arthrodesis to hallux tip; K-wire stabilization of lesser toes

Anatomy
forefoot and toes; metatarsal phalangeal joints; proximal phalangeal bases; interphalangeal joints; metatarsal heads; hallux metatarsal phalangeal joint; hallux valgus; plantar plate; volar capsule; plantar aponeurosis

Equipment
standard surgery equipment, plus power saw; Freer elevator; double-ended, threaded Steinmann pins; K-wire; Band-Aids; wooden shoe

Source
Adapted from Mann RA, Schakel II ME. Surgical correction of rheumatoid forefoot deformities. Foot & Ankle International 1995;16:1-6.

Combitube airway

Description
esophageal tracheal double-lumen airway; AE-5260 Combitube with 2 syringes, 20 ml and 140 ml and 1 suction catheter; prevents aspiration; airtight seal without a mask; gastric fluids can be suctioned; endotracheal intubation can be done around device; can be deflated independently; prevents aspiration of teeth or other oral debris that may occur with esophageal/airway devices

Source
Armstrong Medical Industries Inc. product information. Lincolnshire, IL and San Diego, CA.

Combivent

Generic name
see albuterol sulfate/ipratropium bromide

Come-Orthotic sports replacement insole

Description
three-quarter length insoles; 100% natural wool; for use in athletic shoes

Source
HAPAD Inc. product information. Bethel Park, PA.

Commander angioplasty guidewire

Description
line of guidewires designed for percutaneous transluminal coronary angioplasty (PTCA) procedures; includes SR (stent-ready) series guidewires for coronary stent placement

Source
CR Bard product information. Salt Lake City, UT.

Compat surgical feeding tube

Description
gastrostomy feeding catheter designed specifically for gastrointestinal use; size reduces risk of clogging when feeding whole protein formulas; delivers enteral nutrition into jejunum immediately after surgery

Source
Sandoz Nutrition Corp. product information. Minneapolis, MN.

124

 Compeed Skinprotector dressing

Description
hydrocolloid dressing; acts like an extra layer of protective skin; adheres to the entire skin surface reducing friction at the site of injury; absorbs excessive wound fluid and skin moisture; protects against bacteria and dirt

Source
Bruder Healthcare Co. product information. Marietta, GA.

 complement-mediated tumor cell immunopurging

Synonyms
tumor cell purging; tumor cell negative selection

Use
removal or diminution of tumor cells from patient bone marrow prior to autologous transplant

Method
monoclonal antibody treatment of bone marrow specimen followed by complement treatment to destroy antibody-bound tumor cells

Specimen
autologous bone marrow

Normal range
not applicable

Comments
currently in clinical trials

Source
Adapted from Nimgaonkar M, Kemp A, Lancia J, Ball ED. A combination of CD34 selection and complement-mediated immunopurging (anti-CD15 monoclonal antibody) eliminates tumor cells while sparing normal progenitor cells. Journal of Hematotherapy 1996;5:39-48.

 composite groin fascial free flap

Description
one-stage treatment for injuries with extensive loss of soft tissue, extensor tendon and exposure of bone or joint, dorsum of hand or foot

Anatomy
extensor tendon; fascial flap; external oblique aponeurosis; extensor digitorum longus; extensor digitorum communis; carpi radialis brevis

Equipment
standard surgical equipment

Source
Adapted from Jeng S, Wei F, Noordhoff S. The composite groin fascial free flap. Annals of Plastic Surgery 1995;35:595-600.

computerized bedside transfusion identification system (CBTIS)

Synonyms
automated bedside patient and blood unit matching

Use
pre-transfusion bedside verification of match between patient and blood unit

Method
portable computerized scanner reads and compares barcodes on patient wristband and blood unit

Specimen
patient wristband and blood unit barcodes

Normal range
patient identification has been verified

Comments
can be expected to reduce or eliminate the administration of blood to the wrong patients, the principal cause of fatal transfusion reactions

Source
Adapted from Jensen NJ, Crosson JT. An automated system for bedside verification of the match between patient identification and blood unit identification. Transfusion 1996;36:216-221.

 Comtan

Generic name
see entacapone

 Comvax

Generic name
see haemophilus b (conjugate)/hepatitis B (recombinant) vaccine

 confocal microscope

Description
unique tandem scanning confocal microscope with video attachment for visualization and recording findings

Source
Tandem Scanning Corp. product information. Neston, VA.

confocal microscopy identification of *Acanthamoeba* keratitis

Synonyms
none

Indications
noninvasive study, diagnosis, and treatment of *Acanthamoeba* keratitis

Method
using methyl cellulose as a coupling agent, the confocal microscope objective is applied using a Hamamatsu C2400 SIT video camera to visualize and record findings; able to detect the outline of the amoeba

Normal findings
not applicable

Comments
Acanthamoeba keratitis is a newly recognized and growing infection, especially among contact lens wearers

Source
Adapted from Pfister DR, Cameron JD, Krachmer JH, Holland EJ. Confocal microscopy findings of *Acanthamoeba* keratitis. American Journal of Ophthalmology 1996;121:119-128.

 ## conjugated estrogens/medroxyprogesterone acetate

Brand name
Prempro; Premphase

Use
treatment of moderate to severe vasomotor symptoms associated with menopause; treatment of vulvar and vaginal atrophy; and prevention of osteoporosis in women with an intact uterus

Usual dosage
oral: 28-day cycle packs; one tablet daily

Pharmaceutical company
Wyeth-Ayerst Laboratories. Philadelphia, PA.

Source
University of Pittsburgh Drug Information and Pharmacoepidemiology Center. Pittsburgh, PA.

 ## ConQuest System

Description
provides comfort and security of incontinence management for males without use of Foley catheters, adhesives or absorbents; consists of supporter brief, pressure pad, condom catheter, and leg bag all functioning together

Source
ConvaTec product information. Princeton, NJ.

Consonar

Generic Name
see brofaromine

 Constant-Clens dermal wound cleanser

Description
saline formulated to soften and remove necrotic tissue and debris

Source
Sherwood Medical Co. product information. St. Louis, MO.

 Contimed II

Description
home unit for measuring pelvic floor muscle activity and involuntary loss of urine; provides visual and auditory pelvic floor muscle activity measurement; tracks patient's progress and compliance for 30 days

Source
InCare Medical Products of Hollister Inc. product information. Libertyville, IL.

 continent gastric tube techniques

Description
gastric tissue has been used to create continent catheterizable tubes; diagnoses have included bladder exstrophy, rhabdomyosarcoma, and neurogenic bladder; techniques have been gastrocystoplasty with simultaneous creation of a continent gastric tube from the anterior gastric flap, and creation of a continent gastric tube from an anterior flap raised from the existing gastric bladder (from previous gastrocystoplasty); isolated gastric tubes have also been constructed

Anatomy
antrum; abdominal wall; bladder neck; gastric mucosa; greater curvature of stomach; gastroepiploic arteries; peritoneal cavity; seromuscular layer; transverse colon; umbilicus

Equipment
standard urologic and gastric surgical equipment; GIA 90 stapler

Source
Adapted from Close CE, Mitchell ME. Continent gastric tube: new techniques and long-term follow-up. Journal of Urology 1997;157:51-55.

continuous wave arthroscopy pump

Description
pump that gives even non-pulsing flow and instantaneous response to intra-articular pressure changes; provides surgeon with superior joint visualization by maintenance of precise irrigation and distention

Source
Arthrex Inc. product information. Naples, FL.

 Conveen leg bag strap

Description
latex-free leg bag strap to reduce risk of allergic reactions; made of plush, soft, comfortable materials for optimal patient comfort; straps are easy to size with specialized cutting areas that reduce fraying and provide custom fit; attach easily to the leg bag with reinforced buttons

Source
Coloplast Corp. product information. Marietta, GA.

 ConXn

Generic name
see relaxin H2 (human recombinant)

 COOL TOPS compress

Description
adjustable therapeutic hot/cold breast compress used in postop reconstruction

Source
Corso Enterprises Inc. product information. Sausalito, CA.

 Cooper-Rand intraoral artificial larynx

Description
artificial larynx provides speech for patient with reasonable control of the tongue and jaw; no air-flow required; can be used sitting, lying, or standing as long as jaw movement is not restricted

Source
Luminaud Inc. product information. Mentor, OH.

 Copaxone

Generic Name
copolymer-1

▶ *Copolymer-1 is now known as glatiramer acetate.*

copolymer-1

Brand Name
Copaxone

Use
polypeptide stimulating myelin protein for use in patients with multiple sclerosis

Usual Dosage
injection: 20 µg daily

Pharmaceutical company
Lemmon Company. Kulpsville, PA.

Source
Samford University Global Drug Information Service. Birmingham, AL.

► *Copolymer-1 is now known as glatiramer acetate.*

 core decompression of femoral head

Description
treatment to preserve intact femoral head in patients with Ficat stage I osteonecrosis; coring performed under C-arm control

Anatomy
hip; femur; femoral head

Equipment
standard biopsy equipment; Zimmer 0.95-cm diameter core biopsy needle or Richard 8-mm reamer

Source
Adapted from Smith SW, Fehring TK, Griffin WL, Beaver WB. Core decompression of the osteonecrotic femoral head. The Journal of Bone and Joint Surgery 1995;77-A:674-680.

 Coreg

Generic name
see carvedilol

 Corlopam

Generic name
see fenoldopam

Cortexplorer cerebral blood flow monitor

Description
portable, noninvasive, easily repeatable cerebral blood flow monitor

Source
Adapted from Martin NA, Alsina G, Kordestani R, Lee JH. The Simonsen cerebrograph Cortexplorer. Neurosurgery 1996;39:1059-1061.

 ## cortical cleaving hydrodissector cannula

Description
ophthalmic surgical instrument developed to separate cortex from capsular bag facilitating capsulorrhexis; procedure leaves cleaner capsular bag that requires less irrigation and aspiration during cortical clean-up

Source
Visitec product information. Sarasota, FL.

 ## corticorelin ovine triflutate

Brand name
Acthrel

Use
diagnostic agent used to differentiate pituitary and ectopic production of adrenocorticotropic hormone (ACTH) in patients with ACTH-dependent Cushing syndrome

Usual dosage
injection: maximally-effective study doses were in the range of 3-10 µg/kg in early studies

Pharmaceutical company
Ferring Labs. Suffern, NY.

Source
Stadtlanders Managed Pharmacy Services. Pittsburgh, PA.

 ## Corvert

Generic Name
see ibutilide fumarate

Corydon hydroexpression cannula

Description
ophthalmic surgical instrument designed to express the nucleus with balanced salt solution through a capsulorrhexis during extracapsular cataract extraction (ECCE); designed by Dr. Leif Corydon

Source
Visitec Co. product information. Sarasota, FL.

 ## Covertell composite secondary dressing

Description
layered, absorbent dressing with nonadherent contact layer that contains and maintains hydration within the wound

Source
Gentell Inc. product information. Huntingdon Valley, PA.

 ## Cox II ocular laser shield

Description
eye shield used during application of laser treatment; also available with a suction cup

Source
Oculo-Plastik product information. Montreal, Quebec, Canada.

 ## Cozaar

Generic name
see losartan

 ## CPET (cardiopulmonary exercise testing)

Synonyms
cardiopulmonary exercise testing

Indications
chronic dyspnea

Method
CPET adjusted to reach maximum work load in 10-12 minutes with continuous ECG, blood pressure monitoring, breath-by-breath measurement, analysis of exhaled gases

Normal findings
Not applicable

Comments
CPET can help determine source of dyspnea and by aiding in choosing subsequent tests, it can save unnecessary and expensive further testing

Source
Adapted from Anonymous. A path to the cause of dyspnea. Emergency Medicine 1995;27:47.

 Cragg thrombolytic brush

Description
brush designed to accelerate thrombolytic process in patients with blood clots for treatment of peripheral vascular disease and neurovascular brain disorders associated with strokes

Source
Micro Therapeutics Inc. product information. San Clemente, CA.

 crankshaft clip

Description
modified bayonet aneurysm clip, bent nearly to a right angle with distal blade 5-mm in length and proximal blade or shank portion designed in three lengths; used for clipping aneurysms in the middle cerebral artery in which the aneurysmal neck includes the arterial junction, and for some anterior communicating artery aneurysms

Source
Mizuho Ikakogyo Co. Ltd. product information. Tokyo, Japan.

 Cricket pulse oximetry monitor

Description
lightweight recorder worn for up to 24 hours; designed to monitor pulse rate, movement, and saturated partial pressure of oxygen (SpO_2)

Source
Respironics Inc. product information. Murrysville, PA.

 Crinone

Generic name
see progesterone (natural)

Criss Cross Cradle

Description
device to support abdomen and lower back during pregnancy

Source
Prenatal Cradle product information. Hamburg, MI.

Crixivan

Generic Name
see indinavir sulfate

crossed-screw fixation

Description
crossed-screw fixation involves the shortest segment of spine and results in better stability and less screw pullout, compared to other spinal instrumentation; lateral extracavitary approach through a paramedian linear incision while patient is prone; perform anterior decompression of the dural sac; place screws at 90 degrees to each other; ventral interbody fusion with rib graft completes the stabilization

Anatomy
spinal canal; dural sac; vertebral body; cortex, anterior, and middle column of vertebral body; vertebral interbody; pedicle; transverse process; endplate; neuroforamina; facet joint; paraspinous muscle; segmental intercostal nerve; nerve root origin; epidural vein; radiculomedullary spinal artery

Equipment
standard orthopaedic/neurosurgery equipment; transverse vertebral body screw; unilateral pedicle screw; Texas Scottish Rite Hospital (TSRH) variable-angle bone screw; high-speed drill; crosslink eyebolt; screw eyebolt; variable-angle eyebolt; pliers; rod; rod manipulator; crosslink

Source
Adapted from Benzel EC, Baldwin NG. Crossed-screw fixation of the unstable thoracic and lumbar spine. Journal of Neurosurgery 1995;82:11-16.

C-TUB instrument receptacle

Description
optically clear instrument receptacle that utilizes minimal counter space with tapered base that allows for more solution and instruments

Source
Cetylite Industries Inc. product information. Pennsauken, NJ.

Cueva cranial nerve electrode

Description
cranial nerve electrode featuring atraumatic placement and removal with stable positioning on nerve and high-quality recording

Source
AD-TECH Medical Instrument Corp. product information. Racine, WI.

^{14}C-urea microdose capsule breath test

Synonyms
PY test, microdose ^{14}C-urea *Helicobacter pylori* breath test

Use
diagnosis of *Helicobacter pylori* infection of the stomach

Method
radiometric detection of *Helicobacter pylori* urease enzyme activity utilizing much smaller dose of ^{14}C-urea

Specimen
breath

Normal range
less than 200 dpm

Comments
rapid, noninvasive test for detection of gastric *Helicobacter pylori* infection using microdose of ^{14}C-urea

Source
Adapted from Peura DA, Pambianco DJ, Dye KR, Lind C, Frierson HF, Hoffman SR, Combs MJ, Guilfoyle E, Marshall BJ. Microdose ^{14}C-urea breath test offers diagnosis of *Helicobacter pylori* in 10 minutes. American Journal of Gastroenterology 1996;91:233-238.

Curosurf

Generic name
see pulmonary surfactant

CUSP-LOK bracket

Description
chain and grid for cuspid exposures

Source
Xemax Surgical Products Inc. product information. Napa, CA.

Cyberware 3030RGB digitizer

Description

laser scanning device that features a sensor that rotates around the subject's head as it projects a vertical plane of laser light onto the face to produce 3D full color computer models

Source

Cyberware Laboratories Inc. product information. Monterey, CA.

cyclosporine microemulsion

Brand name

Neoral

Use

used for the prevention of organ rejection in patients who have undergone renal, hepatic, or cardiac transplantation

Usual dosage

oral: initial dose of 2.0 mg/kg/day first 4 days tapered to 1.0 mg/kg/day by 1 week, 0.6 mg/kg/day by 2 weeks, 0.3 mg/kg/day by 1 month, and 0.15 mg/kg/day for 2 months and thereafter as maintenance dose. Note: Dosing should be individualized, depending on the status of the patient and the function of graft. Neoral should not be used interchangeably with Sandimmune

Pharmaceutical company

Sandoz Pharmaceutical Co. East Hanover, NJ.

Source

University of Pittsburgh Drug Information and Pharmacoepidemiology Center. Pittsburgh, PA.

Cystadane

Generic name

see betaine anhydrous

CytoGam

Generic name

see cytomegalovirus immune globulin

cytomegalovirus immune globulin

Brand name
CytoGam

Use
prophylaxis against cytomegalovirus disease in renal transplant patients

Usual dosage
intravenous: 150 mg/kg within 72 hours of transplantation; 100 mg/kg at 2, 4, 6, and 8 weeks post-transplantation; 50 mg/kg at 12 and 16 weeks post-transplantation

Pharmaceutical company
MedImmune Inc. Gaithersburg, MD.

Source
University of Pittsburgh Drug Information and Pharmacoepidemiology Center. Pittsburgh, PA.

daclizumab

Brand name
Zenapax

Use
prevention of acute kidney transplant rejection

Usual dosage
intravenous: doses of 0.5-1.5 mg/kg were used in early clinical trials

Pharmaceutical company
Hoffman LaRoche. Nutley, NJ.

Source
Stadtlanders Managed Pharmacy Services. Pittsburgh, PA.

Dale abdominal binder

Description
provides abdominal support; encourages postoperative mobility; alleviates incisional pain; allows for evenly distributed compression around the abdomen; enhances pulmonary function

Source
Dale Medical Products Inc. product information. Plainville, MA.

Dalla Bona ball and socket abutment

Description
dental prosthesis consisting of titanium alloy ball and socket abutment; provides strong retention both vertically and laterally for overdenture construction

Source
Lifecore Biomedical product information. Chaska, MN.

dalteparin sodium

Brand name
Fragmin

Use
prophylaxis against deep vein thrombosis (DVT) in patients undergoing surgery who are at risk of thromboembolic complications

Usual dosage
subcutaneous: 2,500 IU, which is equivalent to 16 mg, one to two hours prior to abdominal surgery and once daily for 5 to 10 days postoperatively

Pharmaceutical company
Pharmacia Adria Inc. Columbus, OH.

Source
University of Pittsburgh Drug Information and Pharmacoepidemiology Center. Pittsburgh, PA.

danaparoid sodium

Brand name
Orgaran

Use
heparinoid used in the treatment of venous thromboembolism; treatment of acute or progressing ischemic stroke

Usual dosage
subcutaneous: 1250 to 2000 units twice daily have been used in clinical trials

Pharmaceutical company
Organon. West Orange, NJ.

Source
University of Pittsburgh Drug Information and Pharmacoepidemiology Center. Pittsburgh, PA.

DarcoGel ankle brace

Description
ankle brace with removable gel liners that can be refrigerated for cold therapy; stirrup design to support an unstable ankle

Source
Darco product information. Huntington, WV.

Dart pacemaker

Description

implantable, single-chamber, multiprogrammable cardiac pulse generator designed to provide rate-adaptive pacing to atrium or ventricle; using an accelerometer, Dart senses body motions and uses this information to adjust pacing rate

Source

Intermedics Inc. product information. Angleton, TX.

 Datascope true sheathless catheter

Description

intra-aortic balloon catheter with guidewire is specifically designed for use without a plug or sheath, giving better peripheral flow

Source

Datascope Corporation, Cardiac Assist Division product information. Fairfield, NJ.

 daunorubicin liposomal formulation

Brand name

DaunoXome

Use

liposomal formulation used in the treatment of patients with advanced HIV-related Kaposi sarcoma

Usual dosage

intravenous: doses of 40 mg/m^2 every 2 weeks or 100 mg/m^2 every 3 weeks have been used in clinical trials

Pharmaceutical company

Vestar Inc. San Dimas, CA.

Source

University of Pittsburgh Drug Information and Pharmacoepidemiology Center. Pittsburgh, PA.

 DaunoXome

Generic name

see daunorubicin liposomal formulation

David Baker eyelid retractor

Description
retractor for upper eyelid with simultaneous protection of sensitive scleral membranes; especially convenient for laser-assisted blepharoplasty

Source
Byron Medical product information. (*Editor note:* advertising uses byron but company name correctly is Byron) Tucson, AZ.

 ## Davidoff blade

Description
ambidextrous nucleus chopper, used, through paracentesis, for reduced phacoemulsification time; allows for easy fracture of a soft nucleus and epinucleus; double wedge-shaped blades and double-bevel inner blade allows for chopping and manipulating in either hand

Source
Rhein Medical product information. Tampa, FL.

 ## DawSkin prosthetics

Description
below the knee prosthetic featuring seven skin tones; flexible protective "skin system"

Source
Daw Industries product information. San Diego, CA.

 ## Daytimer support

Description
carpal tunnel syndrome support; full finger and hand grasping capability for full productivity at work; provides stable wrist compression

Source:
Brown Medical Industries product information. Hartley, IA.

 ## DDH orthosis

Description
developmental dislocated hip (DDH) orthosis used for infants beyond the Pavlik stage; provides positive abduction positioning; stainless steel thigh bar can be repeatedly formed without fracturing

Source
Fillauer Inc. production information. Chattanooga, TN.

DDV ligator

Description
transurethral approach for ligation of the dorsal vein before trifurcation; reduces significant blood loss during radical retropubic prostatectomy

Source
NAMI product information. Lubbock, TX.

 Debut ear piercing kit

Description
allows precision re-piercing after repair of torn ear lobe; piercing tip automatically disengages after piercing, leaving patient with perfect trainer earring stud

Source
E&A Enterprises product information. Whitestone, NY.

 Decapeptyl

Generic name
see triptorelin

 decay-accelerating factor (DAF) assay

Synonyms
CD55 assay

Use
diagnosis of paroxysmal nocturnal hemoglobinuria (PNH)

Method
immunoassay

Specimen
blood

Normal range
undetermined

Comments
direct measurement of the defective molecule, DAF, in patients suspected of having PNH

Source
Blood 1995;86:3277-3286.

deflazacort

Brand name
Flantadin, Calcort

Use
corticosteroid used in the treatment of allergic rhinitis, asthma, and rheumatoid arthritis

Usual dosage
oral: 6 to 60 mg daily

Pharmaceutical company
Marion Merrell Dow. Kansas City, MO.

Source
University of Pittsburgh Drug Information and Pharmacoepidemiology Center. Pittsburgh, PA.

 Delaprem

Generic name
see hexoprenaline sulfate

 delavirdine mesylate

Brand name
Rescriptor

Use
reverse transcriptase inhibitor for use in HIV patients who have failed other drug therapies; to be used in combination with other antiretroviral agents

Usual dosage
oral: 100 to 400 mg three times daily

Pharmaceutical company
The Upjohn Company. Kalamazoo, MI.

Source
University of Pittsburgh Drug Information and Pharmacoepidemiology Center. Pittsburgh, PA.

 DeltaTrac II metabolic monitor

Description
assesses the energy requirements and nutritional needs of patients on ventilator therapy; measures caloric needs and estimates substrate oxidation by continuously monitoring oxygen consumption and carbon dioxide production; meter can be used with infants, children, and adults; solves problems related to ventilator dependency and weaning

Source
SensorMedics product information. Yorba Linda, CA.

DEMBONE

Description
demineralized freeze-dried bone available in syringes; acts as a soft tissue barrier

Source
Park Dental Research Corp. product information. New York, NY.

 Denavir

Generic name
see penciclovir

 DenLite illuminated hand-held mirror

Description
dental instrument with a disposable mirror head with split-beam illumination

Source
Welch Allyn Inc. product information. Skaneateles Falls, NY.

 density gradient bone marrow progenitor enrichment

Synonyms
CD34 enrichment by density gradient

Use
enrichment of blood-forming stem and progenitor population, prior to transplantation or gene therapy

Method
iso-osmolar Percoll density gradient centrifugation

Specimen
bone marrow; peripheral blood stem cell cytapheresis product; umbilical cord blood

Normal range
investigational

Comments
other methods currently in use include immunoaffinity and immunomagnetic separation

Source
Experimental Hematology 1995;23:1024-1029.

 DentiPatch

Generic name
see lidocaine transoral delivery system

Denver percutaneous access kit (PAK)

Description
ascites shunting system; PAK provides subclavian vein access, reduced surgical time, reduced patient trauma, simplified procedure, easier catheter replacement
Source
Denver Biomaterials Inc. product information. Evergreen, CO.

DeOrio intrauterine insemination catheter

Description
used for introduction of washed spermatozoa into uterine cavity; rigidity of inner cannula facilitates introduction of catheter through the cervix and into the uterus
Source
Cook OB/GYN product information. Spencer, IN.

Deoshoes deodorant

Description
a deodorant system that limits formation of microorganisms in the shoe; each pressure of the heel activates the Deoshoes deodorant
Source
Lemaitre Securite French Co. product information. Chicago, IL.

deoxyspergualin

Brand name
Spanidin
Use
prevention of organ transplant rejection
Usual dosage
intraperitoneal: 5 mg/kg/day
Pharmaceutical company
Bristol-Myers Squibb Co. Princeton, NJ.
Source
Stadtlanders Managed Pharmacy Services. Pittsburgh, PA.

Depacon

Generic name
see valproate sodium

Dermacea alginate gel

Description

forms a moist, stable gel; vertical absorption protects peri-wound skin; use with Viasorb dressing for optimal results

Source

Sherwood Medical product information. St. Louis, MO.

 ## DermaMend foam

Description

second generation hydrophilic polyurethane foam dressing

Source

Dermax Corp. product information. Denver, CO.

 ## Dermanet wound contact layer

Description

protects fragile granulation tissue in burns or chronic wounds; can be used to line deep wounds before application of packing materials

Source

DeRoyal Industries Inc. product information. Powell, TN.

 ## DermaSof sheeting

Description

semi-occlusive reinforced gel sheeting that is slightly adhesive and durable; treatment for flattening and softening hypertrophic and keloid tissue; returns skin to its natural color

Source

McGhan product information. Santa Barbara, CA.

 ## Dermo-Jet injector

Description

needleless high-pressure instrument for automatic injections; achieves painless infiltration when administering anesthetic solutions, parenteral drugs, vaccines, and steroids in aqueous suspension

Source

Robbins Instruments Inc. product information. Chatham, NJ.

DeRoyal laparotomy sponge

Description
domestic-made laparotomy sponge to compete with imported products

Source
DeRoyal Industries Inc. product information. Powell, TN.

 ## desirudin

Brand name
Revase

Use
an adjunct to thrombolytic therapy in acute myocardial infarction

Usual dosage
injectable: intravenous bolus dose of 0.4 to 0.6 mg/kg; followed by continuous infusion ranging from 0.15 to 0.2 mg/kg/hr has been used as an adjunct to thrombolytic therapy

Pharmaceutical company
Ciba-Geigy. Summit, NJ.

Source
University of Pittsburgh Drug Information and Pharmacoepidemiology Center. Pittsburgh, PA.

 ## deslorelin

Brand Name
Somagard

Use
long-acting luteinizing hormone-releasing hormone agonist used for treatment of precocious puberty and endometriosis

Usual Dosage
subcutaneous depot: precocious puberty in children—4 µg/kg/d in children ages ≤ 9.5 years old subcutaneous: endometriosis 100 µg/day starting on day five of cycle and continuing for 28 days

Pharmaceutical company
Roberts Pharmaceutical Corporation. Eatontown, NJ.

Source
University of Pittsburgh Drug Information and Pharmacoepidemiology Center. Pittsburgh, PA.

desogestrel

Brand name
Implanon

Use
long-term hormonal contraceptive

Usual dosage
subdermal implants to last 2 years: contain a total of 68 mg of 3-keto-deso-gestrel with an expected initial release of 67 mcg per day with the amount released decreasing over time to 40 mcg per day at year one and 30 mcg per day at year two

Pharmaceutical company
Organon. West Orange, NJ.

Source
University of Pittsburgh Drug Information and Pharmacoepidemiology Center. Pittsburgh, PA.

 detection of p53, *bcl*-2, and retinoblastoma proteins in follicular lymphoma

Synonyms
p53, *bcl*-2, RB testing

Use
diagnosis and prognostic evaluation of follicular lymphoma

Method
immunohistochemistry using monoclonal antibodies

Specimen
paraffin-embedded tissue biopsy

Normal range
p53 negative, *bcl*-2 negative, RB gene product negative

Comments
correlates well with cytologic grade in follicular lymphoma

Source
Adapted from Nguyen PL, Zukerberg LR, Benedict WF, Harris NL. Immunohistochemical detection of p53, *bcl*-2, and retinoblastoma proteins in follicular lymphoma. American Journal of Clinical Pathology 1996;105:538-543.

 determination of origin of hematuria by immunocytochemical staining

Synonyms
Tamm-Horsfall protein (uromodulin)

Indications
to determine the feasibility of immunocytochemical staining of urinary erythrocytes for Tamm-Horsfall protein to differential renal from nonrenal hematuria

Method
urine samples collected with microscopic or gross hematuria; erythrocyte morphology evaluated; using phase contrast microscopy, erythrocytes were classified as isomorphic or dysmorphic

Normal findings
Tamm-Horsfall protein is a renal epithelial glycoprotein produced by cells of the ascending limbs of the loops of Henle; a normal constituent of urine

Comments
immunocytochemical staining of urine erythrocytes for Tamm-Horsfall protein appears to be a reliable diagnostic tool to determine when hematuria is renal or nonrenal in origin; further studies need to be done

Source
Adapted from Fukusaki A, Kaneto H, Ikeda S, Orikasa S. Determining the origin of hematuria by immunocytochemical staining of erythrocytes in urine for Tamm-Horsfall protein. The Journal of Urology 1996;155:248-251.

 Detrusitol

Generic name
see tolterodine

 dexfenfluramine hydrochloride

Brand name
Redux

Use
treatment of obesity associated with carbohydrate craving

Usual dosage
oral: 15 mg twice daily

Pharmaceutical company
Lederle Laboratories. Wayne, NJ.

Source
University of Pittsburgh Drug Information and Pharmacoepidemiology Center. Pittsburgh, PA.
▶ *As of September 15, 1997, dexfenfluramine hydrochloride has been withdrawn from the market.*

 dexrazoxane

Brand name
Zinecard

Use
cardioprotectant against doxorubicin cardiotoxicity

Usual dosage
intravenous: 1000 mg/m^2 infused 30 minutes before administration of doxorubicin; the maximum tolerated dose is 3500 mg/m^2/day for 3 days in pediatric patients

Pharmaceutical company
Adria Laboratories. Columbus, OH.

Source
University of Pittsburgh Drug Information and Pharmacoepidemiology Center. Pittsburgh, PA.

 DHEA (dehydroepiandrosterone)

Generic name
see prasterone

 DiaPhine trephine

Description
instrument designed for controlled trephination of donor cornea utilizing a diamond blade for precise incision; interchangeable cutting inserts of different sizes and shapes

Source
Storz Ophthalmics product information. St. Louis, MO.

 Diastat

Generic name
see diazepam

 Diastat vascular access graft

Description
Gore-Tex stretch vascular graft provides reduced blood loss, reduced time to hemostasis, reduced incidence of hematomas

Source
W.L. Gore & Associates Inc. product information. Flagstaff, AZ.

 diazepam

Brand name
Diastat

Use
treatment of acute repetitive seizures associated with epilepsy

Usual dosage
topical: viscous solution for rectal administration in concentration of 5 mg/ml in doses of 0.16 mg/kg to 0.5 mg/kg; now being studied in children with status epilepticus seizures

Pharmaceutical company
Athena Neurosciences. San Francisco, CA.

Source
Stadtlanders Managed Pharmacy Services. Pittsburgh, PA.

dibromodulcitol (DBD)

Brand name
Mitolactol

Use
under investigation for orphan drug indication for treatment of recurrent advanced cervical cancer

Usual dosage
injectible: in combination with cisplatin therapy, DBD in doses of 180 mg/m^2 to 270 mg/m^2 intravenously for 5 days, every 3 to 4 weeks used in the clinical trials to determine the efficacy and dose tolerance

Pharmaceutical company
Biopharm Inc. Levittown, PA.

Source
Stadtlanders Managed Pharmacy Services. Pittsburgh, PA.

 # diclofenac sodium and misoprostol

Brand name
Arthrotec

Use
prophylaxis against gastrointestinal ulcers induced by nonsteroidal anti-inflammatory drugs

Usual dosage
oral: 50 mg diclofenac and 200 µg misoprostol, 2 to 3 times a day with food

Pharmaceutical company
G.D. Searle & Co. Chicago, IL.

Source
Stadtlanders Managed Pharmacy Services. Pittsburgh, PA.

 # diethyldithiocarbamate

Brand name
Imuthiol

Use
immunomodulator for use in treating AIDS-related wasting syndrome

Usual dosage
oral: 400 mg/m^2 of body surface area once weekly

Pharmaceutical company
Connaught Labs Inc. Swiftwater, PA.

Source
University of Pittsburgh Drug Information and Pharmacoepidemiology Center. Pittsburgh, PA.

differential display of messenger ribonucleic acid

Synonyms
none

Indications
technique for analyzing differential gene expression in human brain tumors

Method
temporal lobe tissue obtained; temporal lobe tissue and tumor specimens were snap-frozen and stored in nitrogen; tissues histopathologically examined and confirmed by neuropathologists

Normal findings
differential display method for mRNA was successfully used to identify genes of normal brain and malignant glioma tissues

Comments
60 different sequences differentially expressed between normal and malignant tissues; one of the sequences represents a new brain-specific kinesin heavy chain (KHC) gene

Source
Adapted from Uchiyama CM, Zhu J, Carroll RS, et al. Differential display of messenger ribonucleic acid: A useful technique for analyzing differential gene expression in human brain tumors. Neurosurgery Journal 1995;37:464-470.

 Differin

Generic name
see adapalene

 diffusing capacity to evaluate dyspnea

Synonyms
DLCO (carbon monoxide-diffusing capacity)

Indications
interstitial lung disease

Method
21% oxygen, a small amount of carbon monoxide (CO), about 10% helium are inhaled from residual volume; breath shield for 9-11 seconds; mixture is exhaled; washout volume to clear dead space is discarded, alveolar sample is collected

Normal findings
not applicable

Comments
a reduced DLCO may be first pulmonary function abnormality detected in patients with interstitial lung disease

Source
Adapted from Littner MR. The diagnostic value of diffusing capacity. Journal of Respiratory Distress 1995; 16:491-494.

DIGI-FLEX exercise system

Description
color-coded finger and hand exercise system

Source
Digi-Flex product information. Hicksville, NY.

 ## Digital Inflection Rigidometer

Description
device to quantitate the strength of an erection

Source
Southwest Instrument Co. product information. Van Buren, AR.

 ## digital stereotactic core breast biopsy

Indications
assess nonpalpable lesion suspicious for malignancy on mammography; less suspicious lesions may undergo biopsy if physician concern or patient anxiety is high

Method
patient in prone position in a specialized mammography unit; digital computer equipment allows for exact localization of lesion; biopsy performed with multiple passes of 14-gauge needle

Normal findings
post-procedure specimen and in vivo radiographs demonstrate that appropriate specimen material obtained

Comments
more cost-effective than and as accurate as surgical biopsy; streamlines diagnostic work-up of suspicious lesions; no disfigurement or mammographic pseudolesion results

Source
University of Maryland Department of Diagnostic Radiology. Baltimore, MD.

 ## digital x-ray detector

Description
replaces conventional x-ray film by producing instant images on computer screen; allows for easy location and retrieval of images and remote access; eliminates film and chemicals needed for film development; currently in clinical and radiographic trials

Source
EG&G Inc. product and Internet information. Wellesley, MA.

Digitrapper MkIII sleep monitor

Description
monitoring device used to evaluate possible gastroesophageal reflux, reflux asthma, chronic cough, and nocturnal arousals that may result in apnea; single-channel pH meter and standard polysomnograph to identify reflux-related arousals

Source
Synetics Medical Inc. product information. Irving, TX.

 dihydroergotamine mesylate

Brand name
Migranal

Use
nasal spray formulation of an ergot alkaloid for the treatment of migraine headaches

Usual dosage
nasal spray: 2 or 3 mg intranasally for relief of migraine

Pharmaceutical company
Novartis Pharmaceuticals Co. East Hanover, NJ.

Source
Stadtlanders Managed Pharmacy Services. Pittsburgh, PA.

 diltiazem hydrochloride (HCl)

Brand name
Tiazac

Use
calcium channel blocker for hypertension

Usual dosage
oral: once daily 120 mg, 180 mg, 240 mg, 300 mg, 360 mg

Pharmaceutical company
Forest Pharmaceutical Inc. St. Louis, MO.

Source
Internet www.fda.gov.

 diltiazem maleate/enalapril maleate

Brand name
Teczem

Use
extended-release formulation of calcium channel blocker and angiotensin-converting enzyme (ACE) inhibitor, used for the treatment of hypertension

Usual dosage
oral: each extended-release tablet contains diltiazem maleate, equivalent to 180 mg of diltiazem hydrochloride and enalapril maleate 5 mg; as single daily dose

Pharmaceutical company
Merck & Co. Inc. West Point, PA.

Source
Stadtlanders Managed Pharmacy Services. Pittsburgh, PA.

 dinoprostone

Brand Name
Cervidil

Use
synthetic prostaglandin E for initiation and/or induction of labor in pregnant women

Usual Dosage
removable vaginal insert: each pessary contains 10 mg of dinoprostone being released in vivo at a rate of approximately 0.3 mg/hour over a period of 12 hours

Pharmaceutical company
Forest Pharmaceuticals Inc. St. Louis, MO.

Source
University of Pittsburgh Drug Information and Pharmacoepidemiology Center. Pittsburgh PA.

 Diovan

Generic name
see valsartan

 dipalmitoylphosphatidylcholine (also dipalmitoyl phosphatidyl choline) (DPPC or dppc)/phosphatidylglycerol (PG)

Brand name
ALEC

Use
treatment of neonatal respiratory distress syndrome (RDS)

Usual dosage
injection: 1 ml vial containing 25-100 mg in suspension formulation; doses between 50 and 100 mg have been used in the clinical trials

Pharmaceutical company
Britannia Pharmaceuticals Limited. Surrey, UK.

Source
Stadtlanders Managed Pharmacy Services. Pittsburgh, PA.

diphtheria, tetanus toxoids and acellular pertussis absorbed vaccine (DTaP)

Brand name
Infanrix

Use
recommended for FDA (Food and Drug Administration) approval as primary DPT series (diphtheria, pertussis, and tetanus). It is available as three vaccines in one product; to be used in infants to immunize. The pertussis portion is a new form (acellular)

Usual dosage
available as vaccine to be given to infants to immunize against DPT infections

Pharmaceutical company
SmithKline Beecham. Philadelphia, PA.

Source
Internet www.fda.gov.

 ## Dirame

Generic name
see propiram

 ## dirithromycin

Brand name
Dynabac

Use
macrolide antibiotic for use in various infections including acute bronchitis, community-acquired pneumonia, and uncomplicated skin and skin structure infections

Usual dosage
oral: 500 mg daily for 7-14 days

Pharmaceutical company
Eli Lilly Co. Indianapolis, IN.

Source
University of Pittsburgh Drug Information and Pharmacoepidemiology Center. Pittsburgh, PA.

 ## Discover Cryo-Therapy

Description
reusable eye and full face compress for hot and cold therapy; can be sterilized with gas

Source
Corso Enterprises Inc. product information. Sausalito, CA.

Dismutec

Generic name
see pegorgotein

Disten-U-Flo fluid system

Description
device for hysteroscopy; continuous flow removes blood and debris for improved visualization; facilitates diagnosis in presence of heavy bleeding

Source
Circon ACMI product information. Stamford, CT.

diurnal blood pressure study

Synonyms
none

Indications
for evaluation of diurnal BP in normal gravidas and those with preeclampsia

Method
diurnal variation and BP measurement were evaluated using pregnancy-validated SpaceLabs 90207 ambulatory BP monitor for 24 hours, and for which normal references were determined

Normal findings
BP fall was less in preeclamptic than in normotensive women at night; the day-night BP difference decreased as average BP rose

Comments
decrease in day-night BP difference in preeclampsia is inversely related to average BP

Source
Adapted from Halligan A, Shennan A, Lambert PC et al. Diurnal blood pressure in assessment of preeclampsia. Obstetrics & Gynecology 1996;87:205-207

DNA banking

Synonyms
DNA storage

Use
provides purified genetic material that can be used for identification or future diagnostic testing

Method
release and isolate deoxyribonucleic acid (DNA) from white blood cells, tissue, or cultured cells by lysing cells and extracting cell lysate with phenol and chloroform; precipitate purified, intact DNA with salt in presence of alcohol; store indefinitely at 70 degrees C

Specimen
whole blood; tissue; cultured cells

Normal range
not applicable

Comments
none

Source
Lexi-Comp Inc. database. Hudson, OH.

 ## dobutamine-atropine stress echocardiography (DASE)

Synonyms
none

Indications
diagnostic test for detection of coronary heart disease

Method
graded dobutamine infusion given through peripheral arm vein in 3 minute stages; addition of atropine potentiates positive chronotropic and positive inotropic effects of dobutamine

Normal findings
segmental wall motion analysis scored as follows: 0-hyperkinesia, 1-normokinesia, 2-hypokinesia, 3-akinesia, and 4-dyskinesia

Comments
DASE analysis of digitized cineloops was done by computer; study demonstrated that patterns of changes in left ventricular dimensions and wall motion at peak stress are quite different from those observed during maximal exercise

Source
Adapted from Carstensen S, Samir MA, Stensgaard-Hansen FV et al. Does dobutamine simulate exercise in asymptomatic healthy individuals? Stress Echo Update 1996;6:2-6.

 ## docetaxel

Brand name
Taxotere

Use
semisynthetic antineoplastic analog of paclitaxel that has antitumor activity in patients with advanced ovarian, breast, and non-small-cell lung cancer

Usual dosage
intravenous: 100 mg/m² given as a 1 hr infusion every 3 weeks

Pharmaceutical company
Rhone-Poulenc Rorer Pharmaceutical, Inc. Collegeville, PA.

Source
University of Pittsburgh Drug Information and Pharmacoepidemiology Center. Pittsburgh, PA.

docusate sodium

Brand name
Colace Microenema

Use
enema formulation; facilitates rapid bowel evacuation for occasional constipation

Usual dosage
rectal: 5 ml (200 mg/5 ml) inserted into rectum

Pharmaceutical company
Roberts Pharmaceuticals. Eatontown, NJ.

Source
Stadtlanders Managed Pharmacy Services. Pittsburgh, PA.

 ## dofetilide

Brand name
Xelide

Use
antiarrhythmic agent used to terminate sustained atrial fibrillation or flutter

Usual dosage
intravenous: 4 or 8 µg/kg in clinical trials

Pharmaceutical company
Pfizer Laboratories Inc. New York, NY.

Source
Stadtlanders Managed Pharmacy Services. Pittsburgh, PA.

 ## dolasetron mesylate

Brand name
Anzemet

Use
antiemetic; for the treatment of chemotherapy-induced nausea and vomiting

Usual dosage
intravenous: single intravenous dose of 1.8-2.4 mg/kg over 15-20 minutes, beginning 30 minutes prior to chemotherapy

Pharmaceutical company
Hoechst Marion Roussel Pharmaceuticals Inc. Somerville, NJ.

Source
Stadtlanders Managed Pharmacy Services. Pittsburgh, PA.

Dolphin

Description
hysteroscopic fluid intravasation management system
Source
Adapted from Zoler ML. Device monitors fluid intravasation in hysteroscopy. Ob.Gyn. News 1996;31:21.

 domperidone

Brand Name
Motilium
Use
dopamine antagonist used for treating nausea, vomiting, and gastrointestinal disorders
Usual Dosage
oral: 10-30 µg three to four times daily
rectal: 30-60 µg two to four times daily
Pharmaceutical company
Janssen Pharmaceuticals. Titusville, NJ.
Source
University of Pittsburgh Drug Information and Pharmacoepidemiology Center. Pittsburgh, PA.

 donepezil

Brand name
Aricept
Use
treatment of mild to moderate symptoms of Alzheimer disease
Usual dosage
oral: 10 mg per day
Pharmaceutical company
Pfizer Laboratories Inc. New York, NY.
Source
Stadtlanders Managed Pharmacy Services. Pittsburgh, PA.

 Donnez endometrial ablation device

Description
expandable fiberoptic device using Nd-YAG laser; inserts transvaginally in collapsed position into the uterus, expands to triangular shape used for photocoagulation of endometrium for dysfunctional uterine bleeding
Source
Adapted from Donnez J, Polet R, Mathieu P, Konwitz E, Nisolle M, Casanas-Roux F. Endometrial laser interstitial hyperthermy: a potential modality for endometrial ablation. Obstetrics & Gynecology 1996;87:459-464.

D.O.R.C. (Dutch Ophthalmic Research Center) fast freeze cryosurgical system

Description
system operates on either nitrous oxide or carbon dioxide, non-electric, extremely fast freeze/defrost cycle

Source
Dutch Ophthalmic Research Center product information. Kingston, NJ.

D.O.R.C. (Dutch Ophthalmic Research Center) microforceps and microscissors

Description
pressure-sensitive handle design available in titanium, illuminated, subretinal, tapered, and standard models

Source
Dutch Ophthalmic Research Center product information. Kingston, NJ.

dorsal capsulotomy

Description
indications for entering the wrist through a dorsal approach include treatment of fracture, dislocation, ligament rupture, arthritic degeneration, synovectomy, arthrodesis and biopsy; exposure of the carpus through a dorsal approach will require a dorsal wrist capsulotomy; different techniques have limitations including poor tissue coaptation during closure; to avoid limitations, dorsal capsulotomies to the wrist via ligament-sparing, fiber-splitting incisions have been developed

Anatomy
antebrachial fascia; capitate, carpal, hamate, radial, trapezoid, and triquetral bones; capsule; cortex of triquetrum; cortices of scaphoid; carpometacarpal joint; horn of lunate; intercarpal, radiocarpal, lunotriquetral interosseous, radiocarpal and scaphol unate ligaments; Lister tubercle; palmar joint capsule; retinaculum; scaphoid-trapezium-trapezoid joint region; sigmoid notch of radius; extensor pollicis longus and extensor carpiulnaris tendons; triangular fibrocartilage; ulnar styloid process

Equipment
standard hand surgery equipment

Source
Adapted from Berger RA, Bishop AT, Bettinger PC. New dorsal capsulotomy for the surgical exposure of the wrist. Annals of Plastic Surgery 1995;35:54-58.

160

 dorzolamide

Brand name
Trusopt

Use
treatment of ocular hypertension in patients with open-angle glaucoma

Usual dosage
opthalmic: 1 drop into the affected eye three times daily

Pharmaceutical company
Merck. West Point, PA.

Source
University of Pittsburgh Drug Information and Pharmacoepidemiology Center. Pittsburgh, PA.

 Dostinex

Generic name
see cabergoline

 dothiepin

Brand Name
Prothiaden

Use
tricyclic antidepressant for use in depression and various psychotic disorders

Usual Dosage
oral: 75-300 mg/day or divided into three times a day
oral (geriatric): 50-75 mg/day

Pharmaceutical company
Boots Pharmaceuticals Inc. Lincolnshire, IL.

Source
University of Pittsburgh Drug Information and Pharmacoepidemiology Center. Pittsburgh, PA.

 Double Duty cane

Description
sturdy cane with advantage of reacher that extends grasp over three feet

Source
Sammons Preston Inc. product information. Bolingbrook, IL.

double-stapled ileoanal reservoir (DSIAR)

Description
method of operative treatment for ulcerative colitis and familial adenomatous polyposis (FAP) using an ileal pouch-anal anastomosis (first hand-sewn
and later stapled) without mucosal proctectomy leaving the entire anal canal
intact; it has been associated with improved functional outcome, attributed
to the minimal manipulation of anal sphincters, and to the preservation of
the anal transitional zone (ATZ) mucosa

Anatomy
anal canal; anal transitional zone; external sphincter; ileoanal muscle fibers;
internal sphincter muscle; internal anal sphincter; mucosa; rectal cuff

Equipment
standard colorectal surgery equipment

Source
Adapted from Reissman P, Piccirillo M, Ulrich A, Daniel N, Nogueras JJ, Wexner SD. Functional results of the
double-stapled ileoanal reservoir. Journal of American College of Surgeons 1995;181:444-448.

 ## double V-Y plasty with paired inverted Burow triangle excisions

Description
scar revision technique where a V-shaped flap with a wide angle is divided
and each arm is advanced in different directions at an angle of about 60
degrees; paired inverted Burow triangle excisions are used to facilitate
advancement of the flaps and to remove part of the scar

Anatomy
any area of the body that has been burned and needs scar revision

Equipment
standard scar revision equipment

Source
Adapted from Suzuki S, Matsuda K, Nishimura Y. Proposal for a new comprehensive classification of V-Y plasty
and its analogues: the pros and cons of inverted versus ordinary Burow triangle excision. Plastic and
Reconstructive Surgery 1996;98:1016-1022.

 ## Douek-Med ear device

Description
this bioglass middle ear device forms a physiochemical bond with bone and
soft tissue at the implant interface; enables surgeon to reconstruct any portion of the ossicle chain

Source
US Biomaterials Corp. product information. Baltimore, MD.

Dovetail stress broken abutment

Description
dental stress broken abutment; easy-to-cast, stress broken attachment with contoured edges; used when splinting rigid implant restorations to natural dentition

Source
Lifecore Biomedical product information. Chaska, MN.

Dovonex

Generic name
see calcipotriene

Doxil

Generic name
see liposomal doxorubicin

doxofylline

Brand name
Maxivent

Use
derivative of theophylline used in the treatment of asthma and bronchospasm

Usual dosage
oral: doses of 800 mg twice daily have been used in clinical trials; intravenous: 400 mg twice daily

Pharmaceutical company
Roberts Pharmaceutical Corporation. Eatontown, NJ.

Source
University of Pittsburgh Drug Information and Pharmacoepidemiology Center. Pittsburgh, PA.

Dozier radiolucent Bennett retractor

Description
hard plastic surgical instrument designed to be used in hip fractures; can be kept in place while using image intensification or taking x-rays; previously, Bennett retractors had been stainless steel

Source
Innomed Inc. product information. Savannah, GA.

Drake Uroflometer

Description
device for measuring rate of urine flow while obtaining a specimen for urinalysis; useful in determining presence of prostatic or vesical neck obstruction, neurologic bladder dysfunction, meatal stenosis, and stricture of urethra

Source
Grewe Plastics Medical Division product information. Newark, NJ.

 ## drug infusion sleeve

Description
infusion sleeve with proximal drug infusion port and four internal drug delivery tubes; infusion sleeve positioned over a standard balloon angioplasty catheter; after angioplasty, balloon is deflated and infusion sleeve moved forward; balloon reinflated and infusion sleeve inflates to hold position; multiple drugs delivered at angioplasty site to prevent closure or restenosis

Source
LocalMed Inc. product information. Palo Alto, CA.

 ## drug resistance gene transduction

Synonyms
drug resistance gene transfer

Use
during anti-cancer chemotherapy provides patient's benign cells with additional drug resistance

Method
selection of patient's benign marrow stem cells, retroviral-mediated gene transfer into the selected cells, and growth of the genetically-altered cells

Specimen
autologous benign bone marrow stem cells

Normal range
not applicable

Comments
may permit patient's own benign stem cells to survive therapy designed to be lethal to malignant cells

Source
Department of Laboratory Medicine and Pathology, University of Minnesota, Minneapolis, MN.

164

 DryTime for bladder control

Description

moisture sensing system detects first drops of urine, sounding an alarm so someone can tend to the situation immediately; also used as biofeedback device for retraining urinary system

Source

Health Sense International Inc. product information. Coos Bay, OR.

 DS-10 mobile dilator storage tray

Description

lightweight, stackable, protects 11 dilators

Source

EnCompAs Unlimited Inc. product information. Fort Lauderdale, FL.

 dual hinge external pin following mandibulectomy

Description

Marx technique modified by incorporating two hinges over the temporo-mandibular joint region; acts as controlling adjuncts for mandibular function after partial resection of the mandible including the condyle; accurate anatomic positioning can be accomplished following surgery; can be applied prior to surgery, easily disarticulated during surgery, and reassembled after resection

Anatomy

condyle; facial midline; mandible; proximal and distal mandibular segments; temporomandibular joint; zygoma; zygomatic arch

Equipment

two 3/4 inch (or wider) standard brass cabinet hinges joined with bolts, washers, and nuts; acrylic bars

Source

Adapted from Zide MF, Hicks RJ. A dual hinge external pin appliance for stability and function following partial mandibulectomy. Journal of Oral Maxillofacial Surgery 1996;54:236-237.

 DualMesh biomaterial

Description

surgical mesh with open microstructure that allows host tissue incorporation; closed microstructure of smooth surface minimizes tissue attachment; for hernia and soft tissue deficiencies

Source

W L Gore and Associates Inc. product information. Flagstaff, AZ.

dual-scope disinfector (DSD-91) endoscope disinfector

Description
disinfects endoscopes with a possibility of nine different protocols; double-rinses and alcohol purges available

Source
Medivators Inc. (*Editor note:* V is no longer capitalized in company name) product information. Cannon Falls, MN.

 Duckbill voice prosthesis

Description
used in the rehabilitation of patients post total laryngectomy; available in 16 and 20 French sizes; features a thin retention collar for ease of insertion; auxiliary airflow port available

Source
Bivona Medical Technologies product information. Gary, IN.

 Dura-II Concealable penile implant

Description
penile implant

Source
Osbon Medical Systems product information. Augusta, GA.

 Duract

Generic name
see bromfenac

 DURAglide stone removal balloon catheter

Description
tapered design for use with or without guidewire during biliary endoscopy; guaranteed balloon durability

Source
Bard International Products Division product information. Billerica, MA.

Durkan CTS gauge

Description

provides specific and reproducible amount of pressure on the carpal tunnel area for up to 30 seconds; reproduction of symptoms is a positive screening test for carpal tunnel syndrome (CTS)

Source

Gorge Medical product information. Hood River, OR.

Durrani needle

Description

dorsal vein complex ligation needle; flat handle design for simple passage of ligature between dorsal vein complex and urethra during radical prostatectomy

Source

Greenwald Surgical Company Inc. production information. Lake Station, NY.

Dynabac

Generic name

see dirithromycin

Dyna-Care pressure pad system

Description

alternating pressure pad system for beds; helps prevent pressure sores; as pressure is relieved intermittently, the body tolerates even larger pressures

Source

Grant Airmass Corp. product information. Stamford, CT.

DynaGraft bioimplant

Description

dental implant that demonstrates significant osteoinductivity and calcification; available in a variety of delivery formats to accommodate various surgical applications

Source

Biocoll Medical Corp. product information. Vancouver, British Columbia, Canada.

dynamic integrated stabilization chair (DISC)

Description

DISC design concept applies Biomechanical Ankle Platform System (BAPS) principles to back and trunk stabilization programs

Source

Spectrum Therapy Products product information. Jasper, MI.

EarCheck Pro

Description
instrument to detect middle ear effusion and acute otitis media using acoustic reflectometry; manufactured by MDI Instruments

Source
Food and Drug Administration Internet site.

 ## EarPlanes

Description
soft, silicone earplugs containing ceramic pressure regulator that slows the flow of air into and out of the ear canal, lessening the air pressure difference of the middle ear and helping the eustachian tubes to function more normally during air travel; over-the-counter adult and children sizes

Source
Internet www.fda.gov.

 ## EasyStep pressure relief walker

Description
three-layer plantar pad; helps eliminate direct pressure under an ulcer and reduces pressure and shear along the plantar surface of the foot

Source
Kendall Co. product information. Mansfield, MA.

 ## Eccovision acoustic reflection imaging system

Description
for in-office use in quantifying nasal patency; provides cross-sectional analysis of the nasal cavity by directing sound waves into the nares and analyzing the resulting echoes; applications include evaluating for nasal obstruction and congestion such as septal deviation, nasal valve stenosis, turbinate hypertrophy, or nasal polyps; assessing response to allergens and course of treatment including the efficacy of decongestants, and documenting the validity of rhinoplasty, septoplasty, or other nasal procedures

Source
Intercare Technologies Inc. product information. Milwaukee, WI.

 ## echogenic needle

Description
designed to eliminate reflection of excess sound during ultrasound

Source
Accurate Surgical and Scientific Instruments product information. Westbury, NY.

168

 ## Echosight Jansen-Anderson intrauterine catheter set

Description

malleable obturator, guiding catheter, and delivery catheter used for introduction of washed spermatozoa under ultrasound guidance; provides enhanced visualization of catheter

Source

Cook Urological Inc. product information. Spencer, IN.

 ## Echosight Patton coaxial catheter set

Description

gynecologic instrument used for transcervical introduction of washed spermatozoa; design is useful when negotiating a difficult cervix; polyethylene material provides enhanced visualization of catheter when used with ultrasound equipment

Source

Cook OB/GYN product information. Spencer, IN.

 ## Echotip Baker amniocentesis set

Description

needle cannula instrument used with Vacutainer tubes for aspiration of fluid from the amniotic sac; needle design provides enhanced visualization of the needle tip when used with ultrasonic imaging

Source

Cook Urological Inc. product information. Spencer, IN.

 ## Echotip Dominion needle set

Description

surgical instrument set includes stylet, needle cannula, aspiration/extension tubes, and irrigation tube; needle design provides enhanced visualization of needle tip when used with ultrasonic imaging equipment

Source

Cook OB/GYN product information. Spencer, IN.

 ## Echotip Kato-Asch needle set

Description

coaxial surgical instruments; includes needle guide and inner needle; needle guide is used to establish a tract while the inner needle is used through the needle guide; design of each provides enhanced visualization of needle tip when used with ultrasonic imaging equipment

Source

Cook OB/GYN product information. Spencer, IN.

Eckardt Hem-Stopper instrument

Description
ophthalmic surgical instrument for controlling retinal hemorrhages during vitreoretinal surgery

Source
Dutch Ophthalmic product information. Kingston, NH.

 ## EdgeAhead microsurgical knives

Description
crescent, circular, and slit knives for ophthalmologic surgery

Source
Visitec product information. Sarasota, FL.

 ## EDGE blade

Description
coated electrosurgical blade can be wiped clean on sponge or 4x4 gauze; can be bent up to 90 degrees to facilitate access to surgical site (Editor note: also known as The Edge and The Edge Blade)

Source
Valleylab Inc. product information. Boulder, CO.

 ## Edge dilatation catheter

Description
ACS (Advanced Cardiovascular Systems) over-the-wire catheter with low-friction tapered tip, transitionless tapered shaft, and PE-600 balloon material

Source
Guidant Corp. product information. Santa Clara, CA.

 ## edobacomab

Brand Name
XXMEN-0E5

Use
murine monoclonal antibody (Mab), antiendotoxin used in the treatment of Gram-negative sepsis

Usual Dosage
intravenous: 2 mg/kg infused over one hour

Pharmaceutical company
Pfizer Labs Inc. New York, NY.

Source
University of Pittsburgh Drug Information and Pharmacoepidemiology Center. Pittsburgh, PA.

Edwards/Barbaro syringo-peritoneal shunt

Description
shunt device provides continuous drainage of fluid from within a spinal cord
cyst to a site outside spinal canal; shunt includes step-down connector, peritoneal catheter, and Foltz flat-bottom reservoir

Source
Heyer-Schulte NeuroCare product information. Pleasant Prairie, WI.

 Effexor

Generic name
see venlafaxine

 EJ bone marrow biopsy needle

Description
EJ (ergonomically designed Jamshidi) biopsy needle with tapered distal cannula tip; helps hold biopsy specimen during needle removal; unique probe
guide promotes safe removal of specimen for examination

Source
Baxter Healthcare Corp. product information. Waukegan, IL.

 Eklund breast positioning system

Description
aids in positioning the breast for optimal imaging on mammography; reduces
patient discomfort

Source
Instrumentarium Imaging product information. Milwaukee, WI.

 ElastaTrac home lumbar traction unit

Description
allows convenience of patient-controlled management of lumbar pain; adapted for use on bed, treatment table, or floor

Source
Thera-Products Inc. product information. San Jose, CA.

elective lymph node dissection

Description
ELND/lymphadenectomy improves control of regional metastases of malignant melanoma (removes microscopic metastases) with more accurate staging; determine sentinel lymph node (first to show metastasis) by preoperative lymphoscintigraphy or intraoperative lymphatic mapping; mark location of sentinel node with a permanent intradermal tattoo; excise sentinel node and all other lymph nodes from surrounding nodal basins

Anatomy
lymph node; regional lymph nodal basin; sentinel lymph node; non-sentinel lymph node

Equipment
standard surgery equipment; Lymphazurin 1% (radiopaque blue dye)

Source
Adapted from Godellas CV, Berman CG, Lyman G, et al. The identification and mapping of melanoma regional nodal metastases: minimally invasive surgery for the diagnosis of nodal metastases. The American Surgeon 1995;61:97-101.

 Electro-Mesh electrode

Description
fabric socks, gloves, sleeves, and wraps knitted from silver, nylon, and dacron; electrode envelops body part to provide electrotherapy; decreases postoperative pain and disuse atrophy; increases blood circulation

Source
Prizm Medical Inc. product information. Norcross, GA.

 electronic crossmatch

Synonyms
computerized crossmatch

Use
detection of ABO blood group incompatibility prior to transfusion

Method
validated computer system used in place of traditional serologic crossmatch to compare results of blood donor and recipient testing

Specimen
previous blood test results

Normal range
crossmatch compatible

Comments
previous blood test results must meet certain conditions

Source
University of Minnesota Department of Laboratory Medicine and Pathology. Minneapolis, MN.

Elite System rotating resectoscope

Description

rotating continuous flow surgical instrument; working element and telescope rotate within the sheaths; urethral irritation reduced with stationary sheaths; flow ports remain in original position

Source

Circon ACMI product information. Stamford, CT.

 ## Ellipse compact spacer

Description

metered-dose inhaler used in respiratory therapy; clear chamber helps patient identify foreign objects that might otherwise be inhaled; compatible with a variety of respiratory metered-dose inhalers

Source

Allen & Hanburys, Division of Glaxo Inc. product information. Research Triangle Park, NC.

 ## Elmiron

Generic Name

see pentostan polysulfate sodium

 ## Emdogain

Description

amelogenin-based gel used to promote regrowth of tooth-supporting tissue during periodontal flap surgery

Source

Biora Inc. product information. Chicago, IL.

 ## Emitasol

Generic name

see metoclopramide

 ## Enable

Generic name

see tenidap

enalapril maleate/felodipine ER

Brand name
Lexxel

Use
combination of ACE inhibitor and calcium channel blocker for the treatment of hypertension

Usual dosage
oral: doses of 5 mg enalapril and 5 mg felodipine were used in clinical trials

Pharmaceutical company
Astra Merck. Wayne, PA.

Source
Stadtlanders Managed Pharmacy Services. Pittsburgh, PA.

 ## Enbrel

Generic name
see recombinant human tumor necrosis factor receptor fixed chain fusion protein (rhTNFR:Fc)

 ## encapsulated islet cell injection

Description
treatment for type 1 diabetes; transplantation of islets of Langerhans to produce insulin endogenously; encapsulated cells injected into peritoneal cavity through midline incision; encapsulation protects cells from body's immune system and negates need for immunosuppressant drugs; candidates are patients currently awaiting pancreas transplantation

Anatomy
abdominal wall; peritoneal cavity; islets of Langerhans

Equipment
standard surgery equipment

Source
Adapted from Soon-Shiong P, Sandford PA. Encapsulated islet cell therapy for the treatment of diabetes: intraperitoneal injection of islets. Surgical Technology International IV 1995:93-99.

 ## Encapsulon epidural catheter

Description
shear-resistant regional anesthesia catheter devices; incorporate radiopaque stripes within the shaft, leaving clear windows to see fluid flow; available in bullet and open tips; Encapsulon specialty epidural needles are also available

Source
Rusch Inc. product information. Duluth, GA.

Endermologie adipose destruction system

Description

device to reduce the appearance of cellulite noninvasively with motorized rollers and aspiration technique that unclogs and disorganizes adipose tissue over course of weekly sessions, gradually reaching deeper layers of tissue; once a month sessions recommended after completion of sessions for maintenance

Source

LPG USA product information. Fort Lauderdale, FL.

 ## Endocell endometrial cell sampler

Description

device for collecting endometrial cells and/or fluids with no loss or contamination; narrow diameter eliminates dilation of cervix in most cases

Source

Wallach Surgical Devices Inc. product information. Milford, CT.

 ## EndoDynamics glutameter

Description

meter that measures the glutaraldehyde levels in endoscopy and other instrument-cleaning areas; vapors in and near cleaning sites are vacuum-drawn into the instrument by pressing a button

Source

E-Z-EM Inc. product information. Westbury, NY.

 ## EndoLive endoscope

Description

endoscopic stereo instrument; three-dimensional video provides crystal clear and flicker-free images that facilitate procedures traditionally done in flat images

Source

Carl Zeiss Inc. product information. Thornwood, NY.

 ## endometrial laser ablation

Description

treatment of dysfunctional uterine bleeding; endometrium progressively ablated with laser energy monitored by video

Anatomy

uterine cavity; vagina

Equipment
standard laser surgery equipment; Weck-Baggish hysteroscope; CL 100 Nd-YAG laser; Hamou-Hysteromat continuous flow pressure-controlled irrigation system; urinary catheter; central venous line

Source
Adapted from Garry R, Shelley-Jones D, Mooney P, Phillips G. Six hundred endometrial laser ablations. Obstetrics & Gynecology 1995;85:24-29.

 endopancreatic brush cytology

Synonyms
none

Indications
pancreatic stricture; biliary stricture; used to diagnose pancreatic carcinoma

Method
endoscopic retrograde cholangiopancreatography (ERCP) is performed; cholangiograms and pancreatograms and spot films are obtained; a hydrophilic wire is advanced beyond the stricture to the tip of cannula; the cannula is exchanged with a sheath; a pancreatic cytology brush, Wilson-Cook model GRCH-6-220 or GRCH 320, is then advanced to the tip of the sheath; the sheath is withdrawn and multiple brushings are done

Normal findings
not applicable

Comments
the yield of endopancreatic brush cytology is related to the location of the malignancy, with overall yield enhanced by concurrent brushing of bile duct strictures; extremely valuable in planning appropriate therapy and for avoiding additional procedures for tissue diagnosis

Source
Adapted from McGuire DE, Venu RP, Brown RD, Etzkorn KP, Glaws WR, Abu-Hammour A. Brush cytology for pancreatic carcinoma: an analysis of factors influencing results. Gastrointestinal Endoscopy 1996;44:300-304.

 Endopath EZ35 endoscopic linear cutter

Description
stapler for endoscopic procedures

Source
Johnson & Johnson Medical Inc. product information. Arlington, TX.

 Endopath Optiview obturator

Description
optical surgical instrument that allows for visually guided trocar entry; optical lens allows for direct visualization of each tissue layer and possible vessel structures

Source
Ethicon Endo-Surgery Inc. product information. Cincinnati, OH.

Endopath Stealth stapler

Description

circular stapler providing a large lumen; 17%-35% larger diameter than other circular staplers; may help reduce postoperative stenosis

Source

Ethicon Endo-Surgery Inc. product information. Cincinnati, OH.

 Endopore dental implant system

Description

dental implant consisting of titanium alloy beads sintered together to form 3-dimensional latticework that affords 3-dimensional osseointegration

Source

Innova Corp. product information. Toronto, Ontario, Canada.

 endoscope-assisted craniotomy

Description

combination approach to deep brain structures using operating microscope and solid-rod lens endoscope; addition of endoscope allows visualization of structures not otherwise seen; endoscope brings the viewing lens into the center of the operative field and expands the field of vision; use of angled lenses can enlarge field further

Anatomy

brain stem; scalp; optic nerve; carotid artery; opticocarotid triangle; interpeduncular cistern; basilar artery; midbasilar artery; midbrain; pons

Equipment

standard microsurgery and endoscopic equipment; Storz 4-mm diameter solid-rod telescope lens; microchip camera; television monitor; automatic retractors

Source

Adapted from Cohen AR, Perneczky A, Rodziewicz GS, Gingold SI. Endoscope-assisted craniotomy: approach to the rostral brain stem. Neurosurgery 1995;36:1128-1130.

 endoscopic bipolar electrocoagulation and heater probe treatment

Description

endoscopic coagulation of radiation telangiectasia by applying light pressure directly on the telangiectasia and coagulating with low power; control of severe hematochezia due to irradiation treatment of pelvic tumors

Anatomy

colon; rectum; rectosigmoid area

Equipment
flexible sigmoidoscope; Gold probe (bipolar electrocoagulation); heater probe

Source
Adapted from Jensen DM, Machicado GA, Cheng S, Jensen ME, Jutabha R. A randomized study of endoscopic bipolar electrocoagulation and heater probe treatment of chronic rectal bleeding from radiation telangiectasia. Gastrointestinal Endoscopy 1997;45:20-25.

 ## endoscopic forehead-brow rhytidoplasty

Description
forehead-brow rhytidoplasty has evolved from procedure primarily advocated for brow ptosis; surgical results stem from wide undermining and concomitant alteration of forehead muscles; introduction of endoscopically assisted techniques to plastic surgery reduces need for long incisions; unique anatomy of upper face results in different deformities than in lower face providing basis for endoscopically assisted surgery

Anatomy
adipose tissue; cranium; canthus; foramen; glabella; depressor musculature: corrugator supercilii/medial head-approximator, lateral head-depressor; procerus; orbicularis oris; elevator musculature: frontalis muscle; supraorbital and supratrochlear nerves; orbital rim; periosteum; septum; subgaleal plane; temporal and temporoparietal fascia

Equipment
standard surgery equipment for "open" techniques; down-angled and retractor-mounted endoscopes; fibrin glue; standard television, high-resolution video equipment and xenon light source; blunt and sharp periosteal elevators; bolsters; percutaneous screw fixation; retractor; slit knife; angled scissors; punches; insulated electrocoagulating graspers; Takahashi biopsy forceps

Source
Adapted from Matarasso A. Endoscopically assisted forehead-brow rhytidoplasty. Aesthetic Plastic Surgery 1995;19:141-147.

 ## endoscopic intracorporeal laser lithotripsy

Description
endoscopic retrograde intracorporeal lithotripsy with a stone recognition laser system for treatment of difficult bile stones

Anatomy
ampulla of Vater; papilla

Equipment
Lithognost automatic stone recognition laser system; rhodamine 6G dye laser; URF P2 Olympus ultrathin cholangioscope; Rigiflex extractor

Source
Adapted from Schreiber F, Gurakuqi G, Trauner M. Endoscopic intracorporeal laser lithotripsy of difficult common bile duct stones with a stone-recognition pulsed dye laser system. Gastrointestinal Endoscopy 1995;42(5):416-419.

endoscopic intranasal frontal sinusotomy

Description
traditional methods are ablation of frontal sinus, or frontal sinus and frontal outflow tract (FOT) preservation and/or reconstruction; endoscopic intranasal frontal sinusotomy has developed to such a degree that it has become procedure of choice in many centers for management of frontal sinus disease; develops a wide and patent frontonasal communication to prevent recurrent obstruction; provides optimal conditions for reepithelialization of both FOT and sinus endoscopic intranasal frontal sinusotomy (continued)

Anatomy
agger nasi cells; anterior ethmoid artery; cranial fossa; dome of ethmoid complex; ethmoid, frontal, maxillary, and sphenoid sinuses; frontal outflow tract; frontal sinus compartment; infundibulum; mucosa; "nasofrontal beak"; nasal septum; turbinate; uncinate process

Equipment
standard endoscopic surgery equipment; curettes; endotracheal tube; Kerrison rongeur (delicate hypophysectomy type); ostium probe (ostium seeker); curved blunt suction tip; stent; drill; 30-degree and 70-degree telescopes

Source
Adapted from Har-el G, Lucente FE. Endoscopic intranasal frontal sinusotomy. The Laryngoscope 1995;105:440-442.

 ## endoscopic nasogastric-jejunal feeding tube placement

Description
placement of nasogastric-jejunal feeding tubes at the bedside using endoscopy alone without fluoroscopic guidance

Anatomy
nares; mid-esophagus; esophagus; stomach; pylorus; small bowel; duodenum

Equipment
endoscope; Stayput 18F nasogastric-9F jejunal feeding tube; 0.035-inch guidewire; catheter tip syringe

Source
Adapted from Patrick PG, Marulendra S, Kirby DF, DeLegge MH. Endoscopic nasogastric-jejunal feeding tube placement in critically ill patients. Gastrointestinal Endoscopy 1997;45:72-76.

 ## endoscopic resection of duodenal carcinoid tumor

Description
carcinoid tumor is unique neoplasm, being neither completely malignant nor completely benign; described as a malignant neoplasm in slow motion; relatively rare with most cases treated by surgical resection; endoscopic resection by strip biopsy technique with hypertonic solution and epinephrine injection accomplished after endosonographic visualization

Anatomy

duodenum; inferior wall of duodenal bulb; muscularis propria; submucosal layer; submucosal space

Equipment

standard endoscopic surgery equipment; needle forceps; wide-mouthed forceps; semicircular snare; two-channel endoscope; electrosurgical unit with blended current

Source

Adapted from Yoshikane H, Suzuki T, Yoshioka N, Ogawa Y, Hamajima E, Hasegawa N, Hasegawa C. Duodenal carcinoid tumor: endosonographic imaging and endoscopic resection. The American Journal of Gastroenterology 1995;90:642-643.

 endoscopic transrectal drainage of pelvic abscess

Description

endoscopic drainage of a sigmoid diverticular abscess using the transrectal approach

Anatomy

sigmoid colon; rectal wall

Equipment

flexible sigmoidoscope; therapeutic duodenoscope; endoscopic aspiration needle catheter; 10F biliary stent pusher tube; 0.018-inch biliary guidewire; 3F biliary catheter; 0.021-inch guidewire; 5F biliary catheter; 0.035-inch guidewire; 6F biliary stent inner guiding catheter; 10F pigtail nasobiliary tube

Source

Adapted from Baron TH, Morgan DE. Endoscopic transrectal drainage of a diverticular abscess. Gastrointestinal Endoscopy 1997;45:84-87.

 endoscopic ultrasonography

Synonyms

EUS

Indications

aids in diagnosis of gastrointestinal disease

Method

visualizes surface of lesion; provides detailed information about internal structure and peripheral regions

Normal findings

not applicable

Comments

lesions not typically identified by computerized tomography (CT) or magnetic resonance imaging (MRI); useful for diagnosis of esophageal varices

Source

Adapted from Iwase H, Suga S, Morise K et al. Color Doppler endoscopic ultrasonography for the evaluation of gastric varices and endoscopic obliteration with cyanoacrylate glue. Gastrointestinal Endoscopy 1995;41:150-153.

180

 endoscopic ultrasound-assisted band ligation

Description
technique for resection of submucosal tumors (SMTs); technique may be useful for tissue diagnosis of large or infiltrating submucosal lesions and in some cases complete removal of small SMTs

Anatomy
stomach; lesser curvature of duodenum; duodenum

Equipment
a large friction-fit adaptor from a Stiegmann-Goff Endoscopic Ligator kit; standard endoscopy equipment

Source
Adapted from Chang KJ, Yoshinaka R, Nguyen P. Endoscopic ultrasound-assisted band ligation: a new technique for resection of submucosal tumors. Gastrointestinal Endoscopy 1996;44(6):720-722.

 endoscopic ultrasound-directed pancreatography

Synonyms
none

Indications
to obtain pancreatography in a patient whose altered surgical anatomy prevented a complete pancreatogram from being obtained with an ERCP

Method
endoscopic ultrasonography (EUS) was performed with the radial scanning instrument Olympus EUS-20 to evaluate the pancreas and pancreatic duct; a push enteroscopy was performed with an Olympus PCF-20 pediatric colonoscope to inject dye to evaluate for obstruction; a 22-gauge needle inserted under the guidance of linear array instrument, Pentax FG32UA under real-time EUS; contrast material injected

Normal findings
not applicable

Comments
pancreatography is an important diagnostic tool in the evaluation of pancreatic diseases

Source
Adapted from Gress F, Ikenberry S, Sherman S, Lehman G. Endoscopic ultrasound-directed pancreatography. Gastrointestinal Endoscopy 1996;44(6):736-739.

EndoSheath endoscopy system

Description
surgical instruments specially designed for endoscopy with a separate, disposable sheath that contains all air, water, and suction channels; scope remains protected from patient to patient

Source
Vision Sciences Inc. product information. Natick, MA.

 # EndoShield Mask

Description
surgical mask that is lightweight and able to be worn over most prescription eyeware

Source
E-Z-EM Inc. product information. Westbury, NY.

 # endosonography-guided fine-needle aspiration (FNA) biopsy with flow cytometry

Synonyms
none

Indications
staging of non-Hodgkin gastric lymphoma

Method
endoscopic ultrasonography (EUS) was performed with the Olympus EUS-20 instrument; FNA biopsy of the cluster of lymph nodes was performed with the Pentax FG-32UA ultrasound endoscope; under EUS visualization, a 23-gauge 4-cm needle with a full-length stylet was used to obtain cytologic material

Normal findings
not applicable

Comments
flow cytometry is able to confirm nodal involvement that was not apparent from EUS findings and standard cytologic examination

Source
Adapted from Wiersema MJ, Gatzimos K, Nisi R, Wiersema LM. Staging of non-Hodgkin gastric lymphoma with endosonography-guided fine-needle aspiration biopsy with flow cytometry. Gastrointestinal Endoscopy 1996;44(6):734-736.

endosseous dental implant placement for replacement of missing teeth

Description
performed in two stages: during first stage implant is placed into maxilla or mandible and submerged beneath oral mucosa until osseointegration has been achieved; during second stage implant is uncovered and there is placement of a healing abutment that remains supragingival or nonsubmerged

Anatomy
maxilla; mandible; oral mucosa

Equipment
IMZ implants

Source
Adapted from Barber HD, Seckinger RJ, Silverstein K, et al. Comparison of soft tissue healing and osseointegration of IMZ implants placed in one-stage and two-stage techniques: a pilot study. Implant Dentistry 1996;5:11-14.

 Endo Stitch instrument

Description
laparoscopic suturing instrument used to perform sacrospinous ligament colpopexy

Source
United States Surgical Corp. product information. Norwalk, CT.

 Endotrac system for carpal tunnel release

Description
surgical instruments include obturator, cannula, rasp, probe, elevator, retractors, and blade handle; can be used in any two-portal
technique for endoscopic carpal tunnel surgery

Source
Instratek Inc. product information. Houston, TX.

 EndoView

Description
palm-size camera and swivel head monitor that provides high resolution liquid crystal display on a 3-4 inch screen; gives physician wider, clearer view of operative field

Source
UROHEALTH Systems Inc. product information. Costa Mesa, CA.

Energy Plus shoe insert

Description
orthotic device fits into dress shoes and/or shoes and boots with 1-inch heels; provides posture support

Source
Foot Levelers Inc. product information. Roanoke, VA.

enprostil

Brand Name
Gardrin

Use
synthetic prostaglandin E2 used to suppress gastric secretions in peptic ulcer disease

Usual Dosage
oral: 35 µg twice daily

Pharmaceutical company
Syntex Laboratories Inc. Palo Alto, CA.

Source
University of Pittsburgh Drug Information and Pharmacoepidemiology Center. Pittsburgh, PA.

entacapone

Brand name
Comtan

Use
treatment of Parkinson disease in combination with levodopa

Usual dosage
oral: 200 mg taken 4-10 times daily in combination with levodopa in clinical trials

Pharmaceutical company
Novartis. East Hanover, NJ.

Source
Stadtlanders Managed Pharmacy Services. Pittsburgh, PA.

Entos vascular and abdominal intraoperative scanheads

Description
intraoperative ultrasound to help detect, locate, and characterize lesions, guide surgical interventions, and assess procedures prior to closure

Source
ATL Ultrasound product information. Bothell, WA.

Entrease variable depth punch

Description
surgical instrument that makes a controlled depth stab wound for insertion of cannulas; 3 mm-4.5 mm-6 mm stepped punch allows insertion of wound drains without air leakage

Source
Byron Medical product information. (*Editor note:* advertising uses byron but company name correctly is Byron) Tucson, AZ.

EntriStar feeding tube

Description
percutaneous endoscopic gastrostomy (PEG) polyurethane tube with large inner diameter improving flow dynamics; internal bolster design reduces patient and stomal trauma when PEG is removed

Source
Sherwood Medical product information. St. Louis, MO.

Epaq

Generic name
see albuterol sulfate

EPIC functional evaluation system

Description
devices for testing injured clients based on research of Employment Potential Improvement Corporation (EPIC); tests performed: EPIC 1, lift capacity; EPIC 2, motor coordination; EPIC 3, finger and hand dexterity; EPIC 4, range of motion; EPIC 5, balance, carry, and climb

Source
Fred Sammons Inc. product information. Western Springs, IL.

epidermal growth factor receptor detection

Synonyms
tissue growth factor receptor detection

Use
prognostic indicator for breast cancer

Method
enzyme immunoassay (EIA)

Specimen
solid tumor, confirmed as cancer by histologic examination

Normal range
investigational use

Comments
performance characteristics have not been established

Source
Lexi-Comp Inc. database. Hudson. OH.

 EpiLaser system

Description
treats range of cosmetic dermatologic conditions; removal of benign cutaneous pigment located in epidermis or dermis; treatment of facial telangiectasia and other cutaneous vascular lesions; skin resurfacing

Source
Palomar Medical Technologies product information. Lexington, MA.

 epiretinal delamination diamond knife

Description
a one-piece, gem-quality diamond blade with an exquisitely sharp cutting edge

Source
Synergetics Inc. product information. Chesterfield, MO.

 epirubicin

Brand name
Pharmorubicin

Use
anthracycline chemotherapeutic agent being studied for the treatment of solid tumors and breast cancer

Usual dosage
intravenous: international studies have used doses of 50 to 120 mg/m^2 alone or in combination with other agents

Pharmaceutical company
Adria Laboratories. Columbus, OH.

Source
University of Pittsburgh Drug Information and Pharmacoepidemiology Center. Pittsburgh, PA.

 Epitome scalpel

Description
blade-style electrode; technology that focuses the electrosurgical current precisely at the edge of the blade

Source
Utah Medical Products Inc. product information. Midvale, UT.

epoprostenol sodium

Brand name
Flolan

Use
prostacyclin that can be used as long-term treatment of primary pulmonary hypertension; has been used in place of heparin in patients requiring hemodialysis; congestive heart failure; septic shock; fulminant hepatic failure; to prevent platelet aggregation and restenosis following percutaneous transluminal coronary angioplasty (PTCA)

Usual dosage
intravenous: 2 to 4 ng/kg/min; maximum tolerated dose 7 ng/kg/min

Pharmaceutical company
Burroughs Wellcome Co. Research Triangle Park, NC.

Source
University of Pittsburgh Drug Information and Pharmacoepidemiology Center. Pittsburgh, PA.

 eprosartan

Brand name
Teveten

Use
angiotensin II receptor antagonist for the treatment of hypertension

Usual dosage
oral: 200 mg twice daily

Pharmaceutical company
SmithKline Beecham. Philadelphia, PA.

Source
Stadtlanders Managed Pharmacy Services. Pittsburgh, PA.

 eptifibatide

Brand name
Integrilin

Use
platelet aggregation blocking agent used to prevent abrupt closure after coronary angioplasty, coronary stents, and in acute coronary syndromes (editor note: Notice there is only one letter difference between the generic, integrelin, and the brand name, Integrilin.)

Usual dosage
intravenous: 135 µg/kg bolus, then infusion of 0.75 µg/kg/min

Pharmaceutical company
COR Therapeutics. South San Francisco, CA.

Source
Stadtlanders Managed Pharmacy Services. Pittsburgh, PA.

Ergoflex Premiere back support

Description
offers lumbar support and flexibility for reaching, bending, and/or lifting

Source
Lab Safety Supply product information. Janesville, WI.

 ## Ergoset

Generic name
see bromocriptine

 ## ER-MP12 stem cell marker

Synonyms
ER-MP12 stem cell positive selection

Use
isolation of blood-forming stem cells in bone marrow

Method
immunologic isolation of cells expressing the surface antigen recognized by ER-MP12 antibody

Specimen
murine bone marrow

Normal range
not applicable

Comments
investigational, but likely to be frequently discussed and referenced

Source
Experimental Hematology 1995;23:1002-1010.

 ## Ernest nucleus cracker

Description
ophthalmic surgical instrument designed for use through phaco incisions as small as 2.5 mm; cross-action mechanism opens the jaws wide enough to crack the lens nucleus without gaping the incision

Source
Katena Products Inc. product information. Denville, NJ.

EsophaCoil stent

Description
self-expanding esophageal stent; unique tight coil design helps resist tumor ingrowth; designed to minimize dysphagia, and help restore swallowing and nutritional intake for patients with malignant strictures

Source
InStent Inc. product information. Eden Prairie, MN.

 esophageal detection device (EDD)

Description
self-inflating bulb syringe esophageal detector device for assessing tracheal intubation; 1-way flow away from patient prevents risk of inflating the esophagus

Source
ARC Medical Inc. product information. Scottdale, GA.

 esophagojejunostomy, modified stapling technique

Description
modified stapling technique can minimize risk of anastomotic stricture and dysphagia after esophagojejunostomy; esophageal wall dissected into the mucosal, submucosal, and seromuscular layers; stapler fired between esophageal mucosal layer and complete jejunal layer; complete resection of the two "doughnuts" (i.e., the resected tissue between the esophageal mucosal layer and the jejunal wall) was ensured

Anatomy
diaphragm; esophagus; esophageal lumen; esophageal wall; jejunum; jejunal mucosal layer; mucosal, submucosal, and seromuscular layers

Equipment
standard surgical equipment; Premium circular end-to-end anastomosis mechanical stapling device; polypropylene suture

Source
Adapted from Matsushita M, Sugiyama A, Saito H, et al. A modified stapling technique for esophagojejunostomy after total or proximal gastrectomy. Journal of American College of Surgeons 1997;184:513-517.

Espocan combined spinal/epidural needle

Description
surgical needle with an extra lumen in its heel that allows the spinal needle to pass straight through but is too small for passage of epidural catheter; the epidural catheter, when inserted, will be directed away from the dural puncture site

Source
B Braun Medical Inc. product information. Bethlehem, PA.

 ## estradiol

Brand name
Estring

Use
extended release product for treatment of urogenital complications due to estrogen deficiency in postmenopausal women

Usual dosage
ring insert containing a total dosage of 2 mg of estradiol; inserted ring delivers approximately 8 µg/24 hrs for 3 months

Pharmaceutical company
Pharmacia Inc. Columbus, OH.

Source
University of Pittsburgh Drug Information and Pharmacoepidemiology Center. Pittsburgh, PA.

 ## estradiol (patch)

Brand name
Climara

Use
estrogen replacement to be used for moderate-to-severe vasomotor symptoms associated with menopause, vulval and vaginal atrophy, hypoestrogenism, and abnormal uterine bleeding

Usual dosage
12.5 cm^2 or 25 cm^2 transdermal patch; initial dosing recommendation is to apply the 12.5 cm^2 patch once weekly

Pharmaceutical company
Berlex Laboratories. Wayne, NJ.

Source
University of Pittsburgh Drug Information and Pharmacoepidemiology Center. Pittsburgh, PA.

Estring

Generic name
see estradiol

 estrogen receptor immunocytochemistry assay

Synonyms
ER by ICA

Indications
aids in predicting endocrine response in breast cancer patients

Method
frozen tumor tissue or formalin fixed; paraffin embedded tumor tissue is processed with immunoglobulin G1 monoclonal antibody ER1D5; immunoreactivity is detected by the streptavidin-biotin technique

Normal findings
not applicable

Comments
good diagnostic test for tumors less than 1 cm in diameter

Source
Adapted from Pertschuk LP, Feldman JG, Kim YD et al. Estrogen receptor immunocytochemistry in paraffin embedded tissues with ER1D5 predicts breast cancer endocrine response more accurately than H222Spy in frozen sections or cytosol-based ligand-binding assays. Cancer 1996;77:2514-2519.

 Estrostep

Generic name
see norethindrone acetate and ethinyl estradiol

 Ethalloy needle

Description
needle made from a patented alloy specifically developed for peripheral and cardiovascular surgery; resistant to bending

Source
Ethicon Inc. product information. Piscataway, NJ.

 Ethiguard needle

Description
blunt curved suture needle helps reduce HIV transmission

Source
Ethicon/Johnson & Johnson product information. Cincinnati, OH.

Ethyol

Generic name
see amifostine

 Etopophos

Generic name
see etoposide phosphate

 etoposide phosphate

Brand name
Etopophos
Use
treatment of small-cell lung cancer, first-line, and refractory testicular tumors
Usual dosage
injectable: 50-100 mg/m^2/day on days 1 to 5 or up to 100 mg/m^2/day on days 1, 3, and 5 by intravenous infusion for testicular cancer and 35 mg/m^2/day for 4 days or 50 mg/m^2/day for 5 days by intravenous infusion for small-cell cancer
Pharmaceutical company
Bristol-Myers Squibb U.S. Pharmaceuticals. Princeton, NJ.
Source
Stadtlanders Managed Pharmacy Services. Pittsburgh, PA.

 EVAP roller electrode

Description
instrument for use in transurethral resection of the prostate (TURP), uses electrode vaporization to remove tissue over a wider deeper area than cutting loop
Source
Richard Wolf Medical Instruments Corp. product information. Vernon Hills, IL.

 Eve reconstructive procedure

Description
transfer of vascularized rib, fascia, cartilage, and serratus muscle to correct severe hand or facial defects due to trauma; procedure name refers to biblical character Eve created from seventh rib of Adam
Anatomy
seventh rib; costochondral junction; serratus muscle; thoracicus longus nerve; latissimus dorsi muscle; intercostal muscle; neurovascular bundle

Equipment
standard surgery equipment

Source
Adapted from Guelinckx PG, Sinsel NK. The Eve procedure: the transfer of vascularized seventh rib, fascia, cartilage, and serratus muscle to reconstruct difficult defects. Plastic and Reconstructive Surgery 1996;97:527-535.

 ## Evista

Generic name
see raloxifene

 ## Excegran

Generic name
see zonisamide

 ## eXcel DR (disposable/reusable) Glasser laparoscopic needle

Description
device that consists of a reusable needle handle, and disposable suture needle; the "French eye" type needle permits easy threading and suture capture within the abdominal cavity

Source
Advanced Surgical Inc. product information. Princeton, NJ.

 ## Exerball kit

Description
exercise ball fitness package complete with exercise ball and workout video for use in the clinic or at home; 65-cm or 85-cm exercise ball exercises for strengthening the lower back, chest, and arms; to form and tone buttocks, thighs, and abdominals; increases endurance through interval training and innovative Swiss Ball-Aerobix; improves flexibility, balance, coordination, proprioception, and neuromotor learning

Source
OPTP product information. Minneapolis, MN.

 ## eXit puncture closure device

Description
disposable surgical instrument features a "J" shaped suture placement needle which minimizes risk of injury; may be exchanged with the cannula to permit placement of suture with minimal loss of pneumoperitoneum

Source
Advanced Surgical Inc. product information. Princeton, NJ.

Exprin DQI

Description
semiflexible shave biopsy instrument

Source
Exprin LLC product information. Madison, WI.

 extended lateral arm free flap (ELAFF) for head/neck reconstruction

Description
the lateral arm free flap (LAFF) has been used for fasciocutaneous free flap of choice; advantages have been suggested to include its consistent vascular anatomy, its pliable nature, reinnervation capabilities, low donor site morbidity, and ease of closure; ELAFF has also been performed; flap should have large vessels that allow easy anastomosis; sensory cutaneous nerve should be available for reinnervation; vascular pedicle should reach recipient vessels; donor site in location that allows for simultaneous harvesting while ablative surgery is performed

Anatomy
ascending and descending branches of posterior collateral artery; biceps and brachialis muscles; cephalic vein; epicondyle; fascia; intermuscular septum; muscle "bellies"; periosteum; profunda brachii artery; sensory cutaneous nerve; spiral groove of humerus; triceps muscle; venae comitantes vessels; vessel loop; vascular pedicle

Equipment
standard head/neck reconstructive surgery equipment

Source
Adapted from Ross DA, Thomson JG, Restifo R, Tarro JM, Sasaki CT. The extended lateral arm free flap for head and neck reconstruction: the Yale experience. The Laryngoscope 1996;106:14-18.

 external fixation technique in calcaneal fracture

Description
this method takes advantage of the strong superomedial and plantar calcaneonavicular ligaments, which link the sustentaculum to the navicular; traction by pins placed in the first metatarsal indirectly controls the sustentacular fragment; countertraction from medially placed pins in the tuberosity allows derotation of the fragment and correct positioning in relation to the sustentaculum

Anatomy
calcaneus; calcaneonavicular ligaments; cancellous bone; cortices; cuboid; first metatarsal; gastrocsoleus muscle; Gissane angle; navicular bone; neurovascular bundle; posterior facet; peroneal tendons; sustentaculum; superomedial and plantar ligaments; tuberosity; thalamic fragment (inner part of calcaneus) (Editor note: unusual usage of thalamus from thalamos - inner chamber)

Equipment
4-mm Hoffman-type pins; 5-mm half-pins; clamps; connecting bar (rod); external fixator

Source
Adapted from Borowsky KA. Two case reports of a technique of medial external fixation in calcaneal fractures: indirect control of the sustentacular fragment. Foot & Ankle International Journal 1996;17:210-216.

 ## ex vivo cell expansion

Synonyms
in vitro cell growth; ex vivo cell culture

Use
increase number of cells from a rare but critical population required for transplantation or gene therapy

Method
cells cultured for varying periods of time in cytokine-supplemented growth media

Specimen
bone marrow; peripheral blood cytapheresis product; umbilical cord blood

Comments
cells from other specimens are likely to be used as this technology develops

Source
University of Minnesota Department of Laboratory Medicine and Pathology. Minneapolis, MN.

 ## EyeClose external weights

Description
tantalum weights for temporary facial paralysis worn on the outer surface of the upper lid; effective in restoring a voluntary blink mechanism for lubrication of eye

Source
MedDev Corp. product information. Palo Alto, CA.

 ## E-Z Flex

Description
jaw exercising device for temporomandibular joint rehabilitation

Source
E-Z Flex product information. New York, NY.

facet screw system

Description
internal fixation system with beveled-head screws designed for foot and
ankle surgery; various sizes for solid cortical, cannulated cortical, and cannulated cancellous are available; thread pattern on the cortical screws provides improved purchase for increased compression

Source
Orthopaedic Biosystems Ltd. Inc. product information. Scottsdale, AZ.

 facial bone reconstruction with bioactive glass

Description
bones reconstructed with bioactive glass granules and plates; bioactive glass
granules used in facial bone defects in subperiosteal pockets over frontal,
temporal, zygomatic, and maxillary bones, and to obliterate frontal sinuses;
bioactive glass plates were used mostly in orbital wall reconstruction; non-
vascularized bone grafts used for reconstruction of skeletal deformities of the
face are prone to resorption

Anatomy
bones: frontal, maxillary, parietal, temporal, and zygomatic; cortex; endo-
chondral region; frontal sinus; fibrous tissue; orbital floor and roof; subperiosteal region

Equipment
standard plastic surgery equipment; bioactive glass composed of silicon dioxide, calcium oxide, and phosphorus pentoxide (granules and plates)

Source
Adapted from Suominen E, Kinnunen J. Bioactive glass granules and plates in the reconstruction of defects of the
facial bones. Scandinavian Journal of Plastic Reconstructive Hand Surgery 1996;30:281-289.

 facial paralysis reconstruction with
rectus abdominis muscle

Description
paralyzed orbicularis oculi muscle reconstructed through preauricular incision; subcutaneous pockets created in upper and lower eyelids; anterior portion of temporal muscle elevated, and fascial strip fixed to distal portion of
muscle; muscle flap transferred; divided fasciae passed through pockets of eyelids and fixed to inner canthal ligament; recipient vessels prepared; abdominal
rectus muscle dissected and transferred to malar pocket of face and sutured

Anatomy
buccal branches of facial nerve; inferior deep epigastric vessels; inner canthal
ligament; ipsilateral rectus abdominis muscle; branch of intercostal nerve;
orbicularis oculi muscle; temporal muscle; zygomatic major muscle

Equipment
standard plastic surgery equipment

Source
Adapted from Koshima I, Tsuda K, Hamanaka T, Moriguchi T. One-stage construction of established facial paralysis using a rectus abdominis muscle transfer. Plastic and Reconstructive Surgery 1997;99:234-238.

 ## facial plastic surgery scissors

Description
"super-cut" high-precision instruments available in styles such as Castanares, Kaye, Rees, Jameson, Gorney, and Fomon; for face-lift procedures including rhinoplasty, and rhytidectomy

Source
Accurate Surgical and Scientific Instruments Corp. product information. Westbury, NY.

 ## factor V Leiden mutation test

Synonyms
factor V Leiden mutation activated protein C resistance; Leiden mutation APC resistance

Use
identify specific etiology of recurrent thrombosis in patients with activated protein C (APC) resistance

Method
polymerase chain reaction (PCR) to amplify patient's DNA to detect the presence of the mutation

Specimen
blood

Normal range
absence of mutation

Comments
Leiden mutation causes up to 90% of cases of activated protein C resistance

Source
University of Minnesota Department of Laboratory Medicine and Pathology. Minneapolis, MN.

 ## factor VIIa ELISA

Synonyms
enzyme-linked immunosorbent assay for blood coagulation factor VIIa (f VIIa)

Use
measurement of factor VIIa in patients with acute coronary disease and with bleeding disorders

Method
ELISA using neoantigen-specific capture antibody

Specimen
blood

Normal range
0.015-0.035 ng/mL

Comments
provides a simpler alternative to the standard, labor-intensive functional
factor VIIa assay

Source
Adapted from Philippou H, Adami A, Amersey RA, Stubbs PJ, Lane DA. A novel specific immunoassay for plasma
two-chain factor VIIa: investigation of FVIIa levels in normal individuals and in patients with acute coronary
syndromes. Blood 1997;89:767-775.

 factor IX

Brand name
Benefix

Use
recombinant form of human clotting factor IX for the control and prevention
of bleeding episodes in patients with hemophilia B

Usual dosage
intravenous: 9 unit/kg weekly were used in clinical trials

Pharmaceutical company
Genetics Institute. Cambridge, MA.

Source
Stadtlanders Managed Pharmacy Services. Pittsburgh, PA.

 falloposcope

Description
endoscopic instrument used to evaluate the interior of fallopian tube

Source
Adapted from Goldman EL. Diagnostic falloposcopy now a clinical reality. OB.GYN News 1996;31:14.

 famciclovir

Brand name
Famvir

Use
prodrug of the antiviral agent, penciclovir; used in the treatment of uncomplicated herpes zoster infection (shingles) and genital herpes

Usual dosage
oral: 500 mg tablet; 250, 500 or 750 mg every 8 hours for 7 days

Pharmaceutical company
SmithKline Beecham. Philadelphia, PA.

Source
University of Pittsburgh Drug Information and Pharmacoepidemiology Center. Pittsburgh, PA.

fampridine

Brand name
Neurelan

Use
for symptomatic relief of multiple sclerosis

Usual dosage
oral: sustained release capsule formulation will be available in 2.5 mg and 5 mg strength; to be administered as single daily dose of 10 to 25 mg

Pharmaceutical company
Athena Neuroscienes Inc. Ashland, VA.

Source
Stadtlanders Managed Pharmacy Services. Pittsburgh, PA.

 Famvir

Generic name
see famciclovir

 Fareston

Generic name
see toremifene citrate

 Fary anterior chamber maintainer

Description
ophthalmic surgical instrument designed to approximate stab incision in cornea to eliminate rotational movements; side ports direct irrigation above surface of iris to eliminate disturbance of fluid flowing directly into capsule

Source
Storz Ophthalmics product information. St. Louis, MO.

 Feaster radial keratotomy (RK) knife

Description
ophthalmic surgical 2.5-mm diamond blade offers standardized incision length for minimally invasive results; eliminates dragging the blade through tissue

Source
Rhein Medical Inc. product information. Tampa, FL.

FeatherTouch SilkLaser system

Description
FeatherTouch mode for SilkLaser CO_2 laser with variable vaporization depth and SilkTouch modes; optimizes full spectrum of skin resurfacing, from the light laser peel to the most severe sun-damaged cases; also used for endoscopic and incisional procedures, and traditional dermatologic/plastic surgery

Source
Sharplan Lasers Inc. product information. Allendale, NJ.

 ## fecal lactoferrin marker for inflammatory bowel disease

Synonyms
none

Indications
ulcerative colitis and Crohn disease

Method
fecal levels of lactoferrin, fecal hemoglobin, and α_1-antitrypsin were measured

Normal findings
levels not elevated

Comments
clinical and in vitro studies suggest that lactoferrin is most suitable neutrophil-derived fecal marker of inflammation

Source
Adapted from Sugi K, Saitoh O, Hirata I, et al. Fecal lactoferrin as a marker for disease activity in inflammatory bowel disease: comparison with other neutrophil-derived proteins. American Journal of Gastroenterology 1996;91:927-933.

 ## Femara

Generic name
see letrozole

 ## Fem-Flex II femoral cannulae

Description
arterial and venous cannulae have an internal dilator and connector, percutaneous access, and an ultra thin-wall

Source
Research Medical Inc. product information. Midvale, UT.

Femstat One

Generic name
see butoconazole nitrate

 fenoldopam

Brand name
Corlopam

Use
selective dopamine-1 receptor agonist used in the management of severe hypertension, particularly in patients with renal impairment

Usual dosage
intravenous: initial infusion rate of 0.1 mcg/kg/min, increase by increments of 0.05 to 0.2 mcg/kg/min at 15 to 20 minute intervals until target blood pressure is achieved; infusion rates have ranged from 0.25 to 0.5 mcg/kg/min

Pharmaceutical company
SmithKline Beecham. Philadelphia, PA.

Source
University of Pittsburgh Drug Information and Pharmacoepidemiology Center. Pittsburgh, PA.

 fentanyl citrate

Brand name
Actiq

Use
oral transmucosal formulation of a narcotic agonist analgesic for the treatment of breakthrough pain in patients who are already receiving opiate therapy

Usual dosage
oral: initial dose of 200 or 400 µg; then dose is titrated until effective pain relief is achieved

Pharmaceutical company
Anesta Corporation. Salt Lake City, UT.

Source
Stadtlanders Managed Pharmacy Services. Pittsburgh, PA.

 Ferran awl

Description
orthopaedic surgical instrument designed to help create a puncture hole in the piriformis fossa of proximal femur during intramedullary nail fracture fixation

Source
Innomed Inc. product information. Savannah, GA.

Fertinex

Generic name
see urofollitropin

 ferumoxsil

Brand name
GastroMARK

Use
silicone coated iron oxide; magnetic resonance imaging agent used to enhance the delineation of the internal organs, bowel and pelvic lesions

Usual dosage
oral suspension: ingest 600 to 900 ml prior to magnetic resonance imaging (MRI)

Pharmaceutical company
Advance Magnetics. Cambridge, MA.

Source
Stadtlanders Managed Pharmacy Services. Pittsburgh, PA.

 fetal pulse oximetry

Synonyms
none

Indications
diagnostic tool to measure fetal oxygenation

Method
sensor placed along cheek or temple of fetus with sensor held in place by pressure from the uterine wall

Normal findings
normal fetal pulse oximetry

Source
Adapted from Lien JM, Garite TJ. A better way of assessing fetal oxygenation. Contemporary OB/GYN 1997;42:53-65.

 fexofenadine

Brand name
Allegra

Use
active metabolite of terfenadine (Seldane) used in the treatment of seasonal allergic rhinitis

Usual dosage
oral: proposed dosing to FDA is 60 mg twice daily

Pharmaceutical company
Hoechst Roussel Pharmaceuticals Inc. Somerville, NJ.

Source
University of Pittsburgh Drug Information and Pharmacoepidemiology Center. Pittsburgh, PA.

Fibracol dressing

Description
collagen-alginate, nonadhering wound dressing; assists in managing pressure ulcers, diabetic ulcers, venous ulcers, and other chronic wounds

Source
Johnson & Johnson Medical Inc. product information. Arlington, TX.

fibrinopeptide A level

Synonyms
FPA

Use
study hypercoagulable states, procoagulant conditions, and disseminated intravascular coagulation (DIC) in which fibrinopeptide A (FPA) levels are increased

Method
radioimmunoassay (RIA); enzyme immunoassay (EIA)

Specimen
plasma; urine; cerebrospinal fluid; ascitic fluid

Normal range
male 1.5 +/- 1.1 ng/ml; female 1.9 +/- 1.2 ng/ml

Comment
careful attention must be given to proper specimen collection and handling to avoid artifactual elevation of FPA levels as a result of coagulation activation with exogenous conversion of fibrinogen

Source
Lexi-Comp Inc. database. Hudson, OH.

Fillauer prosthesis liner

Description
silicone suspension, hypoallergenic, tear-resistant prosthesis liner; compatible with any shuttle-locking device with set-screw to prevent loosening; metal insert in distal end for maximum strength; limited longitudinal stretch of liner for less pistoning; 7 sizes

Source
Fillauer Inc. product information. Chattanooga, TN.

Filtryzer dialyzer

Description
dialysis device made of biocompatible membrane that is gamma-sterilized; demonstrates significantly less complement-induced leukopenia and provides enhanced middle-molecule clearance

Source
Toray Marketing & Sales Inc. product information. New York, NY.

finasteride

Brand name
Propecia

Use
treatment of male-pattern baldness (alopecia)

Usual dosage
oral: studies using 1 mg daily dose

Pharmaceutical company
Merck & Co. Inc. West Point, PA.

Source
Stadtlanders Managed Pharmacy Services. Pittsburgh, PA.

Fine-Thornton scleral fixation ring

Description
ophthalmic instrument that provides positive fixation of globe without injury; variable angle of handle allows for variations of anatomy including large nose, deep-set eye, and prominent brow

Source
American Surgical Instruments Corp. product information. Westmont, IL.

FIN system

Description
flexible intramedullary nail (FIN) used for fixation of pertrochanteric, intertrochanteric, subtrochanteric fractures, and certain types of femoral shaft fractures; stainless steel implants and instrument set including benders, cortical awl, hook, impactor/extractor, final impactor

Source
DePuy Inc. product information. Warsaw, IN.

First Beat ultrasound stethoscope

Description

early detection mode (EDM) ultrasound stethoscope; increased sensitivity in detecting early pregnancy; allows fetal heart sounds to resonate clearly

Source

Medasonics Inc. product information. Fremont, CA.

FirstQ departure alert system

Description

restrain-free state-of-the-art wanderer patient monitoring system uses digital technology for monitoring with 90-day or 12-month signaling device

Source

WanderGuard Inc. product information. Lincoln, NE.

FirstStep tibial osteotomy system

Description

orthopaedic surgical instruments designed for precise and reproducible wedge cuts; two-piece ratcheted device designed to provide superior fixation and strength and immediate osteotomy stability

Source

Howmedica Inc. product information. Rutherford, NJ.

Flantadin

Generic name

see deflazacort

fleroxacin

Brand name

Megalone

Use

quinolone antibiotic for uncomplicated gonorrhea and as a first-line therapy for uncomplicated urinary tract infection; also used as a second-line therapy for complicated urinary tract infection

Usual dosage

oral: total daily dose of 200-400 mg/day as single or divided doses

Pharmaceutical company

Roche Laboratories. Nutley, NJ.

Source

Stadtlanders Managed Pharmacy Services. Pittsburgh, PA.

Flexderm wound dressing

Description
sterile hydrogel polymer sheet dressing that protects a wound against dehydration and exogenous contamination while providing a moist environment conducive to optimal wound healing

Source
Dow Hickam Pharmaceuticals product information. Sugarland, TX.

 ## Flex Foam orthosis

Description
thoracolumbosacral orthosis that combines the rigidity of a traditional rigid frame with firm exterior foam and soft interior foam; identified for cerebral palsy (seating application), severe scoliosis, muscular dystrophy, cancer patients, geriatric patients, and/or osteoporotic patients

Source
Spinal Technologies Inc. product information. West Yarmouth, MA.

 ## Flex-Foot prostheses

Description
various models (Sure-Flex, Re-Flex VSP, Flex-Walk II) offer smooth and gradual proportional response to load and simulated ankle motion to normalize the gait for amputees

Source
Flex-Foot product information. Aliso Viejo, CA.

 ## Flexiflo Inverta-PEG kit

Description
percutaneous endoscopic gastrostomy (PEG) tube with roll-tip bumper that facilitates external, nonendoscopic removal; designed to resist accidental removal and minimize tissue trauma when pulled

Source
Abbott Laboratories product information. Columbus, OH.

206

 ## Flexiflo tube

Description
Flexiflo Lap J kit for laparoscopic jejunostomy; Flexiflo Lap G kit for laparo-scopic gastrostomy; alternatives to open surgical jejunostomy and/or gas-trostomy; provides access for early enteral feeding; T-Fasteners replace laparoscopic suturing

Source
Ross Laboratory Products Division product information. Columbus, OH.

 ## G5 Fleximatic massage/percussion unit

Description
portable, continuously-variable speed range of 20 to 50 cycles per second; has a directional-stroking motion adapter for machine-assisted physical therapy procedures; manipulates soft tissue to produce effects on nerves and muscu-lar systems; enhances local and general circulation of blood and lymphatic tissues

Source
General Physiotherapy Inc. product information. St. Louis, MO.

 ## Flexi-Seal fecal collector

Description
patient-friendly alternative to diapers; maintains a secure seal for an average wear time of 24 hours; offers security and skin protection to nonambulatory patients with loose-stool fecal incontinence and diarrhea

Source
Bristol-Myers Squibb Co. product information. Princeton, NJ.

 ## Flexi-Therm diabetic diagnostic insole

Description
diagnostic insole for the diabetic/insensate patient; utilizes liquid crystal chemistry to evaluate vascular status on a daily basis; provides a color map of the plantar circulation and shows areas of potential tissue breakdown before they occur

Source
Flexi-Therm product information. Wellington, FL.

Flexi-Therm liquid crystal systems

Description
noninvasive, thermal image analysis to illustrate skin surface temperature in graphic color to aid in the diagnosis and treatment of autonomic nervous dysfunction, especially as it relates to sympathetic pain; also referred to as the Mark III system

Source
Flexi-Therm product information. Wellington, FL.

 ## Flexi-Trak skin anchoring device

Description
designed to secure a variety of tubes, drains and catheters onto the patient's skin; especially suited for anchoring indwelling urinary catheters; helps keep tubes from getting tangled with acrylic adhesive for extended wear time (up to 5 days) without causing skin damage

Source
ConvaTec product information. Princeton, NJ.

 ## Flexxicon catheter

Description
permanent access vascular catheter with precurved shaft and dual lumen; Flexxicon II PC used for outpatient treatment regimens allowing internal jugular vein access

Source
Vas-Cath Inc. product information. Mississauga, Ontario, Canada.

 ## Flip-Flop pillow

Description
dual-purpose pillow, offers cervical support on one side; cutout space for arm rest during sleep on reverse side

Source
TLC Comfort Products product information. Maryville, TN.

FLOAM ankle stirrup brace

Description

ankle brace; provides stability by minimizing ankle rotation; is comprised of two polypropylene outer shells connected with a soft adjustable footpiece; the shells are lined with unique FLOAM bladders that provide uniform compression and customized fit; 50% lighter than most cushioning products and easily flows to conform to body's shape; has no memory prohibiting pressure to be displaced to bony prominences; does not react to changes with hot and cold environments

Source

Johnson & Johnson Orthopaedics product information. New Brunswick, NJ.

 Flolan

Generic name

see epoprostenol sodium

 Flomax

Generic name

see tamsulosin

 Flonase

Generic name

see fluticasone propionate

 Flo-Stat fluid monitor

Description

fluid-management system that monitors distention fluids to prevent excess accumulation within the body

Source

FemRx product information. Sunnyvale, CA.

 flo-Vac safety nozzle

Description

vapor recovery nozzle pulls 360 degree vacuum around exiting fluid and prevents harmful vapors from escaping into breathing zone

Source

The Hampton Group LLC product information. Fishers, IN.

flow cytometric platelet (FCP) crossmatching

Synonyms
none

Use
detection of lymphocyte-reactive and platelet-reactive antibodies

Method
patient serum incubated with platelet and lymphocyte suspensions; followed by fluorescent-labeled anti-IgG (immunoglobulin G) antibody; analyzed by flow cytometry

Specimen
serum

Normal range
negative

Comments
more rapid although less sensitive than current platelet crossmatch methods

Source
Adapted from Kohler M, Dittmann J, Legler TJ, et al. Flow cytometric detection of platelet-reactive antibodies and application in platelet crossmatching. Transfusion 1996;36:250-255.

 flow cytometric quantification of fetomaternal hemorrhage

Synonyms
FACS D+ cell measurement

Use
quantification of the fetal D-positive red blood cell volume in postpartum D-negative women

Method
flow cytometric detection of cells stained with fluorescent-labeled anti-D monoclonal antibody

Specimen
blood

Normal range
no D-positive cells detected

Comments
flow cytometry using directly-labeled anti-D monoclonal antibody is preferable to two-step staining

Source
Adapted from Lloyd-Evans P, Kumpel BM, Bromelow I, Austin E, Taylor E. Use of a directly conjugated monoclonal anti-D (BRAD-3) for quantification of fetomaternal hemorrhage by flow cytometry. Transfusion 1996;36:432-437.

Flowplus pneumatic compression system

Description
pneumatic compression system for treatment of lymphedema, venous insufficiency, and venous stasis ulcers

Source
HNE Healthcare Inc. product information. Manalapan, NJ.

 ## Flowtron thigh-high device

Description
pump device that reduces deep vein thrombosis (DVT) risk biomechanically and biochemically; to be used continuously until patient is fully ambulatory

Source
HNE Healthcare product information. Manalapan, NJ.

 ## FLUFTEX gauze roll

Description
dressing made of fluff-dried gauze, crinkled to give loft and bulk; designed for management of draining wounds

Source
DeRoyal Industries product information. Powell, TN.

 ## flunisolide

Brand name
Nasarel

Use
another formulation of flunisolide for the management of symptoms of seasonal or perennial rhinitis

Usual dosage
topical: 0.025 mg flunisolide/spray with 5% propylene glycol; two sprays in each nostril twice a day

Pharmaceutical company
Roche Laboratories. Nutley, NJ.

Source
Stadtlanders Managed Pharmacy Services. Pittsburgh, PA.

 ## fluorescence in situ hybridization (FISH)

Synonyms
FISH interphase cytogenetics

Use
highly sensitive detection of cytogenetic abnormalities in cells regardless of division rate

Method
fluorescence microscopy of cells bound by fluorescent-labeled DNA probes

Specimen
blood, bone marrow, or other single-cell suspension

Normal range
not applicable

Comments
investigational, but rapidly gaining acceptance

Source
Archives of Pathology and Lab Medicine 1994;118:1196-1200.

 ## fluorouracil/epinephrine

Brand name
Accusite

Use
injectable gel formulation; an intralesional treatment of genital warts in patients who have failed first-line therapy or who have multiple lesions in an extensive area

Usual dosage
injectable: each lesion is injected locally, once a week for up to 6 weeks

Pharmaceutical company
Matrix Pharmaceuticals Inc. Menlo Park, CA.

Source
Stadtlanders Managed Pharmacy Services. Pittsburgh, PA.

 ## flupirtine

Brand Name
Katadolon

Use
nonopioid, centrally-acting analgesic with muscle relaxant properties for pain management

Usual Dosage
oral: 100 mg three times daily; maximum of 600 mg/day rectally: 150 mg three to four times daily; maximum of 900 mg/day

Pharmaceutical company
Carter-Wallace Inc. New York, NY.

Source
University of Pittsburgh Drug Information and Pharmacoepidemiology Center. Pittsburgh, PA.

fluticasone propionate

Brand name
Flonase

Use
corticosteroid used for the management of seasonal and perennial allergic rhinitis

Usual dosage
intranasal: 0.05% nasal spray, two sprays in each nostril once daily

Pharmaceutical company
Glaxo Inc. Research Triangle Park, NC.

Source
University of Pittsburgh Drug Information and Pharmacoepidemiology Center. Pittsburgh, PA.

 Flutter therapeutic device

Description
facilitates sputum expectoration and clearance of mucus from the lungs of cystic fibrosis patients; a hand-held device that the patient blows into causing a steel ball inside to move up and down which creates a vibrating effect in the lungs that causes the mucus to break up and move out

Source
Scandipharm Inc. product information. Birmingham, AL.

 fluvastatin

Brand name
Lescol

Use
hydroxymethylglutaryl coenzyme A (HMG-CoA) reductase inhibitor used as adjunctive therapy of primary hypercholesterolemia

Usual dosage
oral: 20 mg and 40 mg tablets; initial dosage 20 mg once daily at bedtime; can be increased to 40 mg once daily at bedtime

Pharmaceutical company
Sandoz Pharmaceuticals Corp. East Hanover, NJ.

Source
University of Pittsburgh Drug Information and Pharmacoepidemiology Center. Pittsburgh, PA.

 fluvoxamine

Brand name
Luvox

Use
treats depression in patients who fail tricyclic antidepressant therapy; treatment of obsessive-compulsive disorder

Usual dosage
oral: 50 and 100 mg tablet; initial therapy 50 mg daily at bedtime and individually adjusted within the range of 50 to 300 mg daily

Pharmaceutical company
Solvay. Marietta, GA.

Source
University of Pittsburgh Drug Information and Pharmacoepidemiology Center. Pittsburgh, PA.

 ## focused appendix CT (FACT)

Synonyms
none .

Indications
rule out or diagnose appendicitis

Method
insert contrast agent through tube in rectum to highlight appendix area

Normal findings
none

Comments
before this procedure one in five appendectomies were normal while one in five patients were sent home with condition undiagnosed; using this procedure an accurate diagnosis was made before surgery in 98% of cases, while 100% of all true appendicitis cases were accurately identified; cost-effective as exam costs less, it may establish alternative diagnosis, and does not require IV contrast agent

Source
Adapted from Altman L. A better look at appendicitis. New York Times/Reader's Digest April 1997:148 and Rao PM, et al. Presentation at Annual Meeting of Radiological Society of North America (RSNA) Chicago, IL 12/96.

 ## Fogarty catheter extraction of urethral foreign body

Description
an expedient method for the rapid removal and diagnosis of urethral foreign body in the face of acute obstruction; Fogarty catheter under fluoroscopic control is passed beyond the foreign body, the balloon inflated, and the catheter and foreign body withdrawn when cystoscopy not feasible

Anatomy
urethra; penis; vagina; peritoneum

Equipment
Fogarty catheter, fluoroscopy equipment

Source
Adapted from Phillips JL. Fogarty catheter extraction of unusual urethral foreign bodies. Journal of Urology 1996;155:1374-1375.

Foley Cordostat

Description
surgical device used for atraumatic stabilization of cylindrical anatomical structures during endoscopic or ultrasound-guided procedures

Source
Cook OB/GYN product information. Spencer, IN.

Fome-Cuf tracheostomy tube

Description
kit with SidePort, AutoControl airway connector; auto-expanding foam-filled cuff conforms to unique contours of each individual's trachea; Auto-Control connectors ensure lowest possible cuff-to-tracheal wall sealing pressure throughout the ventilatory cycle; provides protection against aspiration

Source
Bivona Medical Technologies product information. Gary, IN.

fomepizole

Brand name
Antizol

Use
an alcohol dehydrogenase inhibitor used in the treatment of methanol and ethylene glycol (antifreeze) poisonings

Usual dosage
intravenous: 10-20 mg/kg have been used in trials

Pharmaceutical company
Orphan Medical. Minnetonka, MN.

Source
Stadtlanders Managed Pharmacy Services. Pittsburgh, PA.

Fonix 6500-CX hearing aid test system

Description
real-time color display instrumentation for hearing aid testing with Quick-Probe operation technology

Source
Frye Electronics Inc. product information. Tigard, OR.

Foradil

Generic name
see formoterol

Force FX generator

Description
surgical device that responds instantly to changes in tissue density; facilitates moving through changing densities in one smooth stroke in multiple surgeries

Source
Valleylab Inc. product information. Boulder, CO.

 ## formoterol

Brand name
Foradil

Use
long-acting beta 2-selective adrenoreceptor agonist used in the treatment of asthma and chronic obstructive pulmonary disease (COPD) as bronchodilator

Usual dosage
inhalation: 12-24 mcg by inhalation twice daily from metered-dose inhaler preferred over oral tablets; orally 40-160 mcg daily in 2-3 divided doses

Pharmaceutical company
Ciba-Geigy. Summit, NJ.

Source
University of Pittsburgh Drug Information and Pharmacoepidemiology Center. Pittsburgh, PA.

 ## Forte ES (electrotherapy system)

Description
instrument used in physical medicine; features customized treatments and capability of real-time alteration of many parameters during treatment when needed; versatility to suit pain management and muscle rehabilitation programs

Source
Chattanooga Group Inc. product information. Hixson, TN.

 ## Forvade

Generic name
see cidofovir (gel)

 ## Fosamax

Generic name
see alendronate sodium

fosfomycin tromethamine

Brand Name
Monurol

Use
anti-infective used in the treatment of uncomplicated lower urinary tract infections and respiratory infections

Usual Dosage
oral: single daily dose of 3 g

Pharmaceutical company
Forest Laboratories Inc. St. Louis, MO.

Source
University of Pittsburgh Drug Information and Pharmacoepidemiology Center. Pittsburgh, PA.

 fosphenytoin

Brand name
Cerebyx

Use
water-soluble prodrug of phenytoin used in the prevention and treatment of seizures

Usual dosage
intravenous: optimal dose regimens have not been established; however, effective intravenous doses will most likely range from 1000 to 1200 mg or 14 to 17 mg/kg; intramuscular: optimal dose regimens have not been established

Pharmaceutical company
DuPont Merck Pharmaceutical Co. Wilmington, DE.

Source
University of Pittsburgh Drug Information and Pharmacoepidemiology Center. Pittsburgh, PA.

 Fourier transform infrared microscopy

Synonyms
FTIRM

Use
identification of crystal deposits in tissue

Method
infrared microscopy coupled with Fourier transform infrared spectrometry

Specimen
tissue biopsy

Normal range
not applicable

Comments
appears superior to polarized light microscopy and histochemical staining

Source
Adapted from Estepa-Maurice L, Hennequin C, Marfisi C, Bader C, Lacour B, Daudon M. Fourier transform infrared microscopy identification of crystal deposits in tissues. American Journal of Clinical Pathology 1996;105:576-582.

 Fragmin

Generic name
see dalteparin sodium

 Freedom Micro Pro stimulator

Description
mini-electrical nerve stimulator (MENS); microcurrent stimulator allows patient self-use to block out pain

Source
Monad Corp. product information. Pomona, CA.

 FreeDop portable Doppler unit

Description
hand-held Doppler with cordless portable base; used to take blood pressure, determine patency of vessel, and locate fetal heartbeat at bedside

Source
Imex Medical Systems product information. Golden, CO.

 Freedox

Generic name
see tirilazad mesylate

 Freestyle aortic root bioprosthesis

Description
stentless bioprosthesis for versatile implant techniques; zero-pressure fixation combined with root-pressure fixation preserves leaflet morphology and maintains valve geometry; in clinical investigations

Source
Medtronic Inc. product information. Minneapolis, MN.

FRIALITE-2 dental implant system

Description
designed for single-tooth replacement

Source
Interpore Dental product information. Irvine, CA.

 ## Friedlander incision marker

Description
ophthalmic surgical dual transverse incision marker places two 3-mm marks on surface of cornea at designated widths for astigmatic keratotomy incisions

Source
Storz Ophthalmics product information. St. Louis, MO.

 ## Fromm triangle orthopaedic device

Description
knee and tibial device designed to position and hold the femur and tibia during intramedullary nailing of tibia, ligament repairs, and extremity fractures

Source
Innomed Inc. product information. Savannah, GA.

 ## Fukasaku pupil snapper hook

Description
ophthalmic surgical instrument designed for the Fukasaku "snap and split" phaco technique through a small pupil

Source
Katena Products Inc. product information. Denville, NJ.

 ## Fullerview iris retractor

Description
ophthalmic surgical flexible translimbal retractor; provides flexibility and maximum retraction capability of disposable retractors; named for Dr. Dwain Fuller

Source
Synergetics Inc. product information. Chesterfield, MO.

fundoplasty, 270 degree posterior

Description
criteria for surgery include esophagitis either resistant to or shortly recurring after medical treatment, Barrett esophagus, pulmonary complications attributed to reflux, paraesophageal hernia, or long history of major clinical symptoms of reflux; laparoscopic operative technique consists of abdominal esophagus mobilization, approximation of the crura, and construction of a 270-degree posterior gastric valve, 5-7 cm in height; posterior fundoplasty avoids the difficulty of having to judge the amount of gastric valve tightening

Anatomy
abdominal esophagus; chondral edge; crura; crus (singular); esophageal body; esophageal sphincter; fundus; hepatic branches; parietal wall; periesophageal veins; pleura; pars flacidalis; stomach; vagus nerve; umbilicus; xiphoid process

Equipment
standard surgery equipment; Digitrapper Mark II; fiberscope; curved needles; nasogastric sump tube No. 16; polyvinyl catheter (four lumen); pH probe; retractors; trocars

Source
Adapted from Mosnier H, LePort J, Aubert A, Kianmanesh R, Sbai Idrissi MS, Guivarc'h M. A 270 degree laparoscopic posterior fundoplasty in the treatment of gastroesophageal reflux. Journal of American College of Surgeons 1995;181:220-224.

 Fungusumungus body soap

Description
all natural antifungal and antibacterial soap; breakthrough soap enables doctors to safely treat various recurrent infections of the skin; keeps infections away because it can be used every day in shower or bath, thus fitting much easier into a person's daily routine; helps treat and prevent tinea pedis, tinea cruris, tinea corporis and others; reduces itching, burning, redness, and edema associated with these diseases; excellent alternative for people sensitive to chemical ingredients found in other antibacterial soaps

Source
Fungusumungus Inc. product information. Media, PA.

Furlow palatoplasty

Description
treatment for submucous cleft palate; superior to standard surgery using pharyngeal flap which can result in postoperative sleep apnea, airway obstruction, and/or hyponasal speech; preoperative diagnosis confirmed by videonasopharyngoscopy and videofluoroscopy

Anatomy
bifid uvula; soft palate; hard palate; levator veli palatini muscle; levator muscle bundle; velopharyngeal gap; nasion point; pharyngeal wall; hamulus; palatal aponeurosis; pharyngeal constrictor muscle; orifice of eustachian tube; Passavant ridge

Equipment
standard surgery equipment

Source
Adapted from Chen PK, Wu JW, Hung KF, Chen YR, Noordhoff MS. Surgical correction of submucous cleft palate with Furlow palatoplasty. Plastic and Reconstructive Surgery 1996;97:1136-1146.

FyBron dressing

Description
calcium alginate dressing for moderately to heavily exudating wounds

Source
B. Braun Medical Inc. product information. Milwaukee, WI.

Gabitril

Generic name
see tiagabine

gadolinium aluminum silicate

Brand Name
Gadolite

Use
contrast imaging agent

Usual Dosage
intravenous: 0.1 mmol/kg; dose varies with procedure

Pharmaceutical company
Pharmacyclics Inc. Sunnyvale, CA.

Source
University of Pittsburgh Drug Information and Pharmacoepidemiology Center. Pittsburgh, PA.

Gadolite

Generic Name
see gadolinium aluminum silicate

 ## Galileo hysteroscope

Description
less invasive hysteroscope to visualize cervical canal and uterine cavity
Source
Leisegang Medical product information. Boca Raton, FL.

 ## Galzin

Generic name
see zinc acetate

 ## ganciclovir

Brand name
Vitrasert
Use
intraocular implant for CMV-retinitis (*Cytomegalovirus*) treatment in people with AIDS
Usual dosage
topical: each implant is designed to release 4.8 mg of ganciclovir over 5 to 8 months
Pharmaceutical company
Chiron Vision. Irvine, CA.
Source
Stadtlanders Managed Pharmacy Services. Pittsburgh, PA.

 ## gap lipase chain reaction (LCR)

Synonyms
none
Use
detection of extremely small amounts of specific DNA sequences
Method
repeated thermal cycles of DNA denaturation and ligation result in an exponential increase in reaction products

Specimen
any biological tissue

Normal range
reaction product detected

Comments
useful in clinical and forensic laboratories; has greater sensitivity and specificity than conventional ligase chain reaction

Source
Adapted from Yajima R. Development of novel clinical tests and their contribution to laboratory diagnosis—ligase chain reaction. Rinsho Byori, Japanese Journal of Clinical Pathology 1997;45:41-46.

 Gardrin

Generic Name
see enprostil

 GastroMARK

Generic name
see ferumoxsil

 Gastronol

Generic name
see proglumide

 Gastro-Port II feeding device

Description
feeding tube with uniquely designed tip that facilitates placement and reduces patient discomfort; designed to expand and contract with patient movement as well as adjust to gastrostomy tract length

Source
Sandoz Nutrition Corp. product information. Minneapolis, MN.

 Gel-Sole shoe insert

Description
free-flowing glycerine gel shoe insert displaces pressure; helps apply weight equally; acts as shock absorber

Source
Pittsburgh Plastics Manufacturing Inc. product information. Pittsburgh, PA.

gemcitabine

Brand name
Gemzar

Use
cytotoxic agent demonstrating activity in advanced breast cancer, non-small-cell lung cancer, pancreatic carcinoma, and ovarian carcinoma

Usual dosage
intravenous: 800 mg/m^2 as a 30-minute intravenous infusion once weekly every 3 or 4 weeks

Pharmaceutical company
Eli Lilly and Company. Indianapolis, IN.

Source
University of Pittsburgh Drug Information and Pharmacoepidemiology Center. Pittsburgh, PA.

Gemzar

Generic name
see gemcitabine

gene rearrangement for leukemia and lymphoma

Synonyms
leukemia gene rearrangement; lymphocyte T-cell receptor gene rearrangement; lymphoma gene rearrangement

Use
gene rearrangement may be used to supplement and complement conventional histopathology and immunophenotyping in the diagnosis of lymphoid leukemia and lymphoma

Method
examine hybridized deoxyribonucleic acid (DNA) probe complexes for bands after autoradiography or color detection to ascertain if germline or unique gene rearrangements are present

Specimen
peripheral whole blood; lymph node biopsies and other tissue such as skin biopsies, gastrointestinal tissue, and bone marrow

Normal range
no unique rearrangement of T- and B-cell receptors found in normal white blood cells; interpretive report is usually included with results

Comments
some tissue yield little DNA or DNA that is degraded; lymph nodes with less than 1% tumor cells cannot provide evidence of gene rearrangement

Source
Lexi-Comp Inc. database. Hudson, OH.

Genesis II total knee system

Description
knee implant; deeper more lateralized trochlear groove improves patellar contact and tracking; anatomically shaped tibial baseplates have an improved fin design and significantly improve coverage of the tibia compared to symmetrical designs

Source
Smith & Nephew Orthopaedics product information. Memphis, TN.

 ## Genesys Vertex variable angle gamma camera

Description
camera with dual detectors that robotically adjust between 90 and 180 degrees, doubling throughput for virtually all nuclear studies; image quality for single photon emission computed tomography (SPECT), total body, and planar imaging procedures

Source
ADAC Laboratories product information. Milpitas, CA.

 ## Genotropin

Generic name
see somatropin (rDNA origin) for injection

 ## Gen-Probe Pace 2 C System

Synonyms
PACE 2C Probe assay

Use
simultaneous screening of endocervical specimens for both *Chlamydia trachomatis* and *Neisseria gonorrhoeae*

Method
direct nucleic acid-based detection of *Chlamydia trachomatis* and *Neisseria gonorrhoeae*

Speciman
endocervical swabs

Normal Range
negative

Comments
sensitivity and specificity equal to or better than culture methods

Source
Iwen PC, Walker RA, Warren KL, Kelly DM, Hinrichs SH, Linder J. Evaluation of nucleic acid-based test (PACE 2 C) for simultaneous detection of Chlamydia trachomatis and Neisseria gonorrhoeae in endocervical specimans. Journal of Clinical Microbiology 1995;33:2587-91.

Gen-Probe Pace-2 direct specimen assay

Description
assay used to diagnose chlamydia and/or gonorrhea, using one swab for both tests; easy sample collection; allows for earlier initiation of treatment

Source
Gen-Probe product information. San Diego, CA.

 ## Geomatrix

Generic name
see nifedipine

 ## Geref

Generic name
see sermorelin acetate

 ## gestodene/ethinyl estradiol

Brand Name
Minulet/Tri-minulet

Use
combination estrogen product used as an estrogen replacement therapy or as oral contraceptives

Usual Dosage
oral: 75 mg gestodene with 30 mg ethinyl estradiol for 28 days

Pharmaceutical company
Berlex Labs Inc. Wayne, NJ.

Source
University of Pittsburgh Drug Information and Pharmacoepidemiology Center. Pittsburgh, PA.

 ## Ghajar guide

Description
for stereotactic intraventricular catheter placement; accurate first pass right angle catheter placement for intracranial pressure monitoring, shunting procedures, external cerebrospinal fluid drainage, or Ommaya reservoir placement; available in all catheter diameters

Source
Neurodynamics Inc. product information. New York, NY.

GII KAFO

Description

knee-ankle-foot orthosis (KAFO), an orthotic device with polyaxial hinge that mechanically follows the biomechanics of the knee to prevent binding under loaded conditions; indicated for varus/valgus deformities, postpolio, unicompartmental osteoarthritic patients with abnormal foot/ankle pathologies; dynamic force strap provides counter-rotational action control

Source

Generation II U.S.A. Inc. product information. Seattle, WA.

 ## GII Unloader ADJ knee brace

Description

Generation II Unloader adjustable (ADJ) orthotic device; hinge adjustment can be made only by those qualified; can be changed as required to "unload" affected arthritic compartment

Source

Generation II USA Inc. product information. Seattle, WA.

 ## G II Unloader knee brace

Description

unique patented Generation II knee brace with dynamic force strap; applies valgus or varus force to "unload" affected part; provides pain relief for degenerative joint disease

Source

Generation II USA Inc. product information. Seattle, WA.

 ## Gladiator shock-suit

Description

for hypovolemic shock; interchangeable gauges are located directly on the suit where they are easy to see while monitoring patient; spine line for quick and proper positioning of the patient; x-ray transparent

Source

Armstrong Medical Industries Inc. product information. Lincolnshire, IL and San Diego, CA.

 ## Glanzmann thrombasthenia platelet phenotyping

Synonyms

human platelet antigen (HPA) phenotyping; Glanzmann thrombasthenia carrier screening

Use

screening families affected with Glanzmann thrombasthenia types I and II

Method
serologic determination of platelet alloantigens on platelet glycoproteins IIb and IIIa
Specimen
blood
Normal range
HPA reactivity present
Comments
screening test, to be followed by molecular testing
Source
Transfusion Medicine 1995;5:123-129.

 ## Glasser fixation screw

Description
5-mm and 10-mm screws to hold uterus in place during laparoscopic-assisted vaginal hysterectomy
Source
J.E.M.D. Medical Sales Associates Inc. product information. Hicksville, NY.

 ## GLASSERS

Description
radiation protection eyeglasses for anyone exposed to radiation; reduced scatter radiation exposure to eye lens up to 90%; provides no less than 0.5 mm lead-equivalent shielding, offers wrap around protection without restricting vision
Source
Nuclear Associates product information. Carle Place, NY.

 ## Gliadel

Generic name
see carmustine

 ## Glidewire Gold surgical guide wire

Description
hydrophilic-coated wire provides maximum radiopacity; allows superselective access in cerebrovascular and general vascular applications; tracks through smaller vessels and slides through bends without kinking
Source
Terumo Medical Corp. product information. Somerset, NJ.

glimepiride

Brand name
Amaryl

Use
oral sulfonylurea used in the treatment of non-insulin-dependent (type II) diabetes

Usual dosage
oral: 1 mg to 8 mg once daily

Pharmaceutical company
The Upjohn Company. Kalamazoo, MI.

Source
University of Pittsburgh Drug Information and Pharmacoepidemiology Center. Pittsburgh, PA.

 Glori pressure earrings

Description
earlobe clips applied to compression plates to reduce formation of keloids and hypertrophic scarring

Source
H&A Enterprises Inc. product information. Whitestone, NY.

 glucagon usage with pancreaticojejunostomy

Description
technique involves administration of one ampule (1 mg) of glucagon intravenously before pancreaticojejunal anastomosis; cessation of jejunal contractions and relaxations can be observed; the anastomosis can be completed before the effect of the drug is dissipated, and the jejunum capable of peristalsis; anastomosis is created with increased technical ease because of the inhibition of motility and the enhanced size of the jejunal lumen

Anatomy
gastrointestinal tract; jejunum; jejunal lumen; pancreas; pancreaticojejunal area

Equipment
standard surgical equipment

Source
Adapted from Jordan PH, Brock PA, Pikoulis E. Glucagon facilitates end-to-end pancreaticojejunostomy. Journal of American College of Surgeons 1997;184:401-402.

 Glucophage

Generic name
see metformin hydrochloride

α-glutathione S-transferase (α-GST) assay

Synonyms
none

Use
monitoring hepatocellular damage in patients undergoing interferon-α therapy for chronic hepatitis C

Method
sandwich enzyme immunoassay

Specimen
blood

Normal range
undetermined

Comments
more reflective of active hepatocellular damage than more conventional AST and ALT tests

Source
American Journal of Clinical Pathology 1995;104:193-198.

 gluteoplasty

Description
surgical repair of the anal sphincter using gluteus muscle transfer

Anatomy
gluteus maximus muscle; anal canal; sciatic nerve; inferior gluteal nerve; rectal mucosa; ischial tuberosity

Equipment
pulse generator; electrodes; vacuum drains

Source
Adapted from Guelincks PJ, Sinsel NK, Gruwez JA. Anal sphincter reconstruction with the gluteus maximus muscle; anatomic and histologic considerations concerning conventional and dynamic gluteoplasty. Plastic and Reconstructive Surgery 1996;98:293-302.

 Glypressin

Generic Name
see terlipressin

 Glyset

Generic name
see miglitol

GM-1 ganglioside

Brand name
Sygen

Use
recovery enhancer for central nervous system damage resulting from stroke and spinal cord injuries

Usual dosage
intravenous: 100 mg per day , 6 days per week for two months, and 100 mg per day for 18 to 32 doses, have been used in clinical trials

Pharmaceutical company
Fidia Pharmaceutical Corporation. Washington, DC.

Source
University of Pittsburgh Drug Information and Pharmacoepidemiology Center. Pittsburgh, PA.

 Godina vessel-fixation system

Description
double hook instrument for microvascular free tissue transfer; replaces time-consuming 3-clamp system; exposes the back edges of the anastomosis so it can be clearly seen and easily sutured

Source
Accurate Surgical & Scientific Instruments Corp. product information. Westbury, NY.

 Gold Series bone drilling system

Description
bone drilling system with a built-in countersink to consistently produce an osteotomy that matches the implant; system includes a 2-mm diameter TiNit-coated, tri-spade, intercooled, non-walking initial starting drill and the final sizing drill in multiple sizes

Source
Osteo-Implant Corp. product information. New Castle, PA.

 Gonostat

Synonyms
none

Indications
rule out gonorrhea

Method
vaginal or penile swab specimens are prepared, inoculated onto chocolate agar plates, and incubated for 48 hours

Normal findings
negative

Comments
easy to perform for the laboratory technician; very reasonable cost for the patient

Source
Adapted from MDDI Reports - The Gray Sheet 1997;23:I&W2-I&W3.

 ## Gore suture passer

Description
surgical instrument allows for facilitation of closure of large port sites, secures prosthetics for laparoscopic incisional and inguinal hernia repairs, and allows ligation of vessels

Source
W.L. Gore & Associates Inc. product information. Flagstaff, AZ.

 ## grading of retinal nerve fiber layer

Synonyms
fundus photography

Indications
quantitative approach for the evaluation of diffuse atrophy of retinal nerve

Method
simultaneous grading system designed, which consisted of set of 25 reference photographs, 64 retinal nerve fiber layer (RNFL) photographs of patients with glaucoma or ocular hypertension, and normal subjects to reference photographs, were evaluated

Normal findings
by using set of reference photographs, a method to derive a quantitative measurement of RNFL was defined; (see comments for elaboration)

Comments
the first photograph was scored as 25, indicating normal, thick nerve fiber bundles; second photograph was numbered 24, and so on; the last photograph was scored as 1, and no fibers were visible

Source
Adapted from Niessen AGJE, van den Berg TJTP, Langerhorst CT, Bossuyt PMM. Grading of retinal nerve fiber layer with a photographic reference set. American Journal of Ophthalmology 1995;120:577-586.

 ## GraftCyte moist dressing

Description
copper peptide gel dressing designed to promote healing and faster hair regrowth in hair transplantation patients

Source
ProCyte Corp. product information. Kirkland, WA.

Grahamizer I exerciser

Description
multi-use exerciser that fits over a door; "wind up" shoulder wheel with rope increases range of motion and reach; for standard rehabilitation exercises; also ideal for post-mastectomy patients

Source
Fred Sammons Inc. product information. Western Springs, IL.

 grepafloxacin

Brand name
Raxar

Use
fluoroquinolone antibiotic for use in acute exacerbation of chronic bronchitis, community-acquired pneumonia, and sexually transmitted disease (STD)

Usual dosage
oral: 400 mg daily was used in clinical trials

Pharmaceutical company
GlaxoWellcome Inc. Research Triangle Park, NC.

Source
Stadtlanders Managed Pharmacy Services. Pittsburgh, PA.

 Grieshaber flexible iris retractor

Description
a disposable iris retractor made of strong, flexible suture material; small in size and ideal for temporal pupillary dilation even in phakic patients

Source
Grieshaber & Co. Inc. product information. Kennesaw, GA.

 Grip-Ease device

Description
individual cylinders are rotated for hand and wrist therapy; assists in early mobilization, edema control, and nerve gliding

Source
Tech Sport Inc. product information. Little Silver, NJ.

growth response-1 messenger ribonucleic acid (mRNA)

Synonyms
early growth response-1 mRNA

Use
recognition of various stages of cancer

Method
polymerase chain reaction, autoradiograph of blot hybridized samples

Specimen
tissue biopsy

Normal range
investigational, presence of factor linked with mutagenesis

Comments
expression of early growth response-1 (mRNA) is associated with stages A2 and B2 adenocarcinoma and intraprostatic primary cancers of patients with D1 disease

Source
Thigpen AE, Cala KM, Guileyardo JM, Molberg KH, McConnell JD, Russell DW. Early growth response expression in prostatic tumors. Journal of Urology 1996;155:994-998.

Guardian DNA system

Synonyms
none

Indications
educational material for parents and DNA collection kit

Method
DNA sample collection kit including documentation stored at a DNA registry

Normal findings
not applicable

Comments
none

Source
In Vitro International product information. Irvine, CA.

Guardsman femoral interference screw

Description
designed for endoscopic femoral placement; double-helix design propels threads for rapid advancement; spiral tip allows for quick initiation

Source
Linvatec Corp. product information. Largo, FL.

Guimaraes ophthalmic spatula

Description

LASIK (laser in situ keratomileusis) multipurpose spatula; blade with semi-sharp edges for dissecting the corneal flap; surfaces designed for entering interface and lifting corneal flap, as well as repositioning flap over stromal bed after ablation

Source

Katena Products Inc. product information. Denville, NJ.

 ## Hadeco intraoperative Doppler

Description

ES1000SPM Smartdop and ES100X Minidop document vessel patency; multiple/variable probe selection

Source

Koven Technology Inc. product information. St. Louis, MO.

 ## haemophilus b (conjugate)/hepatitis B (recombinant) vaccine

Brand name

Comvax

Use

vaccination against invasive disease caused by *Haemophilus influenzae* type b and against infection caused by all known subtypes of hepatitis B virus in infants 6 weeks to 15 months of age

Usual dosage

intramuscular: three 0.5 ml doses given at 2, 4, and 12-15 months of age

Pharmaceutical company

Merck & Co. Inc. West Point, PA.

Source

Stadtlanders Managed Pharmacy Services. Pittsburgh, PA.

 ## hair sample testing for drugs of abuse

Synonyms

hair sample toxicology

Use

testing for amphetamine, methamphetamine, MDA, and MDMA

Method

methods include direct methanol extraction, gas chromatography/mass spectrometry, and hydrolysis using either enzymes, acids, or alkali

Specimen

hair

Normal range
investigational

Comments
relatively drug-testing technique, but an active area of forensic and clinical
research

Source
Adapted from Kintz P, Cirimele V. Interlaboratory comparison of quantitative determination of amphetamine and
related compounds in hair samples. Forensic Science International 1997;84:151-156.

 ## Hallin carotid endarterectomy shunt

Description
surgical device similar to standard endarterectomy shunts using permanent
loop configuration and venting side arm

Source
Heyer-Schulte NeuroCare product information. Pleasant Prairie, WI.

 ## Hall segmental cement extraction system (SEG-CES) for femoral revisions

Description
SEG-CES of orthopaedic instruments; enables complete mantle extraction in
a broad range of revision cases

Source
Hall Surgical division of Zimmer Corp. product information. Largo, FL.

 ## halo cervical traction system

Description
cervical traction vest (model 1223) with 3-way adjustable head block; air bag
relieves pressure on spine; magnetic resonance imaging and computed
tomography (MRI/CT) compatible

Source
PMT Corp. product information. Chanhassen, MN.

 ## Handisol phototherapy device

Description
hand-held phototherapy device for treatment of psoriasis or vitiligo; ultraviolet A or B "light" wands; ideal for treating localized areas

Source
National Biological Corp. product information. Twinsburg, OH.

Hapad shoe insert

Description
natural wool felt foot pad; available orthotics include 3-way heel/arch and metatarsal insole, longitudinal metatarsal arch, metatarsal pads, medial/lateral heel wedges, heel pads, horseshoe heel pads, and heel wedges

Source
Hapad Inc. product information. Bethel Park, PA.

 Hapex bioactive material

Description
homogenous material used in otologic implants; composition results in bioactive material approximating the mechanical properties of cortical bone, yet soft enough to cut with a knife

Source
Smith & Nephew Richards Inc. product information. Memphis, TN.

 Hapset bone graft plaster

Description
bone graft plaster for dental implant; designed to address the need for a moldable hydroxylapatite (HA); Hapset plaster provides initial stabilization of HA particles, and later resorbs, leaving an HA scaffold for bony ingrowth

Source
Lifecore Biomedical product information. Chaska, MN.

 Har-el pharyngeal tube

Description
pharyngeal salivary bypass tube with unique funnel shape that allows anchoring at level of tongue base; for treatment of esophageal fistulas; can be used as prophylactic measure in patients who are at high risk for development of fistula

Source
Boston Medical Products product information. Waltham, MA.

 Hariri-Heifetz microsurgical system

Description
dual-ended instrument system with interlocking feature permitting pairing of instruments; eight different combinations of scissors, forceps, and needle holders

Source
Accurate Surgical & Scientific Instruments Corp. product information. Westbury, NY.

Hasson grasping forceps

Description
laparoscopic forceps with handle that provides 360-degree rotation; distinctive jaw configurations consisting of bullet tip, needle nose, ring, and spike tooth; secures tissue without requiring continuous hand pressure

Source
Cook OB/GYN product information. Spencer, IN.

 ## Haugh ear forceps

Description
microear forceps with serrated jaws; also available in smooth jaws

Source
Accurate Surgical & Scientific Instruments Corp. product information. Westbury, NY.

 ## Havrix

Generic name
see hepatitis A vaccine

 ## Hayek oscillator

Description
noninvasive ventilator alternative to controlled mechanical ventilation (CMV); for the treatment of acute and chronic respiratory insufficiency in both children and adults

Source
Breasy Medical Equipment product information. London, UK.

 ## Heart Aide, Heart Aide Plus and Heart Aide Plus II monitor

Description
Heart Aide is a postsymptomatic event recorder with multiple events; Heart Aide Plus a multiple event looping memory for presymptom and postsymptom event recordings; Heart Aide Plus II is the same as Heart Aide Plus with an additional lead configuration for dual-channel recording of the same event; can be used as a single channel or two channels with up to 135 seconds pretimes and posttimes each channel; all three models record up to 270 seconds total time

Source
TZ Medical Inc. product information. Lake Oswego, OR.

Heelbo decubitus protector

Description
tightly woven fabric offers snug fit and "breathe-ability" to encourage tissue granulation; goes on like a sock; no slippage prevents shearing
Source
Heelbo Inc. product information. Niles, IL.

Heel Hugger therapeutic heel stabilizer

Description
flexible fabric wrap that covers heel and upper foot only; sealed ice gel pads on each side stabilize calcaneus and provide cold therapy; limits lateral and medial movement of heel; absorbs shock to heel; gel pads can be used for cold therapy
Source
Brown Medical Ind. product information. Hartley, IA.

Heel Spur Special

Description
an orthosis designed to resolve specific biomechanical problems
Source
STJ Orthotic Services Inc. product information. Ridgewood, NY.

Helidac

Generic name
see metronidazole/tetracycline, bismuth subsalicylate

hemisection uterine morcellation technique

Description
bisection of the midline anteroposterior division of enlarged uterus to reduce size
Anatomy
cervix; vagina; uterine fundus; uterus
Equipment
knife or heavy scissors; retractors
Source
Adapted from Pelosi MA, Pelosi MA III. A comprehensive approach to morcellation of the large uterus. Contemporary OB/GYN 1997;42:106-125.

hemispherical deafferentation

Description
alternative technique for intractable epilepsy associated with infantile hemi-plegia; deafferentiates (eliminates) afferent nerve pathways connecting the affected hemisphere to contralateral hemisphere; temporofrontal question-mark incision followed by anterior temporal lobectomy, including hip-pocampectomy and amygdalectomy; perisylvian transcortical incision and transventricular callosotomy; dissect down to interhemispherical fissure; remove white matter and cortex to reach previous dissection

Anatomy
splenium and rostrum of corpus callosum; sylvian cortex and fissure; supra-sylvian frontal operculum; superior temporal gyrus; temporal horn and stem; amygdala; hippocampus; uncus; lateral ventricular system; insular and peri-insular cortex; basal ganglia; frontobasal and occipitobasal white matter; ante-rior horn; trigone; frontobasal arachnoid; basofrontal and mediobasal occipi-tal lobes; choroidal fissure; choroid plexus; pericallosal artery; vein of Labbé; calcarine sulcus; falx; cella media; sphenoid wing; interhemispheric fissure; septum pellucidum; hemispherical mantle

Equipment
standard neurosurgery equipment; sucker; Tabotamp R (oxidized cellulose gauze)

Source
Adapted from Schramm J, Behrens E, Entzian W. Hemispherical deafferentation: an alternative to functional hemispherectomy. Neurosurgery 1995;36:509-516.

 ## hemoglobin S rapid assay

Synonyms
sickle hemoglobin rapid assay, Hgb S assay, Quantitative S

Use
determination of hemoglobin S percentage in patients receiving blood trans-fusion therapy

Method
rapid microcolumn chromatographic assay

Specimen
blood

Normal range
not applicable

Comments
investigational, but likely to become more widely used

Source
University of Minnesota Department of Laboratory Medicine and Pathology. Minneapolis, MN.

hepatic cryosurgery studied vs resection in treating hepatic metastases from colorectal adenocarcinoma

Synonyms

colorectal cancer

Indications

patient diagnosed with hepatic metastases; all patients had documented metastatic tumors in liver originating from colorectal adenocarcinoma

Method

anesthesia consisting of endotracheal anesthesia with arterial and pulmonary artery pressure monitoring; liver exposed via extended right subcostal incision, exploration, biopsies, liver scanned, resectable lesions excised; remaining lesions ablated by cryosurgery

Normal findings

not applicable

Source

Adapted from Weaver ML, Atkinson D, Zemel R. Hepatic cryosurgery in treating colorectal metastases. Cancer 1995;76:210-214.

 # hepatic transplantation with aberrant hepatic artery

Description

living-related hepatic transplantation (LRHT) performed as a means of alleviating problem of graft shortage of cadaveric transplant; living donor supplies partial hepatectomy while preserving graft viability; left-sided hepatic graft implanted into recipient by method routinely used for reduced-size or split hepatic transplantation; technical modification is accomplished when donor may have hepatic arterial variant; donors are used with an aberrant left hepatic artery

Anatomy

Arantius ligament; afferent and efferent vessels; Cantlie line; caudate lobe; hepatic hilum; hepatic arteries and veins; lesser omentum; parenchyma; portal vein

Equipment

standard surgical equipment; Doppler ultrasonograph

Source

Adapted from Takayama T, Makuuchi M, Kawarasaki H, et al. Hepatic transplantation using living donors with aberrant hepatic artery. American College of Surgeons 1997;184:525-527.

 # hepatitis A vaccine

Brand name

Havrix

Use

prevention of hepatitis A infection

Usual dosage
intramuscular: 1440 ELISA units/injection; 2 doses required for complete protection; second dose should be administered 6-12 months after the initial dose

Pharmaceutical company
SmithKline Beecham. Philadelphia, PA.

Source
University of Pittsburgh Drug Information and Pharmacoepidemiology Center. Pittsburgh, PA.

 hepatitis B DNA detection

Synonyms
DNA hybridization test; DNA probe test; HBV DNA; HBV DNA probe test; hepatitis B viral DNA assay

Use
diagnose hepatitis B virus (HBV) versus non B hepatitis entities; establish stage of disease

Method
slot-blot deoxyribonucleic acid (DNA) hybridization-based assay using radiolabeled DNA probe

Specimen
blood; liver tissue

Normal range
uninfected serum or tissue contains no hepatitis B viral DNA

Comments
none

Source
Lexi-Comp Inc. database. Hudson, OH.

 hepatitis C RNA detection

Synonyms
quantitative HCV RNA

Use
assess baseline viremia levels before initiation of alpha-interferon therapy for chronic hepatitis C virus (HCV); monitor response during or after therapy; predict and evaluate prognosis of HCV chronically infected patients

Method
chemiluminescent hybridization assay

Specimen
blood

Normal range
uninfected serum contains no hepatitis C viral ribonucleic acid (RNA)

Comments
light emission results are directly proportional to the amount of viral RNA in the sample

Source
Lexi-Comp Inc. database. Hudson, OH.

 hepatitis C virus antibody detection

Synonyms
HCV by RIBA; RIBA HCV

Use
recombinant immunoblot assay (RIBA) identifies 4 recombinant hepatitis C virus (HCV)-coded antigens, 5-1-1, V100-3, C33C, and C22-3; may be used as an aid in the differential diagnosis of patients with clinical evidence of hepatitis

Method
radioimmunoassay (RIA); enzyme-linked immunosorbent assay (ELISA); enzyme immunoassay (EIA)

Specimen
blood

Normal range
negative

Comments
anti-HCV indicates past or present infection but does not necessarily constitute a diagnosis; positive anti-HCV result by EIA but not confirmed by RIBA does not rule out the possibility of infection with HCV

Source
Lexi-Comp Inc. database. Hudson, OH.

 hepatitis C virus (HCV) quantification by in situ reverse transcriptase-polymerase chain reaction (RT-PCR)

Synonyms
HCV measurement by RT-PCR

Use
determination of residual hepatitis C virus in peripheral blood of patients with hepatitis C

Method
reverse transcriptase PCR with fluorescent-tagged primers detected by flow cytometry

Specimen
blood

Normal range
no evidence of HCV-specific fluorescent amplicon

Comments
likely to become widely used in monitoring patients with chronic hepatitis C, particularly those undergoing liver transplant

Source
Adapted from Muratori L, Gibellini D, Lenzi M, Cataleta M, Muratori P, Morelli MC, Bianchi FB. Quantification of hepatitis C virus-infected peripheral blood mononuclear cells by in situ reverse transcriptase-polymerase chain reaction. Blood 1996;88:2768-2774.

 hereditary hemochromatosis genotyping

Synonyms
hereditary hemochromatosis genetic testing; $G_{845}A$ mutation test

Use
early diagnosis of hereditary hemochromatosis

Method
polymerase chain reaction-based amplification of the $G_{845}A$ mutation in the hemochromatosis gene

Specimen
blood

Normal range
$G_{845}A$ mutation absent

Comments
over 83% of patients with hereditary hemochromatosis, a highly treatable autosomal recessive disorder of iron metabolism, have the $G_{845}A$ mutation

Source
Adapted from Jazwinska EC, Powell LW. Hemochromatosis and HLA-H. Hepatology 1997;25:495-496.

 Hermetic external ventricular and lumbar drainage systems

Description
completely closed drainage systems from site to drainage port which provides an instant, sterile path for cerebrospinal fluid (CSF) drainage; the lumbar drainage set provides an alternate route for draining CSF through the lumbar spine

Source
Heyer-Schulte NeuroCare product information. Pleasant Prairie, WI.

 herpes simplex DNA detection

Synonyms
HSV DNA; HSV PCR reaction

Use
less invasive method than biopsy to assist in diagnosis of viral encephalitis or meningitis due to herpes simplex virus (HSV); request viral culture and direct viral detection of all suspected viruses

Method
HSV deoxyribonucleic acid (DNA) amplification by polymerase chain reaction (PCR) and detection using hybridization

Specimen
cerebrospinal fluid; other sterile body fluids

Normal range
negative

Comments
unable to differentiate between HSV 1 and 2; unlike viral culture, HSV DNA does not detect other viral agents

Source
Lexi-Comp Inc. database. Hudson, OH.

 Hexalen

Generic name
see altretamine

 hexoprenaline sulfate

Brand name
Delaprem

Use
selective beta 2 agonist used in the treatment of premature labor and acute fetal distress

Usual dosage
intravenous: initial loading dose of 7.5 to 10 mcg followed by a continuous infusion of 0.15 to 0.3 mcg/min; rate of the infusion may be increased until uterine activity has halted

Pharmaceutical company
Savage Laboratories. Melville, NY.

Source
University of Pittsburgh Drug Information and Pharmacoepidemiology Center. Pittsburgh, PA.

 HGM Spectrum K1 krypton yellow & green laser

Description
laser for vascular and pigmented lesions, removing ectasias caused by skin peels, dermabrasion and CO_2 resurfacing, scar revisions of postoperative cosmetic incisions

Source
HGM Medical Laser Systems Inc. product information. Salt Lake City, UT.

HLA-B2702 peptide

Brand name
Allotrap 2702

Use
a human HLA-derived peptide to promote graft acceptance, following solid organ transplantation

Usual dosage
intravenous: clinical trials have used 7 mg/kg initiated the day of transplantation, followed by an additional 2 to10 days in combination with standard immunosuppressive regimens

Pharmaceutical company
SangStat Medical Corp. Menlo Park, CA.

Source
Stadtlanders Managed Pharmacy Services. Pittsburgh, PA.

HLA-eluted random-donor platelet (RDP) concentrates

Synonyms
HLA-eluted RDP

Use
removal of platelet and mononuclear cell surface HLA class I molecules prior to transfusion into HLA-sensitized, transfusion-refractory patients

Method
brief incubation of platelet-rich plasma with buffered citric acid, followed by neutralization, washing, and transfusion

Specimen
platelet-rich plasma

Normal range
not applicable

Comments
possible alternative to HLA-matched platelet transfusions

Source
Adapted from Novotny VMJ, Huizinga TWJ, van Doorn R, Briët E, Brand A. HLA class I-eluted platelets as an alternative to HLA-matched platelets. Transfusion 1996;36:438-444.

holmium laser lithotriptor (lithotripter)

Description
treats urinary calculi safely and has particular efficacy in complex clinical presentations

Source
Adapted from Grasso M, Ficazzola M. Expanded experience with the holmium laser as an endoscopic lithotrite. American Urological Association 92nd annual meeting 1997; Abstracts.

Horizon nasal CPAP (continuous positive airway pressure) system

Description
innovative breathing activation system for easy start-up with a pressure-delay that makes it more comfortable for patients to fall asleep; micro-processor blower control system automatically adjusts to pressure changes and maintains prescribed pressure level; remote clinical utilization meter provides polysomnographic outputs relating to snoring events, mouth breathing, and mask leaks

Source
DeVilbiss Health Care Inc. product information. Sommerset, PA.

horseshoe LeFort I osteotomy

Description
one-stage surgical technique for reconstruction of the severely atrophic maxilla permits endosteal implant placement, which will secondarily allow for prosthetic attachment and total rehabilitation of the patient

Anatomy
maxilla; hard palate; soft palate; alveolar ridge; sinus mucosa

Equipment
elevator; tension compression screws; endosseous dental implants

Source
Adapted from Ewers R, Kirsch A, Watzinger F et al. Horseshoe LeFort I osteotomy of the maxilla in combination with endosseous dental implants. Implant Dentistry 1996;5:118.

Hoskins-Barkan goniotomy infant lens

Description
lens designed for transverse goniotomy surgery; features a wide aperture anterior surface with magnified view of anterior chamber of eye and angle

Source
Ocular Instruments Inc. product information. Bellevue, WA.

Hosmer voluntary control (VC4) four-bar knee orthosis

Description
orthotic device designed for the amputee; aggressive walker which allows the amputee control over a greater degree of flexion; pneumatic swing phase control allows variable cadence

Source
Hosmer product information. Campbell, CA.

Hosmer weight activated locking knee (W.A.L.K.) prosthesis

Description
available in titanium, aluminum, and stainless steel; includes a patella and an adjustable extension assist

Source
Orthotic Prosthetic Supplies product information. Alpharetta, GA.

 HTLV-1 infectivity assay

Synonyms
HTLV-1 cell-to-cell transmission assay; human T-leukemia virus type 1 cell-to-cell transmission assay

Use
quantitative evaluation of HTLV-1 cell-to-cell transmission in a single round of infection

Method
functional analysis following controlled cell-to-cell HTLV-1 infection

Specimen
isolated viral specimen

Normal range
not applicable

Comments
permits, for the first time, determination of the HTLV-1 molecules required for infectivity

Source
Adapted from Delamarre L, Rosenberg AR, Pique C, Pham D, Dokhélar MC. A novel human T-leukemia virus type 1 cell-to-cell transmission assay permits definition of SU glycoprotein amino acids important for infectivity. Journal of Virology 1997;71:259-266.

 human immunodeficiency virus DNA amplification

Synonyms
HIV DNA amplification assay; HIV DNA PCR test; HIV proviral DNA by polymerase chain reaction amplification; PCR for HIV DNA

Use
identify human immunodeficiency virus (HIV) in patients with unusual or indeterminate HIV serology; useful in patients with immunodeficiency syndromes characterized by a negative HIV serology and Western blot tests

Method
amplification by polymerase chain reaction (PCR) and hybridization with an HIV-specific deoxyribonucleic acid (DNA) probe; hybridization with the HIV DNA probe can be detected using autoradiography or enzymatic detection procedures

Specimen
peripheral blood lymphocytes from 10-20 ml whole blood

Normal range
uninfected serum contains no HIV DNA

Comments
none

Source
Lexi-Comp Inc. database. Hudson, OH.

 # human immunodeficiency virus (HIV) antigen testing

Synonyms
p24 antigen testing

Use
direct viral detection for blood donation screening

Method
reverse transcriptase polymerase chain reaction

Specimen
blood

Normal range
negative

Comments
FDA recently began to require blood banks to perform HIV antigen testing

Source
Adapted from Korelitz JJ, Busch MP, Williams AE, et al. Antigen testing for the human immunodeficiency virus (HIV) and the magnet effect: will the benefit of a new HIV test be offset by the numbers of higher-risk, test-seeking donors attracted to blood centers? Transfusion 1996;36:203-208.

 # human immunodeficiency virus Type 2 antibody detection

Synonyms
HIV-2 antibody detection

Use
document exposure to human immunodeficiency virus-2 (HIV-2); supplemental test for samples which give an indeterminate result on the HIV-1 Western blot and test positive on screening assay

Method
enzyme immunoassay (EIA)

Specimen
blood

Normal range
nonreactive

Comments
cross reactivity exists between HIV-1 and HIV-2 which may cause a false positive result in the HIV-2 test

Source
Lexi-Comp Inc. database. Hudson, OH.

humanized monoclonal antibody (MAb)-cA2

Brand name
CenTNF

Use
tumor necrosis factor (TNF) blocker, controls inflammatory process in Crohn disease

Usual dosage
injectable: a single intravenous infusion in dosage range of 5-20 mg/kg has been studied

Pharmaceutical company
Cetocor, Inc. Malvern, PA.

Source
Stadtlanders Managed Pharmacy Services. Pittsburgh, PA.

human lymphocyte antigen (HLA) class I enzyme-linked immunosorbent assay (ELISA)

Synonyms
HLA ELISA

Use
detection of anti-HLA class I IgG (immunoglobulin G) antibodies in patients being evaluated for kidney transplant

Method
soluble-phase ELISA

Specimen
serum

Normal range
no antibodies detected

Comments
simpler than the current standard, microlymphocytotoxicity testing, and equivalent in sensitivity and specificity.

Source
Adapted from Buelow R, Mercier I, Glanville L, Regan J, Ellingson L, Janda G, Claas F, Colombe B, Gelder F, Grosse-Wilde H et al. Detection of panel-reactive anti-HLA class I antibodies by enzyme-linked immunosorbent assay or lymphocytotoxicity. Results of a blinded, controlled multicenter study. Human Immunology 1995;44:1-11.

human lymphocyte antigen (HLA)-DRB and -DRQ DNA typing

Synonyms
LCR-based HLA typing

Use
typing of prospective tissue donors

Method
differential ligation-based amplification of target DNA (deoxyribonucleic acid)

Specimen
blood
Normal range
not applicable
Comments
simpler and more rapid than differential hybridization methods
Source
Adapted from Fischer GF, Fae I, Petrasek M, Moser S. A combination of two distinct in vitro amplification procedures for DNA typing of HLA-DRB and -DQB alleles. Vox Sanguinis 1995;69:328-335.

 human T-cell leukemia/lymphoma virus (HTLV-1) retrovirus specific antibody testing using dried blood specimens

Synonyms
none
Use
rapid, large-scale screening for HTLV-I
Method
gelatin particle agglutination test
Specimen
dried blood spot samples collected on filter paper
Normal range
no evidence of agglutination
Comments
sensitive, specific and inexpensive method for the detection of HTLV-I antibody
Source
Adapted from Parker SP, Taylor MB, Ades AE, Cubitt WD, Peckham C. Use of dried blood spots for the detection and confirmation of HTLV-I specific antibodies for epidemiological purposes. Journal of Clinical Pathology 1995;48:904-907.

 Humatrix Microclysmic gel

Description
used in treatment of tissue trauma, third degree burns, radiation irritation, mechanical injuries, laser peel, autograft and chronic acute wound therapy; modifies endothermic properties of tissue to reduce surface temperatures 10 to 15 degrees in first three minutes after application; heat reduction capacity achieved by molecular heat transfer with surrounding air
Source
Care-Tech Laboratories product information. St. Louis, MO.

Hunkeler frown incision marker

Description
ophthalmic surgical instrument designed for preparing one-stitch and no-stitch scleral cataract incisions; linear marks leave 10 mm radial curve for incision, as well as for identification of 3.0, 4.0, 5.0, and 6.0 mm incisions

Source
American Surgical Instruments Corp. product information. Westmont, IL.

 Hunstad anesthesia system

Description
variable pressure control for infusion procedures; Pressurefuse automatic constant pressure dual intravenous bags mount behind hinged, transparent unit that plugs into standard air or oxygen outlets to deliver a constant 300 mmHg pressure

Source
Byron product information. Tucson, AZ.

 Hunstad infusion needle

Description
needle with spiral perforations for rapid infusion of anesthesia during the wet technique

Source
Byron Medical product information. (*Editor note:* advertising uses byron but company name correctly is Byron) Tucson, AZ.

 hyaluronic acid

Brand Name
Orthovisc

Use
soft tissue lubricants used in the treatment of temporomandibular joint dysfunction

Usual Dosage
intramuscular: 1% sodium hyaluronate in physiologic saline with a concentration of 10 μg/ml

Pharmaceutical company
MedChem. Woburn, MA.

Source
University of Pittsburgh Drug Information and Pharmacoepidemiology Center. Pittsburgh, PA.

H-Y antigen gene detection

Synonyms
histocompatibility antigen gene detection

Use
evaluation of delayed transplant engraftment, prenatal diagnosis in sex-linked congenital abnormalities, evaluation of minimal residual disease in bone marrow transplantation

Method
polymerase chain reaction

Specimen
blood, tissue biopsy

Normal range
H-Y antigen gene present or absent

Comments
H-Y antigen is thought to inhibit acceptance, by female recipients, of tissue transplanted from male donors

Source
Science 1995;269:1588-1590.

 Hybrid graft

Description
polytetrafluoroethylene (PTFE) vascular graft reduces needle hole bleeding, improves suture time, resists torque compression and anastomotic kinking; latest in "thru-pore" technology; 60/20 micron pore size

Source
Atrium Medical Corp. product information. Hollis, NH.

 hybrid total hip replacement

Description
total hip replacement with insertion of porous-coated acetabular component without cement; femoral component using cement for treatment of painful hip due to osteoarthrosis, rheumatoid arthritis, avascular necrosis, and other causes; addresses postoperative loosening and/or migration of one or both components

Anatomy
hip joint; hip socket; femur; acetabulum; cancellous bone; femoral canal; lower extremities

Equipment
standard surgery equipment; Harris Precoat femoral component implant; Harris-Galante-I acetabular component implant; reamer; titanium screws; surgical drill; Simplex-P methyl methacrylate; suction drains

Source
Adapted from Mohler CG, Kull LR, Martell JM, Rosenberg AG, Galante JO. Total hip replacement with insertion of an acetabular component without cement and a femoral component with cement. The Journal of Bone and Joint Surgery 1995;77-A:86-96.

 Hycamtin

Generic name
see topotecan

 hyCURE wound care product

Description
hydrolyzed powder interacts with wound site as it forms a gel when mixing with wound exudate and provides moist healing environment; wound filler and exudate absorber specifically formulated for chronic wound and dermal ulcer treatment

Source
The Hymed Group product information. Bethlehem, PA.

 Hyde-Osher keratometric ruler

Description
ophthalmic device serves two purposes, location of cylindrical axis and measurement of astigmatism; by rotating the ruler and aligning notches with steepest axis of cylinder, a reflected ring of light appears circular when astigmatism is neutralized

Source
Ocular Instruments Inc. product information. Bellevue, WA.

 hydrocele localization

Description
translabial ultrasound localization and hookwire needle stabilization to excise canal of Nuck (persistent processus vaginalis) hydrocele; technique allows surgical excision of this mobile mass without extensive exploration and trauma

Anatomy
vulva; labia majora; external inguinal ring; canal of Nuck; inguinal canal

Equipment
standard surgery equipment; ultrasonograph; 6.5-cm Homer Mammalok Plus needle

Source
Adapted from Miklos JR, Karram MM, Silver E, Reid R. Ultrasound and hookwire needle placement for localization of a hydrocele of the canal of Nuck. Obstetrics and Gynecology 1995;85:884-886.

 hydrochlorothiazide

Brand name
Microzide

Use
low-dose thiazide diuretic for the treatment of edema and mild-to-moderate hypertension

Usual dosage
oral: 12.5 mg once a day

Pharmaceutical company
Watson Laboratories Inc. Corona, CA.

Source
Stadtlanders Managed Pharmacy Services. Pittsburgh, PA.

 Hydrocol wound dressing

Description
sterile, occlusive hydrocolloid wound dressing designed to optimize moisture management and decrease frequency of dressing changes; unique sacral design features flexible hinge that enhances ease of application

Source
Dow Hickam Pharmaceuticals product information. Sugarland, TX.

 hydrocortisone

Brand name
Sarnol-HC

Use
external preparation containing 1% hydrocortisone, camphor, and menthol for the treatment of steroid responsive dermatoses

Usual dosage
topical: apply 3 to 4 times a day or as directed

Pharmaceutical company
Stiefel Laboratories. Miami, FL.

Source
Stadtlanders Managed Pharmacy Services. Pittsburgh, PA.

hydrocortisone buteprate

Brand name
Pandel

Use
for relief of corticosteroid-responsive dermatosis

Usual dosage
topical: 0.1% cream; apply to the affected areas two to three times per day

Pharmaceutical company
Savage Laboratories. Melville, NY.

Source
Stadtlanders Managed Pharmacy Services. Pittsburgh, PA.

Hydrofloss electronic oral irrigator

Description
dental flossing system that uses tap water and magnetohydrodynamics; alters electrical charges by reversing the polarity of ions; customarily used three times a day for oral hygiene

Source
HYDRO FLOSS INC. product information. Birmingham, AL.

Hyflex X-File instruments

Description
flexible, sharp nickel titanium instruments that cut faster for canal instrumentation; sharp double-fluted design holds debris and transports it out of the canal; durable and damage resistant; sizes 08, 10, and 12.5 in stainless steel for pathfinding

Source
The Hygenic Corp. product information. Akron, OH.

Hygroscopic Condenser Humidifier (HCH)

Description
captures and limits loss of patient's own exhaled moisture and heat; available with and without filtration

Source
Baxter Healthcare Corp. product information. Round Lake, IL.

256

 hypercoagulability testing

Synonyms
none

Indications
test for patients who develop thrombosis in the apparent absence of clinically recognized risk factors

Method
screening tests for hypercoagulable states include natural anticoagulants, fibrinolysis, antiphospholipid protein antibodies, hyperhomocystinemia, and serum homocysteine testing

Normal findings
activity based assays detect loss of function

Comments
as understanding of the coagulation system grows, more abnormalities are recognized in the balance between procoagulant and anticoagulant mechanisms

Source
Adapted from Hassell KL. A practical guide to hypercoagulability testing. Internal Medicine 1996;17:55-64.

 Hyperex thoracic orthosis

Description
lightweight, adjustable orthosis that restricts forward flexion of the thoracolumbar spine; 3-point pressure principle encourages a hyperextended posture; suited for anterior unloading of the thoracic vertebral bodies

Source
United States Manufacturing Co. product information. Pasadena, CA.

 hypospadias repair with urethrocutaneous flap

Description
modification technique for distal hypospadias with minimal or no chordee utilizing advancement of a distally deepithelialized urethrocutaneous flap; procedure incorporates correction of chordee, mobilization of the urethrocutaneous flap, and advancement of the flap through a tunnel until it reaches the tip of the glans; wide tunnel is obtained through the glans over the corpus cavernosum

Anatomy
Buck fascia; corpus spongiosum; coronal sulcus; distal urethra; glans penis; meatal orifice; mucosa; penile shaft; urethra; urethral meatus

Equipment
standard urologic surgery equipment

Source
Adapted from Sensoz O, Celebioglu S, Baran CN, Kocer U, Tellioglu AT. A new technique for distal hypospadias repair: advancement of a distally deepithelialized urethrocutaneous flap. Plastic and Reconstructive Surgery 1997;99:93-97.

Hyzaar

Generic Name
see losartan potassium/hydrochlorothiazide

 # ibutilide fumarate

Brand Name
Corvert

Use
antiarrhythmic for the treatment of atrial fibrillation and atrial flutter as an alternative to electric cardioversion

Usual Dosage
intravenous infusion: 0.125 mg/kg

Pharmaceutical company
Pharmacia & Upjohn. Kalamazoo, MI.

Source
Samford University Global Drug Information Service. Birmingham, AL.

 # Icorel

Generic name
see nicorandil

 # idebenone

Brand Name
Avan

Use
benzoquinone that acts as a free radical scavenger and electron trapping agent used in the treatment of Alzheimer disease

Usual dosage
oral: 30 mg three times daily after meals

Pharmaceutical company
Abbott Labs. Abbott Park, IL.

Source
University of Pittsburgh Drug Information and Pharmacoepidemiology Center. Pittsburgh, PA.

 # Igloo Heatshield system

Description
humidity controlled and warmed environment for low-birth-weight infants

Source
Nascor product information. Crows Nest, Australia.

ileal neobladder in women

Description

urethral support and nerve sparing cystectomy; when used as a reservoir, provides excellent continence; with the nerve and urethral support sparing technique, the urethral closure mechanism rhabdosphincter muscle of the lower urethra, and fibers of the inferior hypogastric plexus supporting the urethra and vagina are left intact; after completion of ureteroileal anastomosis the floor of the neobladder is moderately stretched and anchored to the anterior vaginal wall

Anatomy

autonomic nerve fibers; bladder neck and wall; broad ligament; endopelvic fascia; inferior hypogastric plexus; perivesical vascular plexus; paraurethral vascular and nerve plexus; urethra; rhabdosphincter muscle; ureter; ureterosacral ligaments; urethrovesical junction; vaginal wall; ureteropelvic ligaments

Equipment

standard urologic surgery equipment; Ellis clamp

Source

Adapted from Hautmann RE, Paiss T, de Petriconi R. The ileal neobladder in women: 9 years of experience with 18 patients. The Journal of Urology 1996;155:76-81.

 ## Ile-Sorb absorbent gel packet

Description

absorbent gel packets; transforms liquid in ostomy pouch to semi-solid gel; keeps pouch contents away from stoma; reduces sloshing and pouch noise

Source

Bristol-Myers Squibb Co. product information. Princeton, NJ.

 ## imciromab pentetate

Brand name

Myoscint

Use

diagnosis of myocardial infarction

Usual dosage

injectable available as a two-vial kit with the first containing 0.5 mg of Myoscint and 1 ml of sodium phosphate and is added to the second vial containing sodium citrate; IV injection of full dose is recommended; after mixing, the vial is radiolabeled with Indium III chlorine

Pharmaceutical company

Centocor. Malvern, PA.

Source

University of Pittsburgh Drug Information and Pharmacoepidemiology Center. Pittsburgh, PA.

imiglucerase

Brand name
Cerezyme

Use
long-term enzyme replacement therapy used for Type 1 Gaucher disease

Usual dosage
intravenous: 2.5-60 units/kg infused over 1-2 hours repeated every 2 weeks; can be given as often as 3 times weekly or as infrequently as every 4 weeks, depending upon response

Pharmaceutical company
Genzyme Corp. Cambridge, MA.

Source
University of Pittsburgh Drug Information and Pharmacoepidemiology Center. Pittsburgh, PA.

 imiquimod

Brand name
Aldara

Use
a self-administered cream for the treatment of genital and perianal warts

Usual dosage
topical: 1% cream to be applied three times a week at bedtime for up to 16 weeks

Pharmaceutical company
3M Pharmaceuticals. St. Paul, MN.

Source
Stadtlanders Managed Pharmacy Services. Pittsburgh, PA.

 Imitrex

Generic name
see sumatriptan

 immature oocyte retrieval (IOR)

Description
technique utilizing transvaginal ultrasound retrieval of unstimulated oocytes to be matured in vitro

Anatomy
vagina; cervix; uterus; fallopian tubes

Equipment
transvaginal ultrasound probe; standard OB/GYN in vitro fertilization equipment

Source
Adapted from Scarbeck K. New IVF procedure uses immature oocytes. Ob.Gyn. News 1996;31:14.

Immediate Implant Impression system

Description
surgical system that allows fabrication of a temporary prosthesis for insertion at second-stage surgery

Source
Steri-Oss product information. Yorba Linda, CA.

Immediate Response Mobile Analysis (IRMA) blood analysis system

Description
includes a compact hand-held analyzer; measures blood gases and electrolytes with a turnaround time of less than two minutes

Source
Diametrics Medical Inc. product information. St. Paul, MN.

ImmunoCard *Mycoplasma pneumoniae* test

Synonyms
Mycoplasma ImmunoCard

Use
diagnosis of *Mycoplasma pneumoniae* infection

Method
rapid card-based ELISA for detection of IgM (immunoglobulin M) antibodies to *Mycoplasma pneumoniae*

Specimen
serum

Normal range
no evidence of reactivity

Comments
rapid and simple procedure for laboratories analyzing small numbers of specimens

Source
Adapted from Alexander TS, Gray LD, Kraft JA, Leland DS, Nikaido MT, Willis DH. Performance of Meridian ImmunoCard *Mycoplasma* test in a multicenter clinical trial. Journal of Clinical Microbiology 1996;34:1180-1183.

ImmunoCard used for diagnosis of *Helicobacter pylori*

Synonyms
none

Indications
symptoms of stomach ulcer, stomach cancer and other gastric ailments

Method
detection of IgG antibody to *H. pylori* in serum specimens

Normal findings
not applicable

Comments
credit card-size enzyme immunoassay test can be performed in seven minutes in doctor's office, HMO's, nursing homes and hospital settings

Source
Meridian Diagnostics product information. Cincinnati, OH.

 immunoscintigraphy for detection of recurrent colorectal cancer

Synonyms
111-indium-anti-TAG72 antibody scan; 111-indium-satumomab pendetide scan; OncoScint scan

Indications
suspicion of metastatic or recurrent colorectal cancer based on other radiological studies; elevated serum CEA, liver function tests, or abnormal physical exam

Method
monoclonal antibodies directed against a tumor-associated surface antigen (TAG72) are labeled with the gamma emitting radionuclide indium-111 and intravenously injected; anterior and posterior imaging of chest, abdomen, and pelvis is performed using a standard gamma camera

Normal findings
normal uptake occurs in liver, spleen, and bone marrow; kidneys, bladder, and male genitalia may be faintly seen; increased activity may also be seen at colostomy sites, degenerated joints, abdominal aneurysms, and local inflammatory lesions

Comments
extrahepatic areas of increased activity not associated with normal structures or along the expected distribution of lymph nodes are likely to represent tumor recurrence or metastatic deposits; recent studies indicate this method may be more sensitive than computed tomography (CT) or magnetic resonance imaging (MRI)

Source
University of Maryland Department of Diagnostic Radiology. Baltimore, MD.

 Implanon

Generic name
see desogestrel

Implantaid Di-Lock cardiac lead introducer

Description

peel-away introducers designed for rapid insertion of transvenous leads and catheters with minimal venous trauma; easy to use with single- or dual-chamber pacing systems

Source

Intermedics Inc. product information. Angleton, TX.

 ## Implantech facial implants

Description

facial implants constructed using 3D scanning to create precise matching components for aesthetic and reconstructive facial surgery

Source

Implantech product information. Ventura, CA.

 ## implant site dilator

Description

dilator used in conjunction with the Sinus Lift osteotome to enlarge the osteotomy site to the desired implant diameter and height

Source

ACE Surgical Supply Company Inc. product information. Brockton, MA.

 ## Implatome dental tomography system

Description

instrument for dental tomography; constant magnification provides accurate diagnostic measurements directly from films and cross-sectional visualization of potential implant sites

Source

Steri-Oss Bausch & Lomb Co. product information. Yorba Linda, CA.

 ## Impress Softpatch

Description

single-use, prescription foam pad coated with adhesive on one side; creates a seal helping block urine leakage; external, noninvasive treatment for women with mild to moderate urinary incontinence

Source

UroMed Corp. product information. Needham, MA.

Impulse oxygen conserving device

Description
designed for use with portable oxygen cylinders; equipped with audible and visible alarms that alert users of no inspiration or low battery situations

Source
AirSep Corp. product information. Buffalo, NY.

 ## Imuthiol

Generic name
see diethyldithiocarbamate

 ## IMx CA 15-3 assay

Synonyms
Abbott 15-3 assay

Use
ongoing evaluation of patients with known malignancies

Method
microparticle automated enzyme immunoassay

Specimen
blood

Normal range
25 U/ml

Comments
adds automation to an otherwise complex assay now in use

Source
Adapted from van Kamp GJ, Bon GG, Verstraeten RA et al. Multicenter evaluation of the Abbott IMx CA 15-3 assay. Clinical Chemistry 1996;42:28-33.

 ## Incavo wire passer

Description
orthopaedic surgical instrument designed to pass multiple cerclage wires around a bone during a multiple wire wrap procedure

Source
Innomed Inc. product information. Savannah, GA.

INCERT sponge

Description
bioabsorbable, implantable sponge to prevent formation of postsurgical adhesions; not yet FDA approved; in preclinical trials

Source
Anika Therapeutics product information. Woburn, MA.

Indiana tome carpal tunnel release system

Description
device used for direct canal visualization and division of distal ligament without endoscope; divides only the transverse carpal ligament with minimal disturbance of other palmar structures

Source
Biomet Inc. product information. Warsaw, IN.

indinavir sulfate

Brand Name
Crixivan

Use
protease inhibitor for use in HIV-infected patients; to be used in combination with other antiretroviral agents

Usual Dosage
oral: 800 mg three times a day was used in clinical trials

Pharmaceutical company
Merck. West Point, PA.

Source
University of Pittsburgh Drug Information and Pharmacoepidemiology Center. Pittsburgh, PA.

indirect enzyme immunoassay (EIA) for anti-*Mycoplasma pneumoniae* IgM (immunoglobulin M)

Synonyms
M. pneumoniae IgM EIA

Use
serodiagnosis of acute *Mycoplasma pneumoniae* infection

Method
chromogenic indirect enzyme immunoassay using *Mycoplasma pneumoniae* glycolipid antigen and peroxidase-conjugated goat anti-human IgM

Specimen
serum

Normal range
must be determined for a specific population

Comments
normal or reference ranges may vary to optimize predictive value in different populations

Source
Adapted from Cimolai N, Cheong ACH. An assessment of a new diagnostic indirect enzyme immunoassay for the detection of anti-*Mycoplasma pneumoniae* IgM. American Journal of Clinical Pathology 1996;105:205-209.

 ## In-Exsufflator respiratory device

Description
assists patients in clearing retained bronchopulmonary secretions by gradually applying positive pressure to the airway then rapidly shifting to negative pressure; delivered via face mask or mouthpiece; produces a high expiratory flow rate from the lungs, simulating a cough; for any patient with ineffective cough due to poliomyelitis, spinal cord injuries, or other neurologic disorders accompanied by some paralysis of the respiratory muscle; particularly important for patients using noninvasive ventilation since performing suction is difficult without a tracheostomy tube

Source
JH Emerson Co. product information. Cambridge, MA.

 ## Infanrix

Generic name
see diphtheria and tetanus toxoids and acellular pertussis vaccine absorbed/DTaP

 ## Infiniti catheter introducer system

Description
Avanti 0S5 and 5F introducer systems minimize site trauma, ensure ease of entry, and provide excellent angiographic quality; patients are able to receive same-day catheterization surgery

Source
Cordis Corp. product information. Miami, FL.

 ## Infinity stirrups

Description
stirrups featuring remote-release handle; allows patient's leg to float weightlessly

Source
NuMED Surgical Inc. product information. Orange Village, OH.

infrared thermometry for detection of reflux of spermatic vein in varicocele

Synonyms
none

Indications
varicocele

Method
infrared thermometer measurement of scrotal temperatures

Normal findings
no increase in temperature

Comments
scrotal neck temperature increased with Valsalva maneuver with upright position; no significant increase in controls; two weeks after high ligation of internal spermatic vein scrotal temperature in patients decreased to same level

Source
Adapted from Takada T, Kitamura M, Matsumiya K. Infrared thermometry for rapid, noninvasive detection of reflux of spermatic vein in varicocele. The Journal of Urology 1996;156:1652-1654.

 INFUSET T

Description
fluid delivery system designed for use in liposuction, tissue expansion, and other tumescent related procedures

Source
Ackrad Laboratories Inc. product information. Cranford, NJ.

 Inhibace

Generic name
see cilazapril

 Inosiplex

Generic name
see isoprinosine

 Input PS (percutaneous sheath) introducer

Description
a sheath that allows patients to sit up comfortably postprocedure without compromise on insertion, catheter movement, or hemostasis

Source
C.R. Bard Inc. product information. Billerica, MA.

"inside-out" technique for establishing ankle portal

Description
surgical arthroscopy is used in the treatment of various anomalies of foot and ankle; traditionally, three main portals have been used; "inside-out" is used to establish one posterolateral portal, an adaptation of the Wissinger rod technique; portal usually established by measuring a fixed distance (2.5 cm) from tip of fibula and making an incision just lateral to the Achilles tendon; when using a 2.7-mm arthroscope, a separate inflow portal is helpful, especially if any shaving or burring is performed

Anatomy
Achilles tendon; capsule of ankle joint; fibula; tibialis anterior tendon; tibiotalar joint

Equipment
arthroscope; cannula dilator and introducer; inflow cannula; K-wire; tourniquet; well-leg holder; Zimmer distractor

Source
Adapted from Katchis SD, Smith RW. A simple way to establish the posterolateral portal in ankle arthroscopy. Foot and Ankle International Journal 1997;18:178-179.

 Insta-Nerve device

Description
noninvasive, pass measuring device for the diagnosis of carpal tunnel syndrome; provides monitoring of median nerve conduction latency for early detection of developing compression neuropathy and repetitive motion injury

Source
Insta-Nerve product information. Champlain, NY.

 INSTRA-mate instrument-holding spring

Description
surgical device for allowing safe and convenient positioning of microinstruments within the operating field; instruments can be easily placed onto the spring

Source
Accurate Surgical & Scientific Instruments Corp. product information. Westbury, NY.

 Integra artificial skin

Description
biological skin replacement system that advances the care of thermal injury; provides for immediate physiological wound closure for burns; donor sites can be reserved for optimal cosmetic or functional repair

Source
Integra LifeSciences Corp. product information. Plainsboro, NJ.

Integra tissue expander

Description
designed for more anatomical expansion and has a unique, low-profile design

Source
PMT Corp. product information. Chanhassen, MN.

 Integrilin

Generic name
see eptifibatide

 Intellicath pulmonary artery catheter

Description
catheter capable of automatic and continuous cardiac output (CCO) by thermodilution determination; involves release of heat from a thermal filament incorporated into the pulmonary artery catheter (PAC)

Source
Baxter Healthcare Corp. product information. Irvine, CA.

 Inteq small joint suturing system

Description
system includes cannulated curved and straight needle, suture retriever, and small joint suture hook handle; facilitates suturing of triangular fibrocartilage complex to dorsal capsule when peripheral separation has occurred

Source
Linvatec Corp. product information. Largo, FL.

 interferon beta-1a

Brand Name
Avonex

Use
recombinant interferon for use in multiple sclerosis

Usual Dosage
intramuscular: 30 µg once weekly

Pharmaceutical company
Biogen. Cambridge, MA.

Source
Samford University Global Drug Information Service. Birmingham, AL.

interleukin-3/granulocyte macrophage-colony stimulating factor fusion protein

Brand name
Pixykine

Use
used to treat neutropenia and thrombocytopenia in bone marrow transplant patients

Usual dosage
injectable: 750 μg/m² administered in 2 divided doses daily has been used in clinical trials

Pharmaceutical company
Immunex. Seattle, WA.

Source
University of Pittsburgh Drug Information and Pharmacoepidemiology Center. Pittsburgh, PA.

 interleukin-6

Brand name
Sigosix

Use
recombinant human interleukin-6 (IL-6) used in the treatment of thrombocytopenia caused by radiotherapy and chemotherapy, autologous bone marrow transplant, and malignant diseases

Usual dosage
subcutaneous: doses of 10 mcg/kg/day have been used in clinical trials

Pharmaceutical company
Serono Laboratories Inc. Norwell, MA.

Source
University of Pittsburgh Drug Information and Pharmacoepidemiology Center. Pittsburgh, PA.

 interleukin-8 (IL-8)/creatinine ratio

Synonyms
none

Use
altered ratio is indicative of peptic ulcer disease

Method
radioimmunoassay used to determine IL-8 and creatinine measurements

Specimen
fasting urine specimen

Normal range
greater than 0.6

Comments
low urinary excretion of the proinflammatory agent IL-8 as measured by IL-8/creatinine ratio is associated with increased gastric IL-8 levels and higher activity of gastritis

Source
Adapted from Taha AS, Kelly RW, Carr G et al. Altered urinary interleukin-8/creatinine ratio in peptic ulcer disease: pathological and diagnostic implications. The American Journal of Gastroenterology 1996;91:2528-2531.

 internal fixation of spine using braided titanium cable

Description
braided titanium cable has the advantage of producing minimal magnetic resonance imaging artifact as compared to steel cable or monofilament wire, and is an instrument for segmental spine fixation; the cable consists of a 49-strand wire (seven groups of seven titanium wires braided together); the free end of the cable is inserted through an integral crimp; a provisional crimp prevents cable slippage while the cable loop is tightened by the tensioner

Anatomy
atlantoaxial vertebrae; cervicothoracic area; cervical spine; cranial base; interspinous region; intervertebral disk; lamina; occipitocervical area; spinal canal; suboccipital region; sublaminar area; thoracic spine

Equipment
braided titanium cable; tensioner; lateral mass plates; contoured 5-mm rod; transarticular screws; Luque rectangle or rod

Source
Adapted from Doran SE, Papadopoulos SM, Miller LD. Internal fixation of the spine using a braided titanium cable: clinical results and postoperative magnetic resonance imaging. Neurosurgery Journal 1996;38:493-497.

 internal mastopexy

Description
procedure to resculpt breast tissue following removal of silicone gel breast implant; corrects laxity, ptosis, and parenchymal maldistribution; inframammary incision; skin flap elevated from nipple-areola complex to inframammary fold; breast tissue invaginated; breast parenchyma plicated in layers with sutures

Anatomy
breast mound; breast parenchyma; nipple-areola complex; inframammary fold

Equipment
standard surgery equipment

Source
Adapted from Scioscia PJ, Hagerty RC. Internal mastopexy following explantation. Plastic and Reconstructive Surgery 1996;97:1014-1019.

interstitial laser coagulation (ILC)

Description
ILC necrotizes well-defined tissue volumes interstitially, leading to subsequent resorption and tumor or benign tissue reduction; designed to minimize complications associated with more invasive structures while preserving healthy structures

Anatomy
urological tissue

Equipment
830 nanometer (nm) portable diode laser

Source
Adapted from Muschter R, Delarosette J, Whitfield H, Pellerin JP, Madersbacher S, Gillatt D. Initial human clinical experience with diode-laser interstitial treatment of benign prostatic hyperplasia. Urology 1996;48:223-228.

 INTRACELL mechanical muscle device

Description
allows rehabilitating patient to self-perform general and segmental therapeutic procedures with precision; nonmotorized biomechanical device is composed of semirigid core around which smooth independent 1-inch modules freely revolve; rolling, stretching, twisting, and compressing of muscle tissue converts noncompliant into compliant muscle

Source
Scrip Inc. product information. Peoria, IL.

 intracranial meningioma resection

Description
intracranial meningioma resection by means of an interactive surgical navigation (ISN) system ("frameless stereotaxy"); ISN system locates minimal craniotomy and optimizes bone flap design; location of parasagittal draining veins and carotid or basilar arteries identified; traditional frame-based stereotaxy with intricate computer-assisted systems provides surgical guidance for primary intra-axial brain tumors and metastases to brain; reduces wound and neurologic morbidity

Anatomy
skull; brain; superior sagittal sinus; basilar artery intracranial meningioma resection

Equipment
standard neurosurgery equipment; interactive neurosurgical navigation device; 3-D sonic digitizer, ISN wand

Source
Adapted from Barnett GH, Steiner CP, Weisenberger J. Intracranial meningioma resection using frameless stereotaxy. Journal of Image Guided Surgery 1995;1:46-52.

intracranial pressure (ICP) Express digital monitor

Description
provides a continuous digital display of systolic, diastolic, and mean intracranial pressure

Source
Johnson & Johnson Professional Inc. product information. Raynham, MA.

 intramyometrial coring uterine morcellation technique

Description
coring technique for removing enlarged uterus vaginally

Anatomy
cervix; vagina; uterine fundus; uterus; isthmus; uterine corpus

Equipment
knife or heavy scissors; retractors

Source
Adapted from Pelosi MA, Pelosi MA III. A comprehensive approach to morcellation of the large uterus. Contemporary OB/GYN 1997;42:106-125.

 intraspinal drug infusion system

Description
implantable pump and spinal catheter; pump placed under skin stores and releases prescribed morphine; spinal catheter inserted through needle into spinal canal; for chronic pain when conservative treatment fails

Source
Medtronic Inc. product information. Minneapolis, MN.

 intravelar veloplasty

Description
surgical dissection and relocation of the levator muscle complex to improve speech

Anatomy
levator muscle complex; hard palate; oral mucosa

Equipment
retractor; stripper

Source
Adapted from Rohrich RJ, Rowsell A, Johns DF et al. Timing of hard palate closure: a critical long-term analysis. Plastic and Reconstructive Surgery 1996;98:236-246.

Introl bladder neck support prosthesis

Description
prosthesis for urinary stress incontinence; can be used as a temporary alternative to surgery, as a diagnostic test prior to surgery, in conjunction with behavioral modification techniques, or as permanent solution where surgery may not be an option; made of flexible silicone in 25 sizes; inserts into vagina; supports vagina and bladder neck

Source
Johnson & Johnson Medical Inc. product information. Piscataway, NJ.

inverse polymerase chain reaction (PCR)-based detection of frataxin gene

Synonyms
X25 PCR; frataxin gene PCR

Use
diagnosis of Friedreich ataxia

Method
polymerase chain reaction with inverse primer pairs

Specimen
blood

Normal range
X25-specific PCR product not detected

Comments
investigational

Source
Adapted from Campuzano V, Montermini L, Molto MD, et al. Friedreich ataxia: autosomal recessive disease caused by an intronic GAA triplet repeat expansion. Science 1996;271:1423-1427.

Invirase

Generic name
see saquinavir

in vitro fertilization micropipette

Description
specially designed micropipettes for intracytoplasmic sperm insertion (ICSI), subzonal insertion (SUZI), partial zonal dissection (PZD), assisted hatching, blastomere biopsy, and holding

Source
Humagen Fertility Diagnostics Inc. product information. Charlottesville, VA.

INVOS transcranial cerebral oximeter

Description
noninvasive sensor device used to evaluate regional cerebral oxygen saturation in the underlying area of the brain using in vivo optical spectroscopy (INVOS)

Source
Somanetics Corp. product information. Troy, MI.

 iodixanol

Brand name
Visipaque

Use
nonionic radiographic contrast medium

Usual dosage
not given

Pharmaceutical company
Nycomed Inc. Princeton, NJ.

Source
Nycomed Inc. product information. Princeton, NJ.

 iopromide

Brand Name
Ultravist

Use
nonionic contrast agent for radiographic imaging

Usual Dosage
intravenous: doses range from 31.2% to 76.9% iopromide. Dose varies with procedures

Pharmaceutical company
Berlex Labs/Schering AG. Wayne, NJ/Germany.

Source
University of Pittsburgh Drug Information and Pharmacoepidemiology Center. Pittsburgh, PA.

 irbesartan

Brand name
Avapro

Use
an angiotensin II receptor antagonist for the treatment of hypertension

Usual dosage
oral: 10 or 50 mg daily has been used in clinical trials

Pharmaceutical company
Bristol-Myers Squibb Co. Princeton, NJ.

Source
Stadtlanders Managed Pharmacy Services. Pittsburgh, PA.

 irinotecan hydrochloride (HCl)

Brand name
Camptosar

Use
for patients with metastatic carcinoma of the colon and rectum whose disease has progressed following 5-FU (5-fluorouracil)-based therapy

Usual dosage
injection: 125 mg/m² starting dose

Pharmaceutical company
Pharmacia & Upjohn. Kalamazoo, MI.

Source
Internet www.fda.gov.

 Irox endocardial pacing leads

Description
cardiac pacing leads provide direct connection to a broad variety of pulse generators; four models: ventricular bipolar, ventricular unipolar, atrial bipolar, and atrial unipolar

Source
Intermedics Inc. product information. Angleton, TX.

 irregular antibody detection by magnetic force solid-phase assay

Synonyms
magnetic-mixed passive hemagglutination (M-MPHA)

Use
detection of irregular antibodies to blood group antigens

Method
M-MPHA using anti-human globulin magnetic indicator particles

Specimen
plasma or serum

Normal range
negative

Comments
may evolve into an automated screening test

Source
Adapted from Ohgama J, Yabe R, Tamai T, Nakamura M, Mazda T. A new solid-phase assay system using magnetic force on blood group serology. Transfusion Medicine 1996;6:351-359.

Irri-Cath suction system

Description
dual-lumen continuous irrigating suction system created by the insertion of an irrigation line through the lumen of a standard-sized suction catheter; isotonic normal saline solution is continuously fed into the irrigation line and simultaneously aspirated by the coaxial catheter; vortex created by similar suction/irrigation creates a low-velocity, liquid-medium siphoning field; allows recovery of large amounts of secretions with minute removal of tidal air, no damage to bronchial mucosa, and minimal interference with respiratory dynamics and gas exchange

Source
Smiths Industries Medical Systems Inc. product information. Keene, NH.

 ## Isepacin

Generic Name
see isepamicin

 ## isepamicin

Brand Name
Isepacin

Use
antibacterial agent for use in the treatment of urinary tract infections

Usual Dosage
oral: 7.5 mg/kg

Pharmaceutical company
Schering-Plough Research Institute. Kenilworth, NJ.

Source
University of Pittsburgh Drug Information and Pharmacoepidemiology Center. Pittsburgh, PA.

 ## island adipofascial flap in Achilles tendon resurfacing

Description
flap design based on the most distal perforators of the posterior tibial artery

Anatomy
Achilles tendon; subdermal plexus; posterior tibial artery; medial malleolus

Equipment
magnifying loupe; retractors; scalpel; tourniquet; drain

Source
Adapted from El-Khatib H. Island adipofascial flap for resurfacing of the Achilles tendon. Plastic and Reconstructive Surgery 1996;98:1034-1038.

islet cell antigen 512/IA-2 autoantibody combined radioimmunoassay

Synonyms
ICA 512/IA-2 combined RIA

Use
detection of autoantibodies against islet cell antigen 512, or IA-2, in patients with type 1 diabetes

Method
radioimmunoassay for combined islet cell antigen 512/IA-2 autoantibodies using two radiolabels

Specimen
blood

Normal range
no detectable autoantibody activity

Comments
should facilitate large-scale autoantibody screening

Source
Adapted from Kawasaki E, Yu L, Gianani R, et al. Evaluation of islet cell antigen (ICA) 512/IA-2 autoantibody radioassays using overlapping ICA512/IA-2 constructs. Journal of Clinical Endocrinology and Metabolism 1997;82:375-380.

Isolator blood culture system

Synonyms
none

Use
detect aerobic and anaerobic microorganisms in blood

Method
incubates, agitates, and monitors blood in each bottle with continuous readings

Specimen
blood

Normal range
no growth

Comments
rapid detection of microorganism growth

Source
Adapted from Engler HD, Fahle GA, Gill VJ. Clinical evaluation of the BacT/Alert and Isolator aerobic blood culture systems. American Journal of Clinical Pathology 1996;105:774-781.

isoprinosine

Brand name
Inosiplex

Use
restoration of depressed lymphocyte functions associated with HIV/AIDS

Usual dosage
oral: 4 g per day for 4 weeks in clinical trials

Pharmaceutical company
Newport Pharmaceuticals. Laguna Hills, CA.

Source
Stadtlanders Managed Pharmacy Services. Pittsburgh, PA.

 isoproterenol tilt table test

Synonyms
none

Indications
syncope in the setting of structural heart disease

Method
patient restrained on an electric tilt table; instrumentation consisted of peripheral intravenous cannula, automatic and manual sphygmomanometric cuffs, sequential head-up tilt, infusion of isoproterenol, application of defibrillator pads

Normal findings
not applicable

Comments
tilt table testing provides a diagnosis of neuromediated syncope

Source
Adapted from Sheldon R, Rose S, Flanagan P, Koshman ML, Killam S. Effect of beta blockers on the time to first syncope recurrence in patients after a positive isoproterenol tilt table test. The American Journal of Cardiology 1996;78:536-539.

 itraconazole

Brand name
Sporanox

Use
oral formulation and indication for the treatment of oropharyngeal and esophageal candidiasis

Usual dosage
oral: swish and swallow 10 ml (100 mg/10 ml) twice, for a total dose of 200 mg, once daily *(Editor note: Note new oral solution; previously only capsule form)*

Pharmaceutical company
Janssen Pharmaceutical Inc. Titusville, NJ.

Source
Stadtlanders Managed Pharmacy Services. Pittsburgh, PA.

IVEC-10 neurotransmitter analyzer

Description
computer-based system for measuring monoamine neurotransmitters; i.e., dopamine, serotonin, or norepinephrine in "real-time"; applications include measurements with cultured cells, in vitro and in vivo tissue

Source
Medical Systems Corp. product information. Greenvale, NY.

ivermectin

Brand name
Stromectol

Use
antiparasitic agent for the treatment of strongyloidiasis and onchocerciasis

Usual dosage
oral: single dose treatment of 150 µg/kg (in onchocerciasis) or 200 µg/kg (in strongyloidiasis)

Pharmaceutical company
Merck & Company Inc. West Point, PA.

Source
Stadtlanders Managed Pharmacy Services. Pittsburgh, PA.

IvyBlock

Generic name
see bentoquatam

Jace hand continuous passive motion unit

Description
continuous passive motion (CPM) device ensures full composite motion of the digits; H440 CPM gradually progresses to full range of programmed motion; dual finger drive-bar simultaneously distributes force to the proximal and distal phalanx

Source
Jace Systems Inc. Thera-Kinetics product information. Moorestown, NJ.

Jackson-Pratt Gold wound drain

Description
wound drains with Duraflo treatment; heparin and binding agent applied to internal and external surfaces; inhibits formation of blood clots

Source
Allegiance Healthcare Corp. product information. McGaw Park, IL.

 ## JedMed TRI-GEM microscope

Description
microscope that illuminates the operative field with three beams of light, reducing shadows; magnification of x 6, x 10, and x 16 possible; improves on the illumination of a treatment light, the magnification of loupes, and the documentation capability of an intraoral camera

Source
JedMed Instrument Co. product information. St. Louis, MO.

 ## Jettmobile

Description
(positioning and tumble forms) develop neck, shoulder, and arm muscle coordination while maintaining child in an extension position; features protective fenders, hip strap for positioning, and concealed ball casters for protection; includes three positioning shapes and an abductor wedge

Source
J.A. Preston Corp. product information. Jackson, MI.

 ## Jewel pacer-cardioverter-defibrillator

Description
implantable cardiac device released from clinical trials March 1995; on as-needed basis, delivers less uncomfortable therapies before resorting to cardiac shock

Source
Medtronic Inc. product information. Minneapolis, MN.

 ## J-59 Florida brace

Description
spinal control orthosis for postoperative lumbar fusion, lumbosacral spine stabilization, and protection of thoracolumbar junction injuries

Source
Florida Brace Corp. product information. Winter Park, FL.

J-needle

Description
instrument has curved distal aspect that presents smooth surface of contact to any closely underlying organ; using a few basic suturing moves, can be ready to tie off

Source
Unimar Inc. product information. Wilton, CT.

Jobst athrombic pump system

Description
pneumatic noninvasive device with tubing connected to calf- or thigh-high stockings; graduated compression inflation which increases venous velocity and retards clot formation

Source
Jobst product information. Charlotte, NC.

Judet view to assess complex acetabular fractures

Synonyms
none

Indications
acetabular fracture with need for treatment planning

Method
anteroposterior and Judet oblique views are initial means of assessing fracture; rotational digital subtraction angiography for imaging complex pelvic and acetabular fractures

Normal findings
none

Comments
assessment of orientation, location, and exact number of fracture fragments as well as status of joint space requires computed tomography

Source
Adapted from Patel NH, Hunter JC, Routt Jr ML. Rotational imaging of complex acetabular fractures: the dynamic Judet view. Emergency Radiology 1995;2:384-386.

jugular bulb catheter placement assessment

Synonyms
none

Indications
bedside placement of oxygen saturation catheter into jugular bulb

Method
portable over-penetrated Stenver view and companion over-penetrated lateral radiograph as well as computed tomographic scans of neck or skull base are used to detect malpositioning of catheter

Normal findings
catheter in jugular bulb

Comments
many radiologists are not familiar with jugular bulb catheters; it is important to ensure that catheter is advanced into the jugular bulb

Source
Adapted from Hayman LA, Fahr LM, Taber KH, et al. Radiographic assessment of jugular bulb catheters. Emergency Radiology 1995;2:331-338.

 Jux-A-Cisor exerciser

Description
wire tree device for arm exercises; exercise can be timed, forearm weights added, and other variations for maximum benefit

Source
Fred Sammons Inc. product information. Western Springs, IL.

 Kadian

Generic name
see morphine sulfate

 Kamdar microscissors

Description
ophthalmic microscissors with a curved tip that follows the curve of the retina, allowing cutting in the vertical plane and minimizing the risk of engaging the retina

Source
Dutch Ophthalmic USA product information. Kingston, NH.

 Kangaroo gastrostomy feeding tube

Description
biocompatible medical grade silicone feeding tube; trifunnel design allows easy irrigation and medication delivery; external skin disc helps prevent tube migration

Source
Sherwood Medical Co. product information. St. Louis, MO.

Karl Storz lithotriptor (lithotripter)

Description
instrument for extracorporeal lithotripsy

Source
Karl Storz product information. Culver City, CA.

Katadolon

Generic Name
see flupirtine

Kazanjian vestibuloplasty

Description
surgical repair of an atrophic mandible with an implant-supported prosthesis helps to gain fixed mucosa around implants with little resorption of the underlying bone

Anatomy
mandible; buccal mucosa; mandibular bone

Equipment
implant-supported prosthesis; cylindrical and screw implants

Source
Adapted from Kreusch T. Implantation in the atrophic mandible — cylinder or screw type implants. Implant Dentistry 1996;5:122-123.

Kenicef

Generic Name
see cefodizime

Keradiscs

Description
highly absorbent cellulose placed in contact with eye and with easy finger tip depression, releases apical anesthetic during excimer laser procedures

Source
John Weiss & Son Ltd. product information. Milton Keynes, England.

284

 ketotifen

Brand name
Zaditen

Use
mast cell stabilizer used primarily in the treatment of asthma

Usual dosage
oral: 1 to 2 mg twice daily

Pharmaceutical company
Sandoz Pharmaceuticals Corp. East Hanover, NJ.

Source
University of Pittsburgh Drug Information and Pharmacoepidemiology Center. Pittsburgh, PA.

 Keystone Plus oxygenator concentrator

Description
six liter concentrator designed to handle the needs of high-liter flow oxygen patients; minimizes deliveries, equipment, and service calls

Source
DeVilbiss Health Care Inc. product information. Somerset, PA.

 K-Fix Fixator system

Description
external stabilization device that provides effective alternative to casting and internal fixation in the reconstruction of compound wrist fractures

Source
Kinetikos Medical Inc. product information. San Diego, CA.

 Ki-67 marker detection

Synonyms
Ki-67 immunohistochemistry

Use
detection of Ki-67, the nuclear proliferation-associated antigen, in human tissue sections

Method
immunohistochemical staining

Specimen
tissue biopsy

Normal range
staining pattern consistent with normal cell proliferation

Comments
investigational

Source
Analytical Cellular Pathology 1992;4:181-185.

Kinder Design pedo forceps

Description
small, light surgical stainless steel forceps designed to provide a firm grasp of primary teeth; its small design enables the surgeon to hide the instrument from pediatric patients

Source
Hu-Friedy Manufacturing Inc. product information. Chicago, IL.

kinetic fibrinogen assay (KFA)

Synonyms
kinetic Fgn assay

Use
determination of fibrinogen concentration in disease states associated with coagulopathies

Method
thrombin-catalyzed conversion of fibrinogen to fibrin, followed by turbidimetric determination of fibrin polymerization rate

Specimen
blood

Normal range
greater than 100 mg/dL

Comments
more closely related to physiologic blood coagulation than other fibrinogen assays

Source
American Journal of Clinical Pathology 1995;104:455-462.

Kingsley Steplite foot

Description
a prosthesis designed specifically for the moderately active amputee desiring maximum comfort while walking; available in three styles, the Low Profile 3/4", Strider 1/4", and Flattie 3/8"; the Steplite is also available as a KC09 Litefoot

Source
Kingsley Mfg Co. product information. Costa Mesa, CA.

Kirschenbaum retractor

Description
acromioplasty surgical instrument designed to fit under posterior edge of
acromion; levers humeral head down out of the way; helps to protect shoulder, and articular surface of humeral head

Source
Innomed Inc. product information. Savannah, GA.

Klaron

Generic name
see sodium sulfacetamide

Klippel retractor set

Description
polygonal retractor surgical instrument for certain operations in the perineal
area and for reconstructive surgery of penis

Source
Accurate Surgical & Scientific Instruments Corp. product information. Westbury, NY.

KLS centre-drive screw

Description
craniomaxillofacial plating system designed with centre-drive screws and
screwdrivers; enhances visualization and eliminates obscured views in the
surgical field

Source
KLS Martin L.P. product information. Jacksonville, FL.

Knead-A-Ball exerciser

Description
hand exerciser; arthritis sufferers can take this breathable foam polymer ball
with them wherever they go to squeeze in helpful hand exercises; also good
for working off everyday stress

Source
Fred Sammons Inc. product information. Western Springs, IL.

KOH Colpotomizer system

Description
patented component of RUMI System manipulator; can also be used with most surgical power sources

Source
CooperSurgical Inc. product information. Shelton, CT.

Kollagen dressing

Description
wound dressing and gel made of collagen, providing the natural environment for the body to heal itself

Source
BioCore Inc. product information. Topeka, KS.

Kramp scissors

Description
ophthalmic surgical scissors mounted on an instrument at a 45-degree angle to the shaft to permit dissection of epiretinal membranes

Source
Storz Ophthalmics product information. St. Louis, MO.

KRD L2000 rehab device

Description
kinetic rehab device (KRD) delivers controlled motion exercise of lumbar region of spine; microprocessor-controlled motion; enhances spinal rehabilitation

Source
Physicians Consulting Inc. product information. Austin, TX.

lacidipine

Brand name
Lacipil

Use
calcium channel-blocking agent used in the treatment of hypertension

Usual dosage
oral: 4 to 6 mg once daily

288

Pharmaceutical company
Glaxo Inc. Research Triangle Park, NC.

Source
University of Pittsburgh Drug Information and Pharmacoepidemiology Center. Pittsburgh, PA.

 Lacipil

Generic name
see lacidipine

 Lalonde hook forceps

Description
forceps with double opposing hooks that grasp the skin with a gentle over-lapping pincher action that permits atraumatic eversion and exposure of the dermis; also speeds running intradermal (subcuticular) sutures and facilitates double instrument tying; available with baby and/or standard hooks

Source
Accurate Surgical & Scientific Instruments Corp. product information. Westbury, NY.

 lambda sign

Synonyms
twin-peak sign

Indications
undetermined chorionicity in multiple pregnancy

Method
ultrasound evaluation for the presence or absence of a triangular projection of placental tissue extending between the layers of the intertwin membrane in multiple pregnancy

Normal findings
not applicable

Comments
none

Source
Adapted from Wood SL, St. Onge R, Connors G, Elliott PD. Evaluation of the twin peak or lambda sign in determining chorionicity in multiple pregnancy. Obstetrics & Gynecology 1996;88:6-9.

 Lambert-Heiman scissors

Description
ophthalmic straight vitreous scissors; 20-gauge shaft with straight 3-mm scissors blades

Source
Storz Ophthalmics product information. St. Louis, MO.

lamellar keratectomy for nontuberculous mycobacterial keratitis

Description
lamellar keratectomy is reported as treatment for nontuberculous keratitis for unresponsiveness to medical therapy; corneal lesions were outlined; perpendicular cut made at clear cornea close to margin of keratitis; tissue to be excised was grasped and stretched with fine corneal forceps; lamellar dissection performed with a spatula knife; dissector directed parallel to stromal lamella; entire specimen removed with corneal scissors

Anatomy
anterior chamber; bed of stromal lamella; conjunctiva; conjunctival epithelium; cornea; corneal stroma; epithelium; lamella; stromal bed

Equipment
standard ophthalmic surgery equipment; Beaver blade; spatula knife; specimen removed placed in brain-heart infusion and Tenbroek tissue grinders for cultures

Source
Adapted from Hu FR. Extensive lamellar keratectomy for treatment of nontuberculous mycobacterial keratitis. American Journal of Ophthalmology 1995;120:47-53.

 Lamictal

Generic name
see lamotrigine

 laminoplasty with extended foraminotomy for cervical myelopathy

Description
advantages of anterior cervical approach for cervical myelopathy caused by ossification of posterior longitudinal ligament or spondylosis gives the ability to address the lesion completely; when the lesion is long or multiple in nature, posterior approaches are the procedures of choice; an extended foraminotomy added to the standard laminoplasty procedure, reduces the incidence of resistant postoperative radiculopathy; the dorsal component of the internal surface of the intervertebral foramina is removed as far laterally as possible; the external surface of the facet joints are spared as much as possible

Anatomy
articular facets; dural sac; dorsal aspect of lamina; facet joints; intervertebral foramina; lamina; nerve roots; osseous cord; posterior longitudinal ligament; spinous processes, C3-C7 and C7-T1; spinal canal; venous plexus

Equipment
standard neurosurgery equipment; high-speed air drill; hydroxyapatite spacer stabilized with titanium wires and/or silk suture; Mayfield apparatus; microscope

Source
Adapted from Koshu K, Tominaga T, Yoshimoto T. Spinous process-splitting laminoplasty with an extended foraminotomy for cervical myelopathy. Neurosurgery Journal 1995;37:430-435.

LaminOss implant

Description
one-stage endosseous implant to support fixed or removable prostheses
Source
Impladent Inc. product information. Holliswood, NY.

 Lamisil

Generic name
see terbinafine hydrochloride

 lamivudine

Brand name
3TC
Use
reverse transcriptase inhibitor used for the treatment of advanced acquired immunodeficiency syndrome (AIDS) and AIDS-related complex (ARC)
Usual dosage
oral: 150 to 300 mg twice daily has been used in clinical trials
Pharmaceutical company
Glaxo Inc. Research Triangle Park, NC.
Source
University of Pittsburgh Drug Information and Pharmacoepidemiology Center. Pittsburgh, PA.

 lamotrigine

Brand name
Lamictal
Use
treatment of adults with partial epilepsy
Usual dosage
oral: 100, 150, 200, and 250 mg tablets; in clinical trials dosage ranged from 50 to 500 mg daily; as much as 1300 mg being well tolerated in life-threatening epilepsy
Pharmaceutical company
Burroughs Wellcome Co. Research Triangle Park, NC.
Source
University of Pittsburgh Drug Information and Pharmacoepidemiology Center. Pittsburgh, PA.

Langerman diamond knife system

Description
ophthalmic surgical instruments that includes a trifacet step knife to make a groove and angled keratome knife for a 2-mm tunnel; all knives necessary to construct any incision

Source
Rhein Medical Inc. product information. Tampa, FL.

 lanreotide

Brand name
Angiopeptin

Use
tested to treat metastatic hormone refractory prostate cancer and advanced breast cancer

Usual dosage
injectable: 30 mg intramuscular injection (depot formulation) once weekly was tested in the clinical studies

Pharmaceutical company
Biomeasure Inc. Milford, MA.

Source
Stadtlanders Managed Pharmacy Services. Pittsburgh, PA.

 lansoprazole

Brand name
Prevacid

Use
proton-pump inhibitor used in the treatment of peptic ulcer, reflux esophagitis, and Zollinger-Ellison syndrome

Usual dosage
oral: 30 mg once daily for 4 weeks in the treatment of duodenal ulcer; 30 mg once daily for 8 weeks in the treatment of gastric ulcer and gastrointestinal reflux disease; 60 to 120 mg daily for Zollinger-Ellison syndrome

Pharmaceutical company
Abbott Laboratories. Abbott Park, IL.

Source
University of Pittsburgh Drug Information and Pharmacoepidemiology Center. Pittsburgh, PA.

292

 laparoelytrotomy

Description
anterior vaginotomy that avoids uterine incision with abdominal delivery
Anatomy
vagina; cervix; vesicouterine fold; uterus
Equipment
standard low transverse cesarean section equipment
Source
Adapted from Goodlin RC. Anterior vaginotomy: abdominal delivery without a uterine incision. Obstetrics & Gynecology 1996;88:467-469.

 laparoscopic adrenalectomy

Description
widespread use of noninvasive adrenal imaging with ultrasound, computed tomography, and magnetic resonance imaging has greatly increased the detection of adrenal masses; surgery remains the basis of treatment; meticulous hemostasis and delicate tissue handling are mandatory; the most used route on laparoscopy adrenalectomy is the transperitoneal or semilateral approach
Anatomy
accessory hepatic vein; Gerota fascia; pericapsular venous plexus; perinephric fat; retropancreatic, para-aortic, and parasplenic areas
Equipment
standard laparoscopic surgical equipment
Source
Adapted from Weisnagel SJ, Gagner M, Breton G, Pomp A, Pharand D, Lacroix A. Laparoscopic adrenalectomy. The Endocrinologist 1996;6:169-177.

 laparoscopically assisted colpoceliotomy

Description
vaginal removal of adnexally mobile dermoid cysts; videolaparoscopy improves visualization of cyst and uterine structures; laparoscopic forceps assist in grasping ligaments; laparoscopy used for postexcision evaluation of operative site
Anatomy
peritoneum; utero-ovarian ligament; Douglas cul-de-sac; ovary; abdominal cavity; vascular pedicles; infundibulopelvic ligament

Equipment

standard laparoscopic surgery equipment; Allis forceps; Duval forceps; laparoscopic forceps; absorbable suture

Source

Adapted from Pardi G, Carminati R, Ferrari MM, Ferrazzi E, Bulfoni G, Marcozzi S. Laparoscopically assisted vaginal removal of ovarian dermoid cysts. Obstetrics & Gynecology 1995;85:129-134.

 ## laparoscopically assisted distal partial gastrectomy (LADPG)

Description

treatment for gastric carcinoma when lymph nodes and distal stomach must be removed; pneumoperitoneum created through subumbilical cannula; laparoscope inserted through cannula; four additional trocars inserted as operating ports

Anatomy

umbilicus; abdominal wall; greater curvature of stomach; greater omentum; epiploic arcade; gastrocolic ligament; pole of spleen; pylorus; gastric artery; gastroepiploic artery; pancreatic head; cardiac lymph node; superior gastric lymph node; suprapyloric lymph node; celiac lymph node; retropyloric lymph node; xiphoid; duodenum; celiac trunk

Equipment

standard surgery equipment; Hasson cannula; angled laparoscope; trocar; grasping forceps; Babcock grasper; ultrasonic dissector; clamping forceps; U-shaped retractor; Proximate linear stapler

Source

Adapted from Kitano S, Maeo S, Shiraishi N, Shimoda K, Miyahara M, Bandoh T, et al. Laparoscopically assisted distal partial gastrectomy for early-stage gastric carcinomas. Surgical Technology International IV 1995:115-119.

 ## laparoscopically assisted penile revascularization

Description

inferior epigastric vessels, visualized during intraperitoneal and preperitoneal laparoscopic procedures, are mobilized and tunneled into the operative field at the base of the penis for subsequent microvascular anastomosis with penile vessels; used to treat vasculogenic impotence due to trauma or cavernous arterial insufficiency

Anatomy

male genitalia; pubic symphysis (symphysis pubis); pelvis; inferior epigastric vessels; dorsal vein; dorsal penile artery

Equipment

standard laparoscopic and microsurgery equipment; Hasson cannula

Source

Adapted from Lund GO, Winfield HN, Donovan JF. Laparoscopically assisted penile revascularization for vasculogenic impotence. The Journal of Urology 1995;153:1923-1926.

laparoscopic cholecystectomy

Description
laparoscopic cholecystectomy (LC) performed by four-trocar technique; common bile duct examined by routine cholangiography during conventional cholecystectomy (CC) and not during LC; laparoscopic approach compares favorably with CC in terms of hospital stay, weight loss, postoperative pain, and pulmonary function; affords diminished operative trauma; patients with acute cholecystitis, pancreatitis, choledocholithiasis, and malignant disease excluded from LC

Anatomy
antecubital vein; cystic pedicle; common bile duct

Equipment
standard laparoscopic surgery equipment; enzyme-linked immunosorbent assay kit

Source
Adapted from Glaser F, Sannwald GA, Heinz JB, et al.General stress response to conventional and laparoscopic cholecystectomy. Annals of Surgery 1995;221:372-379.

 ## laparoscopic esophageal hiatus mesh repair

Description
defects of the esophageal hiatus (on rare occasions) are too large to be closed primarily without excessive tension; use of prosthetic mesh is the logical choice for a tension-free diaphragmatic closure in these instances; in cases of esophagogastric erosion in obesity operations, and the Angelchik ring, the mesh should not be in proximity to the esophagus or stomach; laparoscopic mesh repair interposes the right diaphragmatic crus between the implanted mesh and the esophagus

Anatomy
crura; diaphragm; diaphragmatic muscle and fascia; esophagogastric area; esophagus; pleura

Equipment
standard surgical equipment; Ethibond suture; trapezoidal-shaped polypropylene mesh; Ethibond stapler; Angelchik ring

Source
Adapted from Huntington TR. Laparoscopic mesh repair of the esophageal hiatus. Journal of American College of Surgeons 1997;184:399-400.

laparoscopic esophagectomy with esophagogastroplasty

Description
procedure indicated for advanced achalasia of esophagus, severe reflux stenosis, squamous cell carcinoma, and adenocarcinoma of esophagus; esophageal resection and esophagogastrostomy through cervical and videolaparoscopic approach without opening abdominal or pleural cavity; stomach and lower two-thirds of esophagus mobilized laparoscopically, upper third of esophageal dissection through cervical incision

Anatomy
aortic arch; cervical esophagus; crus; esophagus; gastric vessels; gastrocolic omentum; gastroepiploic artery; gastric fundus; lumen; laryngeal nerve; mediastinum; prethyroid muscles; phrenoesophageal membrane; stomach; sternomastoid muscle; thoracic esophagus; umbilicus

Equipment
standard laparoscopic surgery equipment; camera; catheter; clip; blunt dissector; GIA stapler; ligature; videolaparoscope; Veress needle; trocar

Source
Adapted from dePaula AL, Hashiba K, Ferreira EAB, dePaula RA, Grecco E. Laparoscopic transhiatal esophagectomy with esophagogastroplasty. Surgical Laparoscopy & Endoscopy 1995;1:1-3.

 ## laparoscopic laser assisted auto-augmentation for pediatric neurogenic bladder

Description
removal of detrusor muscle in dome of bladder to expand bladder capacity allowing underlying mucosa to bulge outward as a wide-mouthed diverticulum to increase bladder capacity and compliance

Anatomy
pelvic area; urethra; bladder; bladder neck; dome; detrusor muscle; peritoneum; trigone

Equipment
standard surgical equipment plus KTP/532 laser

Source
Adapted from Poppas DP, Uzzo RG, Britanisky RG, Mininberg DT. Laparoscopic laser assisted auto-augmentation of the pediatric neurogenic bladder: early experience with urodynamic follow-up. Journal of Urology 1996;155:1057-1060.

laparoscopic liver resection of tumors

Description
during laparoscopy, exact localization and surgical limits of benign tumors were determined by ultrasonography and visualization; dissection was performed using the endoscopic cavitational ultrasonic surgical aspiration (CUSA); this achieved resection of tumors with minimal blood loss; adequate control of the vessels and ducts of bleeding during liver surgery can be accomplished using ultrasonic dissector devices; the probe of the CUSA dissector is introduced through a cannula when used in endoscopic surgery

Anatomy
abdomen; common bile duct; costal margin; falciform ligament; gallbladder; Blisson capsule; hepatic vein; left triangular ligament; left lobe of liver; pancreas; parenchyma; retroperitoneal space; subxiphoid area; umbilicus

Equipment
accessory probe; clips; cannula; CUSA; electrocautery; "endobag"; Endo GIA stapler; enhanced argon coagulation system; trocar; ultrasonographic flexible transducer; ultrasonic dissector devices

Source
Adapted from Cuesta MA, Meijer S, Paul MA, de Brauw LM. Limited laparoscopic liver resection of benign tumors guided by laparoscopic ultrasonography: report of two cases. Surgical Laparoscopy and Endoscopy 1995;5:396-401.

 laparoscopic nephropexy

Description
laparoscopic nephropexy is performed for symptomatic, documented nephroptosis; Gerota fascia was secured to the peritoneal reflection of the line of Toldt using tacking clips in one patient; in the subsequent patients the lateral border of the kidney was sutured to the overlying fascia of the quadratus lumborum muscle; the superior edge of the incised infrahepatic triangular ligament was sutured to the anterior mid portion of the renal capsule, creating a vertical and horizontal means of fixation

Anatomy
abdomen; anterior axillary line; external oblique fascia; Gerota fascia; infrahepatic triangular ligament; kidney; mesocolon; midclavicular line; psoas muscle; peritoneal cavity; quadratus lumborum muscle; renal capsule; renal parenchyma; retroperitoneum; subcostal area; umbilicus

Equipment
standard laparoscopic equipment; absorbable suture clips; dilation balloon; looped suture; Veress needle; tacking clips

Source
Adapted from Elashry OM, Nakada SY, McDougall EM, Clayman RV. Laparoscopic nephropexy: Washington University experience. Journal of Urology 1995;154:1655-1659.

laparoscopic orchiopexy

Description
treatment of intra-abdominal undescended testis with reduced morbidity and length of stay

Anatomy
gubernaculum; processus vaginalis; spermatic vessels; vas; epididymis; ureters; umbilical ligament; renal hilum; vas deferens

Equipment
zero-degree laparoscope; Endoshears; grasping forceps; dissecting tips

Source
Adapted from Poppas D, Lemack G, Miniberg D. Laparoscopic orchiopexy, clinical experience and description of technique. The Journal of Urology 1996;5(2):708-711.

laparoscopic paraesophageal hernia repair

Description
Type II paraesophageal hernia occurs when distal esophagus is in its anatomic position, anchored by phrenoesophageal ligament, and a defect in the diaphragm causes stomach and hernia sac to travel into chest; surgical correction is universally advised because of risk of catastrophic gastric volvulus; operation reduces hernia, eliminates hernia sac, and repairs opening in diaphragm hiatus

Anatomy
abdominal wall; arcuate ligament; cardia; colon; crura; diaphragm; esophagus; falciform ligament; peritoneum; liver; midclavicular line; midepigastrium; pericardium; phrenoesophageal ligament; spleen; triangular ligament; subxiphoid

Equipment
standard laparoscopic surgery equipment; Babcock grasper; 12, 14, and 16F dilators; dissector; Endohernia stapler; Foley catheter; French bougie; fan retractor; guide wire; Metzenbaum scissors; laparoscope; orogastric tube; Prolene mesh; reducer; Veress needle; Russell gastrostomy kit; 15F Silastic balloon tube

Source
Adapted from Edelman, DS. Laparoscopic paraesophageal hernia repair with mesh. Surgical Laparoscopy & Endoscopy 1995;1:32-36.

laparoscopic peritoneal dialysis catheter placement

Description
placement of catheter under laparoscope through an infraumbilical port; Tenckhoff catheter placed through abdominal wall via suprapubic port; in seven procedures the suprapubic port was replaced by percutaneous introducing kit including needle, guidewire, dilator, and splitting sheath; two other ports used for passage of grasping and suturing instruments to site the catheter tip deep in the pelvis; catheter is secured to back wall of uterus in females, or peritoneum overlying back wall of bladder in males

Anatomy
abdominal wall; back wall of uterus; bladder; iliac fossa; infraumbilical area; peritoneum; suprapubic area

Equipment
percutaneous introducing kit; laparoscope; laparoscopic grasper; Tenckhoff catheter

Source
Adapted from Watson DI, Paterson D, Bannister K. Secure placement of peritoneal dialysis catheters using a laparoscopic technique. Surgical Laparoscopy and Endoscopy 1996;6:35-37.

 laparoscopic radical nephrectomy

Description
laparoscopic approach to radical nephrectomy offers significantly less postoperative pain, shorter hospital stay, and earlier return to activity than standard laparoscopic method

Anatomy
pelvic area; peritoneum; Gerota fascia; kidney; ureter; renal artery; renal vein; aorta; vena cava

Equipment
standard laparoscopic equipment; vascular endogastrointestinal anastomosis device

Source
Adapted from McDougall EM, Clayman RV, Elashry OM. Laparoscopic radical nephrectomy for renal tumor: the Washington University experience. Journal of Urology 1996;155:1265-1267.

 laparoscopic Taylor procedure, modified technique

Description
surgery performed for duodenal ulcer when conservative treatment fails; seromyotomy is performed first; left lobe of liver retracted away from stomach; posterior truncal vagotomy performed at level of diaphragmatic hiatus; laparoscopic technique allows approach to posterior vagus with minimal dissection; right diaphragmatic crus unmistakably recognizable through a posterior approach; further advantages of this approach are that the anatomy of the esophagogastric junction is minimally disturbed, and there is no risk of damaging the trunk of the anterior vagus nerve

Anatomy

angle of His; anterior vagus nerve; aponeurosis; cardia; caudate lobe of liver; crow's foot; diaphragmatic crus; esophagogastric junction; esophageal wall; gastric fundus, mucosa, and serosa; inferior vena cava; lesser omentum; lesser and greater curvature of stomach; nerve of Latarjet; pars flaccida; posterior mediastinum; posterior vagus nerve; peritoneum, xiphoid process

Equipment

Veress needle; Endo Retract (retractor); Babcock forceps; clip applicator; Endo Mini-Retract; gastrofibroscope; 30-degree viewing laparoscope; 5-mm and 10-mm trocars; right-angle dissecting hook; needle holder; aspirator-irrigator; titanium clip (LT 300, Ethicon); methylene blue

Source

Adapted from Gertsch P, Wing-Cheong Chow L, Boon-Hua Lim. Laparoscopic Taylor procedure in Chinese patients. Gastrointestinal Endoscopy 1996;43:243-246.

 ## laparoscopy for diagnosis of pneumatosis cystoides intestinalis (PCI)

Synonyms

Indications

epigastric discomfort, weight loss, diarrhea

Method

standard diagnostic laparoscopic technique used to detect gas-filled cysts in the submucosa or subserosa of the gastrointestinal tract that is indicative of PCI

Normal findings

no evidence of gas-filled cysts in the submucosa or subserosa of the gastrointestinal tract

Comments

pneumatosis cystoides intestinalis is an uncommon condition usually incidentally detected on plain radiography films, barium x-ray film, or computed tomography scan; laparoscopy provides a more accurate diagnostic method

Source

Adapted from Mehta SN, Friedman G, Fried GM, Mayrand S. Pneumatosis cystoides intestinalis: laparoscopic features. The American Journal of Gastroenterology 1996;91:2610-2612.

 ## LaparoSonic coagulating shears

Description

ultrasonic scissors powered by generator; has a scissor-like handle, an ultrasonic three-sided blade that vibrates at 55,500 cycles/second, flat edge for coagulation and grasping, a sharp edge for cutting, and a blunt edge for dissection; causes less damage to tissue and decreases postoperative adhesions

Source

UltraCision product information.Smithfield, RI.

Lap-Band gastric banding system

Description
for treatment of severe obesity; laparoscopically placed flexible device; access port for postoperative adjustment of inflatable band; replaces gastric stapling procedures
Source
BioEnterics Corp. product information. Carpinteria, CA.

lapping tool

Description
diamond-coated dental lapping tool consisting of three parts: two white Delrin lapping guides and diamond-coated stainless steel lapping tool
Source
Steri-Oss Bausch & Lomb Co. product information. Yorba Linda, CA.

Laqua black line retinal hook

Description
ophthalmic surgical instrument with ebonized nonglare finish; hook allows for atraumatic elevation and dissection of distinct epiretinal membranes
Source
Storz Ophthalmics product information. St. Louis, MO.

Laryngoflex reinforced endotracheal tube

Description
siliconized, stainless steel spiral reinforced endotracheal tubes using high volume/low pressure cuff and permanent connector; x-ray opaque; 26-cm, 28-cm, and 29-cm length and size 7 to 11 mm
Source
Rusch Inc. product information. Duluth, GA.

Laschal precision suture tome (PST)

Description
surgical scissors engineered with a suture guide-channel through which the knot cannot pass; acts as a stop at which point the cut is made; cut can be made above or on the knot
Source
Laschal Surgical Inc. product information. Purchase, NY.

LaseAway ruby and Q-switched neodymium:yttrium-aluminum-garnet (Nd:YAG) lasers

Description
lasers used to remove pigmented lesions and tattoos

Source
Polytec PI product information. Costa Mesa, CA.

laser dermal implant

Description
surgery to correct scars, "plump up" facial folds and augment lips; especially effective in correcting acne scars; selectively removes epidermis while maintaining integrity of dermis

Anatomy
area to be revised and donor site for skin graft, inner arm or behind ear

Equipment
carbon dioxide laser; tunable pulsed-dye laser or Nd:YAG laser; scanner; topical anesthetic

Source
Adapted from Abergel RP. New cosmetic dermal implant. Plastic Surgery Products 1996;30.

Laseredge microsurgical knife

Description
microsurgical knife for ophthalmic procedures; produces a consistently sharp knife; yields a nonreflective surface to improve visibility

Source
Storz Ophthalmics product information. St. Louis, MO.

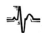

laser-induced autofluorescence

Synonyms
none

Indications
need for differentiation of neoplastic urothelial bladder lesions versus normal or nonspecific inflammatory mucosa

Method
three different pulsed laser excitation wavelengths were used successively: xenium chloride excimer, nitrogen, and coumarin dye lasers; fluorescent light was captured and channeled; definite diagnosis could be established based on fluorescent intensity ratio

Indications
not applicable

Normal findings
fluorescence intensity is decreased in bladder tumors

Comments
effective for detection of occult urothelial neoplasms

Source
Adapted from Anidjar M, Ettori D, Cussenot O. Laser-induced autofluorescence diagnosis of bladder tumors: dependence on the excitation wavelength. The Journal of Urology 1996;156:1590-1596.

 ## laser Raman microprobe identification of calcium oxalate deposits

Synonyms
nondestructive spectroscopic calcium oxalate identification

Use
nondestructive identification of calcium oxalate deposits in cases of oxalosis

Method
Raman microprobe spectroscopy of paraffin-embedded tissue specimens using focused argon-ion laser excitation

Specimen
paraffin-embedded tissue biopsies

Normal range
no evidence of calcium oxalate spectra

Comments
investigational

Source
Adapted from Pestaner JP, Mullick FG, Johnson FB, Centeno JA. Calcium oxalate crystals in human pathology: molecular analysis with the laser Raman microprobe. Archives of Pathology and Laboratory Medicine 1996;120:537-540.

 ## Lasertubus

Description
laser-resistant tracheal tube for laryngeal surgery with 2-way stopcock; a white Merocel sponge dissipates the laser light and prevents back scatters, resulting in protection of the tube shaft; inner-diameters measure 4, 5, and 6 mm

Source
Rusch Inc. product information. Duluth, GA.

 ## Lasette

Description
laser finger perforator designed for capillary blood sampling of glucose and other chemistries; opens small hole in fingertip by vaporizing water molecules in the skin providing less painful monitoring for patient; eliminates the possibility of accidental needle pricks of health workers

Source
Cell Robotics International product and Internet information. Albuquerque, NM.

latanoprost

Brand name
Xalatan

Use
for the treatment of high intraocular pressure in patients with glaucoma

Usual dosage
opthalmic: one drop every evening in both eyes

Pharmaceutical company
Pharmacia Inc. Columbus, OH.

Source
University of Pittsburgh Drug Information and Pharmacoepidemiology Center. Pittsburgh, PA.

 lateral patellar autologous graft

Description
open surgical repair of large osteochondral knee defects using patellar autologous graft; patella is identified as a ready source of graft material, yielding grafts ranging from 720 to 1290 m² from the lateral facet alone; use of autologous material eliminates expenses related to harvesting and preservation, as well as reducing risk of hepatitis and infection associated with use of allograft

Anatomy
patella; lateral facet; medial and lateral femoral condyle; patellofemoral joint; retinacular fibers; retinaculum; cancellous bone; articular cartilage

Equipment
standard surgery equipment; sandbag; tourniquet; paper template; osteotome; surgical drill; calipers; oscillating saw; sponge-covered punch; absorbable pins; subcutaneous suction drains

Source
Adapted from Outerbridge HK, Outerbridge AR, Outerbridge RE. The use of a lateral patellar autologous graft for the repair of a large osteochondral defect of the knee. The Journal of Bone and Joint Surgery 1995;77-A:65-72.

 Lat pull down

Description
freestanding device with overhead pulley and isotonic weights; pulley adjusts to desired line of tension; strengthens latissimus (Lat) and related muscles; unit of Alliance rehabilitation system

Source
Chattanooga Group Inc. product information. Hixson, TN.

Laurus ND-260 needle driver

Description
surgical instrument that combines needle driving, knot pushing, and suture material in one device; provides access to difficult suturing areas
Source
Ethicon Endo-Surgery Inc. product information. Cincinnati, OH.

 Lea shield contraceptive

Description
vaginal barrier contraceptive in phase II trial; design consists of elliptical bowl that fits over cervix; valve that extends towards outside of vagina prevents a pocket of air from existing between cervix and inside of device
Source
Ultracision product information. Smithfield, RI.

 leech mobile home

Description
two-chamber, transparent plexiglas storage and transport apparatus for medicinal leeches
Source
Leeches USA LTD. product information. Westbury, NY.

 Leica vibrating knife microtome

Description
used for suctioning fresh tissue or fixed tissue immersed in a cooled buffer solution to preserve enzymatic activity; semiautomatic Leica VT 1000 M and fully automatic Leica VT 1000 E have multiple applications; produces sections down to a thickness of approximately 0.10 mcg
Source
Leica Inc. product information. Willowdale, Ontario, Canada.

 Lema strap

Description
lightweight leg strap designed as an aid in rehabilitating the stroke patient; assists the following movements: ankle dorsiflexion, knee extension, hip hiking, flexion, and internal or external rotation
Source
Fred Sammons Inc. product information. Western Springs, IL.

leprosin A nasal provocation test

Synonyms
leprosin A stimulation

Use
detection of mucosal immunity in leprosy

Method
measurement of salivary anti-*Mycobacterium leprae* immunoglobulin A (IgA) following stimulation with nasal leprosin A

Specimen
saliva

Normal range
no detectable anti-*Mycobacterium leprae* IgA

Comments
investigational

Source
Adapted from Ramaprasad P, Cree IA, Oluwole M, Samson PD. Development of a mucosal challenge test for leprosy using leprosin A. Journal of Immunologic Methods 1995;188:239-246.

 Lere bone mill

Description
small device with two blades for crushing of fine and coarse bone; provides uniform bone particles for bone graft used in revision surgery, spinal fusing, trauma bone loss, and defect filling

Source
DePuy Inc. product information. Warsaw, IN.

 Lescol

Generic name
see fluvastatin

 letrozole

Brand name
Femara

Use
aromatase inhibitor; chemotherapeutic for the treatment of advanced breast cancer in postmenopausal women when prior therapy with antiestrogen fails

Usual dosage
oral: 2.5 mg/day has been used in phase III clinical trials

Pharmaceutical company
Ciba-Geigy Pharmaceuticals. Summit, NJ.

Source
Stadtlanders Managed Pharmacy Services. Pittsburgh, PA.

 Leucomax

Generic name
see molgramostim

 Leutrol

Generic name
see zileuton

 levacecarnine

Brand name
Alcar

Use
naturally occurring substance related to acetylcholine that has been studied in connection with treatment of Alzheimer disease and diabetic peripheral neuropathy

Usual dosage
oral: doses of 2 g daily have been used in clinical trials

Pharmaceutical company
Roche Laboratories. Nutley, NJ.

Source
University of Pittsburgh Drug Information and Pharmacoepidemiology Center. Pittsburgh, PA.

 Levaquin

Generic name
see levofloxacin

 Level I normothermic irrigating system

Description
warming device that delivers consistent body temperature irrigating solutions; keeps patients warm; used for hysteroscopy, laparoscopy, arthroscopy, cystoscopy and other procedures; reduces incidence of hypothermia

Source
Level I Technologies Inc. product information. Rockland, MA.

Levin drill guide

Description
orthopaedic instrument designed to help simplify the procedure of locating and starting portal for femoral intramedullary rodding

Source
Innomed Inc. product information. Savannah, GA.

 levofloxacin

Brand name
Levaquin

Use
antibacterial for respiratory infections, skin, urinary tract, and kidney infections (Editor note: This has been incorrectly spelled as Levoquin on several Internet sites including Johnson & Johnson; Ortho-McNeil is a division of Johnson & Johnson)

Usual dosage
tablet and intravenous forms, once a day

Pharmaceutical company
Ortho-McNeil Pharmaceutical. Raritan, NJ.

Source
Ortho-McNeil Pharmaceutical press release on Internet.

 Lewis blood group system genotyping

Synonyms
Le system genotyping; FUT3 genotyping; Lewis system PCR

Use
blood group subtyping, particularly of Lewis-negative individuals

Method
sequence-specific primed polymerase chain reaction

Specimen
blood

Normal range
not applicable, multiple FUT3 gene mutation patterns exist in Lewis-negative individuals

Comments
investigational

Source
Adapted from Elmgren A, Börjeson C, Svensson L, Rydberg L, Larson G. DNA sequencing and screening for point mutations in the human Lewis (FUT3) gene enables molecular genotyping of the human Lewis blood group system. Vox Sanguinis 1996;70:97-103.

308

 Lexxel

Generic name
see enalapril maleate/felodipine ER

 liarozole fumarate

Brand name
Liazal

Use
under investigation for the treatment of hormone refractory prostate cancer and for the treatment of severe psoriasis

Usual dosage
oral: caplet formulation; in clinical trials, doses of 37.5 mg to maximum of 300 mg twice daily dosing were used to treat prostate cancer, and doses of 75 mg to 150 mg twice daily dosing were used to treat severe psoriasis

Pharmaceutical company
Janssen Pharmaceutical. Titusville, NJ.

Source
Stadtlanders Managed Pharmacy Services. Pittsburgh, PA.

 Liazal

Generic name
see liarozole fumarate

 Lidakol

Generic name
see n-docosanol

 lidocaine transoral delivery system

Brand name
DentiPatch

Use
first transoral patch used as local anesthetic during soft-tissue dental procedures; duration of anesthesia activity may last up to 45 minutes

Usual dosage
small adhesive patch placed transorally for approximately two minutes

Pharmaceutical company
Noven Pharmaceuticals Inc. Miami, FL.

Source
Internet www.fda.gov.

LiftALERT

Description
lightweight electronic device; lifting monitor clips on the back of a shirt collar; internal sensor sounds an audible alert when the wearer bends over into an incorrect lifting position; reinforces proper lifting habits and helps make proper lifting a subconscious habit

Source
OPTP product information. Minneapolis, MN.

 ## LighTouch Neonate thermometer

Description
infrared thermometer recommended for axilla; can be used on wet skin, in incubators, during phototherapy, and in presence of heaters

Source
Exergen product information. Newton, MA.

 ## Lim Broth concentrate

Description
screening concentrate for detecting group B streptococcal disease

Source
Becton Dickinson product information. Sparks, MD.

 ## limited toxicology screening

Synonyms
LIM

Use
detection of multiple pharmaceutical agents, emphasizing drugs of abuse

Method
automated enzyme immunoassays in combination with colorimetric spot tests

Specimen
urine

Normal range
negative

Comments
due to cost effectiveness may replace more costly comprehensive toxicology screening in many cases

Source
Adapted from Bailey DN. Results of limited versus comprehensive toxicology screening in a university medical center. American Journal of Clinical Pathology 1996;105:572-575.

Lindstrom arcuate incision marker

Description
ophthalmologic surgery incision marker

Source
ASSI product information. Westbury, NY.

 Lindstrom Star nucleus manipulator

Description
ophthalmic surgical instrument designed to fit through a paracentesis or phaco incision for easy manipulation of nucleus; unique star-shaped tip is ideal for rotating and fracturing nucleus when used with phaco tip

Source
Rhein Medical Inc. product information. Tampa, FL.

 Lingeman drape

Description
surgical drape for abdominal perineal procedures; pre-attached bag for total fluid control

Source
Lingeman Medical Products Inc. product information. Indianapolis, IN.

 Linomide

Generic name
see roquinimex

 Lion's Claw grasper

Description
reusable toothed forceps for aggressive grasping of hardened tissue during endoscopic procedures

Source
Aslan Medical Technologies product information. Kalamazoo, MI.

 Lion's Paw grasper

Description
reusable forceps for non-aggressive grasping of hardened tissue during endoscopic procedures

Source
Aslan Medical Technologies product information. Kalamazoo, MI.

Lipitor

Generic name
see atorvastatin

liposomal doxorubicin

Brand name
Doxil

Use
treatment of Kaposi sarcoma in AIDS patients

Usual dosage
injectable: 20 mg/m² intravenously every two to three weeks has been used in clinical trials

Pharmaceutical company
SEQUUS Pharmaceuticals Inc. Menlo Park, CA.

Source
University of Pittsburgh Drug Information and Pharmacoepidemiology Center. Pittsburgh, PA.

Liposorber cholesterol filtering system

Description
filters low density lipoprotein (LDL "bad" cholesterol) in patients with extremely high cholesterol levels unable to be lowered by low-fat diet and cholesterol-lowering medications; process similar to kidney dialysis and must be repeated every one to two weeks

Source
Kaneka America Corp. product information. New York, NY.

Liquid Embolic System (LES)

Description
nonadhesive liquid embolic material for treatment of arteriovenous malformations and aneurysms; delivered to site via microcatheter under continuous fluoroscopic monitoring; human clinical trials have started outside the United States

Source
Micro Therapeutics Inc. product information. San Clemente, CA.

LiquiVent

Generic name
see perflubron

lisofylline (LSF)

Brand name
Protec

Use
toxicity modifier for patients receiving radiation and/or chemotherapy in phase III studies; also phase II studies for treatment of acute myeloid leukemia; also studies with adult respiratory distress syndrome following multiple trauma pending; inhibits cytokine-induced phosphatidic acid production; also known as CT 1501-R

Usual dosage
not given at this time

Pharmaceutical company
Cell Therapeutics Inc. Seattle, WA. with Johnson & Johnson Inc. Arlington, TX.

Source
Food and Drug Administration Internet site.

 Lite Blade

Description
disposable laryngoscope system that fits on a standard handle; offers the rigidity of a metal blade and a bright white light for better visualization; sizes include pediatric short, small/penlight, stubby short, and medium standard; Howland lock handle adjusts to different angles, including 180 degrees, 135 degrees, 90 degrees, or 45 degrees

Source
Rusch Inc. product information. Duluth, GA.

 Lite-Gait therapy device

Description
partial weightbearing gait therapy device; harness promotes balance and posture for walking therapy; facilitates proper gait patterns early in rehabilitation process; provides supported gait training to patients with all impairment levels; lifts patients out of wheelchair into an upright walking position; also Lite-Gait Jr., which provides supported gait training for pediatric population

Source
Mobility Research LLC product information. Tempe, AZ.

Lithospec lithotriptor (lithotripter)

Description
intracorporeal lithotriptor using electromagnetic energy to deliver high-impact mechanical fragmentation power directly to urinary tract stone

Source
Medispec Ltd. product information. Rockville, MD.

Littman Master Classic II stethoscope

Description
has a single-sided chest piece that responds to finger pressure to mimic the bell side and diaphragm side of a traditional chest piece; also features single lumen tube that folds without kinking

Source
3M Health Care product information. St. Paul, MN.

live oral polio vaccine

Brand name
OPOL

Use
vaccine to prevent polio

Usual dosage
oral: 0.5 ml placed directly into the mouth; recommended schedule of 3 doses with the first being at age 2 months followed by the second dose at age 4 months and the third dose at age 15-18 months

Pharmaceutical company
Lederle Laboratories. Wayne, NJ.

Source
University of Pittsburgh Drug Information and Pharmacoepidemiology Center. Pittsburgh, PA.

Livernois pickup and folding forceps

Description
L-shaped winged forceps used to engage and pick up intraocular lens; uniquely shaped concave jaw surfaces followed the lower edges of the convex lens optic for maximum exposure allowing central placement of the inserting forceps; broad tips make it easy to insert the leading haptic into the folding lens

Source
Katena Products Inc. product information. Denville, NJ.

Livial

Generic name
see tibolone

 LMA-Unique (laryngeal mask airway-Unique)

Description
single-use, disposable airway device

Source
Gensia Sicor product information. San Diego, CA.

 Logiparin

Generic name
see tinzaparin

 logistic discriminant analysis

Synonyms
none

Indications
interpretation of initial visual field defects

Method
retrospective study of visual field defects; fields visualized at least twice with program G1 of Octopus 500; data base information created and logistic discriminant analysis (SAS Logistic Procedures) applied

Normal findings
classification rules of qualifying visual field defects as glaucomatous or nonglaucomatous obtained and tested with an independent sample

Comments
logistic discriminant analysis is a useful tool to aid in interpretation of early glaucomatous and nonglaucomatous visual field defects

Source
Adapted from Anton A, Maquet JA, Mayo A, Tapia J, Pastor JC. Value of logistic discriminant analysis for interpreting initial visual field defects. Ophthalmology Journal 1997;104:525-531.

long-term culture-cobblestone-area-forming cells

Synonyms
LTC-CAFC

Use
long-term culture-cobblestone-area-forming cells (LTC-CAFC) detect and enumerate true functional blood stem cells in bone marrow, peripheral blood stem cell cytapheresis products, and umbilical cord blood

Method
prolonged liquid co-culture of cells on a stromal cell monolayer followed by enumeration of hemopoietic cobblestone areas long-term culture-cobblestone-area-forming cells

Specimen
bone marrow; peripheral blood stem cell cytapheresis product; umbilical cord blood

Normal range
investigational use

Comments
results expressed as number of LTC-CAFC

Source
University of Minnesota Department of Laboratory Medicine and Pathology. Minneapolis, MN.

 long-term culture initiating cell assay

Synonyms
LTC-IC assay; long-term bone marrow culture assay; LT-BMC assay

Use
long-term culture initiating cell (LTC-IC) assay detects and enumerates true functional blood stem cells in bone marrow culture (BMC), peripheral blood stem cell cytapheresis products, and umbilical cord blood

Method
prolonged liquid co-culture of cells on stromal cell monolayer, followed by progenitor assay to detect colony-forming units (CFUs)

Specimen
bone marrow; peripheral blood stem cell cytapheresis product; umbilical cord blood

Normal range
investigational use

Comments
results reported as numbers of colony-forming unit-granulocyte/macrophage (CFU-GM), burst-forming unit-erythroid (BFU-e), and colony-forming unit-granulocyte/erythrocyte/megakaryocyte/macrophage (CFU-GEMM)

Source
University of Minnesota Department of Laboratory Medicine and Pathology. Minneapolis, MN.

long-term repopulating ability assay

Synonyms
LTRA assay

Use
long-term repopulating ability (LTRA) assay detects and enumerates true functional blood stem cells in bone marrow, peripheral blood stem cell cytapheresis products, and umbilical cord blood

Method
transplantation of genetically marked cells into recipients, commonly mice

Specimen
bone marrow; peripheral blood stem cell cytapheresis product; umbilical cord blood

Normal range
investigational use

Comments
performance characteristics and appropriate interpretation of results have not been established

Source
University of Minnesota Department of Laboratory Medicine and Pathology. Minneapolis, MN.

 losartan

Brand name
Cozaar

Use
angiotensin II receptor antagonist used for the treatment of hypertension and congestive heart failure

Usual dosage
oral: 50 mg once daily

Pharmaceutical company
Merck & Co. West Point, PA.

Source
University of Pittsburgh Drug Information and Pharmacoepidemiology Center. Pittsburgh, PA.

 losartan potassium/hydrochlorothiazide

Brand Name
Hyzaar

Use
combination of angiotensin converting enzyme inhibitor and thiazide diuretic for the treatment of hypertension

Usual Dosage
oral: one tablet daily which contains 50 mg of losartan, 12.5 mg of hydrochlorothiazide, and 4.24 mg of potassium

Pharmaceutical company
Merck. West Point, PA.

Source
University of Pittsburgh Drug Information and Pharmacoepidemiology Center. Pittsburgh, PA.

 ## Lotemax Tm

Generic name
see loteprednol etabonate

 ## loteprednol etabonate

Brand name
Lotemax Tm

Use
topical steroid for the treatment of seasonal allergic conjunctivitis

Usual dosage
ophthalmic: 0.5% suspension, 1 drop to eye(s) 4 times a day in clinical trials

Pharmaceutical company
Bausch & Lomb Pharmaceuticals. Tampa, FL.

Source
Stadtlanders Managed Pharmacy Services. Pittsburgh, PA.

 ## Lotrel

Generic Name
see amlodipine/benazepril

 ## low margin standard abutment

Description
one-piece abutment designed for externally hexed implants making it compatible with most standard implants; its low occlusal height and small diameter allow it to be used where a standard abutment would not fit

Source
Sterngold-ImplaMed product information. Attleboro, MA.

 ## Low Profile Port vascular access

Description
implantable port for vascular access

Source
Arrow International product information. Reading, PA.

lubeluzole

Brand name
Prosynap

Use
treatment of ischemic stroke or intracerebral hemorrhage

Usual dosage
injectable: 7.5-15 mg over 1 hour, then 10-20 mg/day

Pharmaceutical company
Janssen Pharmaceuticals. Titusville, NJ.

Source
Stadtlanders Managed Pharmacy Services. Pittsburgh, PA.

 Luhr pan fixation system

Description
oral maxillofacial pan fixation system includes plate and screw; 0.5 mm
micro and pan plate thickness; 0.7 mm mini-plate thickness

Source
Howmedica Inc. product information. Rutherford, NJ.

 lumbar periosteal turnover flap

Description
surgical method that provides a secure and watertight closure over a primary repair of the spinal cord; adds additional autologous layer to standard skin
or muscle flap repairs

Anatomy
spinal cord; latissimus dorsi; thoracolumbar fascia; bony pedicle; periosteum; paraspinous muscles; cerebrospinal fluid

Equipment
standard neurosurgical equipment

Source
Adapted from Fiala GS, Buchman SR, Muraszko KM. Use of lumbar periosteal turnover flaps in myelome-
ningocele closure. Neurosurgery 1996;39:522-526.

 lunch-box type umbilical reconstruction

Description
method of reconstruction of the umbilicus using cartilage from patient's ear

Anatomy
omphalocele; umbilicus; conchal cartilage graft

Equipment
standard surgical equipment

Source
Adapted from Onishi K, Yang Y, Maruyama Y. A new lunch-box type method in umbilical reconstruction. Annals of Plastic Surgery 1995;35:654-656.

 lung injury score (LIS)

Synonyms
none

Indications
a method to assess the extent of lung injury, as a predictor of outcome in adult respiratory distress syndrome (ARDS)

Method
scoring on C-4 scale from best to worst, based on the following parameters: 1) chest roentgenogram score: alveolar consolidation 0 equals none, 4 equals four quadrant consolidation; 2) hypoxemia score PaO_2/FIO_2: >300 to <100; 3) PEEP score when intubated: >5 cm H_2O to >15 cm H_2O; 4) respiratory system compliance score (RSCS): >8 ml/cm H_2O to <19 ml/cm H_2O

Normal findings
score equals 0

Comments
LIS is a short, practical method of assessment with a continuum of severity within the index

Source
Adapted from Meduri G, Kohler G, Headley S, Tolley E, Stentz F, Postlewaite A. Inflammatory cytokines in the BAL of patients with ARDS. Chest 1995;108(5):1303-1314.

 Luntz-Dodick punch

Description
ophthalmic surgical instrument designed to perform trabeculectomy through the sclerocorneal tunnel; used for small or large trabeculectomies

Source
Katena Products Inc. product information. Denville, NY.

 Luvox

Generic name
see fluvoxamine

Luxtec surgical telescope

Description
illuminated telescope for hand surgery, microsurgery, and aesthetic surgery;
provides direct light to operative site
Source
Luxtec Corp. product information. Worcester, MA.

Lyme disease DNA detection

Synonyms
Borrelia burgdorferi DNA assay; *Borrelia burgdorferi* DNA probe test; DNA
hybridization test for *Borrelia burgdorferi*; DNA probe test for Lyme disease
Use
detect presence of deoxyribonucleic acid (DNA) from spirochete *Borrelia
burgdorferi* in patients with signs and symptoms of Lyme disease
Method
treat specimens to isolate DNA and rid the sample of substances that inhibit amplification of DNA; amplify DNA using specific primers for *Borrelia
burgdorferi* sequences; confirm amplified DNA as *Borrelia burgdorferi* by
hybridization with DNA probe
Specimen
blood; cerebrospinal fluid; synovial fluid; urine
Normal range
uninfected specimen contains no *Borrelia burgdorferi* DNA
Comments
none
Source
Lexi-Comp Inc. database. Hudson, OH.

Lym-1 monoclonal antibody with radioisotope iodine-131

Brand name
Oncolym
Use
treatment of refractory B-cell lymphoma
Usual dosage
injectable: doses of 5-50 mg/day were studied in clinical trials
Pharmaceutical company
Techniclone/Alpha Therapeutics. Los Angeles, CA.
Source
Stadtlanders Managed Pharmacy Services. Pittsburgh, PA.

LYOfoam dressing

Description
semipermeable polyurethane foam dressing that promotes healing of light-to-moderate exuding wounds; LYOfoam A is water resistant; LYOfoam C has activated carbon to absorb and neutralize offensive odors; and LYOfoam T has cross-cut design to fit around tubes, cannulas, or pins

Source
Acme United Corp. product information. Fairfield, CT.

 lysophosphatidylcholine (lysoPC)

Synonyms
none

Use
diagnostic ovarian cancer test

Method
not given

Specimen
plasma

Normal range
not reported

Comments
component of normal blood found to be elevated in patients with ovarian cancer

Source
Adapted from Okita M, Gaudette DC, Mills GB, Holub BJ. Elevated levels and altered fatty acid composition of plasma lysophosphatidylcholine (lysoPC) in ovarian cancer patients. International Journal of Cancer 1997;71:31-34.

 Madajet XL local anesthesia

Description
podiatric model eliminates the needle and overcomes much of the physical and psychological trauma associated with traditional needle and syringe injection; provides instant local anesthesia for treatment of incurvated nails, nail evulsions, removal of viral verrucae, and other podiatry procedures; can also be used as a pre-injection site for deep needle insertion or the infiltration of steroids for dermatological lesions

Source
Mada Equipment Co. product information. Carlstadt, NJ.

Maddacare child bath seat

Description

aluminum frame, support surface is open mesh polyester knit, rustproof, knobs to adjust angles and backrest, suction cup feet to prevent scratching of tub

Source

Maddak Inc. product information. Pequanock, NJ.

Maddapult Asissto-Seat

Description

assistive device for patients with arthritis or other disabilities to easily sit down and rise through spring action lever

Source

Maddak Inc. product information. Pequanock, NJ.

Magill Safety Clear & Safety Clear Plus endotracheal tube

Description

high volume, low pressure cuff with black positioning ring with x-ray opaque line; available in 3.5 mm size increasing to 4.5 mm in 0.5-mm increments

Source

Rusch Inc. product information. Duluth, GA.

Magnassager massage tool

Description

hand-held device simulates natural hand massage with stainless steel balls suspended by a natural permanent magnet

Source

Optimum Health Technologies Inc. product information. Rocklin, CA.

Magnatherm and Magnatherm SSP electromagnet therapy unit

Description

portable, electromagnetic therapy unit with 2 interdependent treatment sources; allows therapy to 2 areas simultaneously or to treat 1 site synergistically; designed to increase blood flow, improve oxygenation, and increase metabolic rate; relieves pain and edema and speeds healing of such conditions as low back pain and muscle spasms, arthritis, sprains, strains, and other debilitative musculoskeletal conditions, as well as wound healing

Source

Medical Electronics Ltd. product information. Kansas City, MO.

magnetic resonance neurography (MRN)

Description
technique used to image fascicular structure of peripheral nerves and its distortion by mass lesions or trauma in the lower extremity

Source
Adapted from Kuntz C, Blake L, Britz G et al. Magnetic resonance neurography of peripheral nerve lesions in the lower extremity. Neurosurgery 1996;39:750-757.

magnetic source imaging

Indications
preoperative mapping of sensorimotor cortex in neurosurgical patients; characterization and localization of epileptiform activity; characterizes abnormal spontaneous rhythms prominent in a wide range of neurologic disorders

Method
biomagnetometer is used to measure the neuromagnetic field generated by parts of the brain; mathematical models are used to integrate this information with structural magnetic resonance (MR) imaging data, identifying those brain structures responsible for the detected currents magnetic source imaging

Normal findings
selectively stimulated neurons or epileptic foci produce a detectable signal within the brain which allows exact localization of the brain structures responsible for the signal

Comments
completely noninvasive, preoperative localization of sensorimotor cortex; provides better risk assessment and craniotomy site selection

Source
University of Maryland Department of Diagnostic Radiology. Baltimore, MD.

Mahurkar curved extension catheter

Description
180-degree extensions improve patient comfort and help promote patient acceptance of the jugular route for peripheral vascular access

Source
Quinton Instrument Co. product information. Seattle, WA.

Maidera-Stern suture hook

Description

ophthalmic surgical instrument designed to assist in suture placement around the iris for manual retraction; particularly useful in small pupil retinal procedures

Source

Storz Ophthalmics product information. St. Louis, MO.

Malarone

Generic name

see atovaquone/proguanil

mammalian cell-derived recombinant human growth hormone

Brand name

Serostim

Use

treatment of AIDS-related wasting syndrome

Usual dosage

injectable: 6 mg/day given as a subcuntaneous injection

Pharmaceutical company

Serono Labs Inc. Norwell, MA.

Source

University of Pittsburgh Drug Information and Pharmacoepidemiology Center. Pittsburgh, PA.

Mammopatch gel self adhesive

Description

breast scar treatment that is washable, reusable, and soft; covers scars around the areola, extending vertically down the breast and underneath the breast for any type of breast surgery

Source

Medical Z Corp. product information. San Antonio, TX.

Mandelkorn suture lysis lens

Description

ophthalmic lens developed to cut subconjunctival nylon sutures following trabeculectomy surgery to improve outflow through scleral flap, and/or cataract surgery for astigmatism control through release of tight sutures

Source

Ocular Instruments Inc. product information. Bellevue, WA.

mangafodipir trisodium

Brand name
Teslascan

Use
magnetic resonance imaging (MRI) enhancer for the evaluation of hepatocellular carcinoma and cirrhotic livers

Usual dosage
injectable: 5 μmol/kg in clinical trials

Pharmaceutical company
Nycomed Inc. Princeton, NJ.

Source
Stadtlanders Managed Pharmacy Services. Pittsburgh, PA.

 ## Mangum knot pusher

Description
surgical instrument that allows surgeon to tie multiple extracorporeal surgical knots quickly and simply; design of distal tip securely holds knots without having to thread suture through knot pusher

Source
Innovative Surgical Inc. product information. West Palm Beach, FL.

 ## marking clips for positioning of esophageal stents

Description
stents are frequently used for palliation of dysphagia caused by inoperable esophageal carcinoma; self-expandable metallic stents were developed to allow less traumatic insertion; a metallic clip with a marking clip was used to facilitate accurate positioning of the stent under fluoroscopic control; stents are placed via small-diameter delivery systems; they are introduced over a guide wire that is placed endoscopically

Anatomy
esophagus; esophageal wall; lumen

Equipment
standard surgery equipment; 12-mm balloon; endoscope; guide wire; HX-3L clip fixing device; Microvasive Ultraflex self-expandable stent; small-diameter delivery system

Source
Adapted from deBoer WA, van Haren F, Driessen WMM. Marking clips for the accurate positioning of self-expandable esophageal stents. Gastrointestinal Endoscopy 1995;42:73-76.

Marquette Responder 1500 multifunctional defibrillator

Description

emergency cardiac device serves as a defibrillator and electrocardiograph monitor; offers noninvasive pacing and computerized 12-lead electrocardiogram analysis

Source

Marquette Electronics Inc. product information. Milwaukee, WI.

 Marritt dilator

Description

surgical dilator used specifically in hair transplantation procedures

Source

Robbins Instruments Inc. product information. Chatham, NJ.

 Marrs intrauterine catheter

Description

gynecologic instrument for introduction of washed spermatozoa into the uterine cavity; closed-end catheter with side opening features an adjustable positioner for optimal catheter placement

Source

Cook OB/GYN product information. Spencer, IN.

 mask lift with facial aesthetic sculpting

Description

surgical approach reduces appearance of aging or corrects deformity; facial mask lifted subperiosteally, allowing aesthetic sculpture of underlying structures; includes contour burring to smooth forehead and orbital rims and/or bone grafting to chin and/or malar region; may involve lateral canthopexy, galea-frontalis muscle resection with corrugator excision, and lip augmentation

Anatomy

facial soft tissue; periosteum; skin; adipose tissue; fascia; frontal bone; orbital margins; orbital cavity; zygomatic arch; malar prominences; maxilla; palpebral fissure

Equipment

standard surgery equipment, with periosteal elevator

Source

Adapted from Krastnova-Lolov D. Mask lift and facial aesthetic sculpturing. Plastic and Reconstructive Surgery 1995;95:21-36.

Matritech nuclear matrix protein (NMP) 22 test kit

Description
quantitative, noninvasive urine test for bladder cancer based on protein marker

Source
Matritech Inc. product information. Newton, MA.

 Mavik

Generic name
see trandolapril

 Maxalt

Generic name
see rizatriptan benzoate

 Maxamine

Brand name
none given

Use
cytokine therapy for adjuvant treatment of cancer and infectious diseases including acute myelogenous leukemia, multiple myeloma, renal cell carcinoma, and hepatitis; in phase III trials

Usual dosage
not given

Pharmaceutical company
Maxim Pharmaceuticals. San Diego, CA.

Source
Food and Drug Administration Internet site.

 MaxForce TTS balloon dilatation catheter

Description
esophageal dilatation catheter; provides fast, effective approach to through-the-scope (TTS) dilatation; reduced procedure time due to inflation and deflation in seconds

Source
Microvasive Boston Scientific Corp. product information. Natick, MA.

MaxiFloat wheelchair cushion

Description
cushions provide therapy, comfort, positioning, and passive restraint for wheelchair-bound patients; pressure reduction

Source
BG Industries product information. McGaw Park, IL.

 maxillomandibular advancement for treatment of obstructive sleep apnea

Description
mandibular advancement by bilateral retromolar sagittal split osteotomy and maxillary advancement by Le Fort I osteotomy that enlarges the pharyngeal opening

Anatomy
mandible; maxilla; suprahyoid muscle; velopharyngeal muscle; hard palate; soft palate

Equipment
standard oral surgery instruments

Source
Adapted from Hochban W, Conradt R, Brandenburg U, et al. Surgical maxillofacial treatment of obstructive sleep apnea. Plastic and Reconstructive Surgery 1997;99:619-626.

 Maxima Plus plasma resistant fiber (PRF) oxygenator

Description
surgical device for oxygen transfer during procedure; has a hollow fiber oxygenator with plasma resistant fiber; improves hemostasis management and reduces the whole inflammatory response

Source
Medtronic Inc. product information. Minneapolis, MN.

 Maxima II transcutaneous electrical nerve stimulator

Description
multimode transcutaneous electrical nerve stimulator (TENS) unit; programmed treatment mode works like patient-controlled analgesia (PCA) pump

Source
Staodyn Inc. product information. Longmont, CO.

Maxipime

Generic name
see cefepime

 Maxivent

Generic name
see doxofylline

 Maxum reusable endoscopic forceps

Description
tough reusable forceps used with gastroscopes and colonoscopes; forceps guarantee consistent bite; acuMax forceps cups close evenly along the rim for a clean cut; no tearing or crushing of sample tissue

Source
Wilson-Cook Medical product information. Winston-Salem, NC.

 Mayfield/ACCISS stereotactic device

Description
interactive image-guided surgical navigation and planning system

Source
Ohio Medical Instrument Co. product information. Cincinnati, OH.

 MB-900 AC machine

Description
dedicated foot and ankle x-ray machine with adjustable kv selection from 50 to 90 kVp; state-of-the-art microprocessor-controlled timer with digital read-out and keypad entry; includes a 6-inch high-power box which allows x-rays without special lead-lined walls

Source
X-Cel X-Ray Corp. product information. Crystal Lake, IL.

McBride procedure, further modification

Description
procedure for hallux valgus using Acufex tag system to reattach adductor hallucis; adductor tendon exposed through separate incision proximal to dorsal aspect of web space; released from both insertions; suture passed through tendon; lateral capsule released to allow correction of valgus angle at metatarsophalangeal joint; medial capsular reefing then performed; Acufex tag suture attached to neck of first metatarsal using the hand awl; adductor suture tied to tag suture that attaches the adductor to neck of metatarsal

Anatomy
adductor hallucis; adductor tendon; dorsal aspect of web space; flexor hallucis brevis; hallux valgus; intertarsal ligament; lateral and medial capsules; metatarsophalangeal joint; metatarsal neck

Equipment
standard orthopaedic equipment; Acufex tag suture and hand awl

Source
Adapted from Harris NJ, Scott B, Smith TWD. A further modification to the McBride procedure for hallux valgus using the Acufex tag system to reattach the adductor hallucis. Foot and Ankle International Journal 1997;18:57-58.

 McDonald optic zone marker

Description
ophthalmologic incision marker

Source
ASSI product information. Westbury, NY.

 McDougal prostatectomy clamps

Description
secures the dorsal vein complex during radical retropubic prostatectomy; made of stainless steel with 2-cm jaw length; useful for other deep retropubic or deep pelvic work during abdominal approach procedure; allows easy access when operative site obstructed by the pubis or other structures

Source
Rusch Inc. product information. Duluth, GA.

 M-cup vacuum device

Description
vacuum extraction device featuring both stainless steel and disposable cups

Source
Adapted from Bofill JA, Rust OA, Schorr SJ, Brown RC, Roberts WE, Morrison JC. A randomized trial of two vacuum extraction techniques. Obstetrics and Gynecology 1997;89:758-762.

MedaSonics ultrasound stethoscope model BF4B and model BF5A

Description
ideal for locating vessels, taking weak pulses, and assessing vessel patency; superior alternative to using stethoscopes for systolic pressures of shock patients, infants, obese patients, and others with weak pulses

Source
MedaSonics product information. Fremont, CA.

Mediflow pillow

Description
pillow containing a thermal reflector blanket and water sac

Source
Mediflow Inc. product information. Markham, Ontario, Canada.

Medipore H surgical tape

Description
soft cloth surgical tape that is more adhesive than regular Medipore tape, suitable to use in situations when increased movement or swelling may affect tape's ability to hold dressings in place

Source
3M Health Care product information. St. Paul, MN.

MediSkin

Description
skin care product for incontinence and general quality skin care

Source
Benjamin Ansehl Co. product information. St. Louis, MO.

MedMorph III

Description
computer package that allows the plastic surgeon to graphically perform changes directly on patient's computerized image for blepharoplasty, rhinoplasty, chin augmentation/reduction, facelift, browlift, breast augmentation, liposuction

Source
MedMorph product information. Slidell, LA.

Medpor surgical implants

Description

high density porous polyethylene product line of 70 facial, malar, and chin implants for augmentation and reconstruction; chin shapes have a 2-piece split design which enables the surgeon to place the implant sections through a small incision and then bring the sections together

Source

Porex Surgical Inc. product information. College Park, GA.

 Megalone

Generic name

see fleroxacin

 Melacine

Generic name

see melanoma theraccine

 melanoma theraccine

Brand name

Melacine

Use

therapeutic melanoma vaccine for the treatment of malignant melanoma or adjunctive therapy for melanoma in patients with no evidence of disease

Usual dosage

subcutaneous: one weekly injection of 20 million tumor cell-equivalents on weeks 1, 2, 3, 4, and 6 for 1 to 2 courses followed by monthly injections

Pharmaceutical company

Ribi ImmunoChem Research Inc. Hamilton, MT.

Source

University of Pittsburgh Drug Information and Pharmacoepidemiology Center. Pittsburgh, PA.

 Mentane

Generic name

see velnacrine maleate

 Mentax

Generic name

see butenafine hydrochloride

Mentor Self-Cath soft catheter

Description
latex-free line of self-catheters

Source
Mentor Urology product information. Mentor, OH.

 ## Menuet Compact urodynamic testing device

Description
electrodiagnostic device performs all standard urodynamic tests; provides diagnosis of lower urinary tract disorders; offers optional plotting to diagnose obstructions and to analyze stress urethral pressure profiles

Source
Dantec Medical Inc. product information. Campbell, CA.

 ## Mepitel dressing

Description
dressing that protects moist wounds without adhering to it; indicated for post-trauma/postsurgery wounds, graft recipient sites, first- and second-degree burns, freshly debrided wounds, wounds with friable or excoriated surrounding skin, or wounds where current dressings tend to stick

Source
Medwest Surgical Inc. product information. Fair Oaks, CA.

 ## Mepron

Generic Name
see atovaquone

 ## Meridia

Generic name
see sibutramine

 ## Merlin arthroscopy blade

Description
bendable arthroscopy blade can be bent while in the sterile field and if necessary bent again offering a specialized instrument for each patient

Source
Linvatec Corp. product information. Largo, FL.

meropenem

Brand name
Merrem

Use
carbapenem antibiotic used in intra-abdominal and soft tissue infections, febrile neutropenia, urinary tract infections, and Pseudomonas meningitis

Usual dosage
intravenous: 0.5 to 1 g every 8 hours; 2 g every 8 hours has been administered in meningitis

Pharmaceutical company
Zeneca Pharmaceuticals Group. Wilmington, DE.

Source
University of Pittsburgh Drug Information and Pharmacoepidemiology Center. Pittsburgh, PA.

 Merrem

Generic name
see meropenem

 mesorectal excision of the rectum

Description
total mesorectal excision (TME) is reported to reduce local recurrence in patients with carcinoma of rectum; a large percentage of patients have either full-thickness penetration of the rectal wall or involvement of mesorectal lymph nodes; TME provides local control through resection of the entire unit of regional spread that is excised, intact and with negative circumferential margins; TME is compatible with autonomic nerve preservation and with sphincter preservation

Anatomy
adventitia; autonomic nerves; Denonvilliers fascia; internal iliac artery; inferior mesenteric artery and vein; levator ani; levator fascia; mesorectal lymph nodes; mesorectum; parietal plane of pelvic fascia; pelvic sidewall; pelvic peritoneum; pelvic auton omic, sympathetic, and parasympathetic nerves; nerve plexus; piriformis muscles; pouch of Douglas; rectovaginal septum; rectum; superior hypogastric nerves; sphincter; true pelvis

Equipment
standard surgery equipment

Source
Adapted from Enker WE, Thaler HT, Cranor ML, Polyak T. Total mesorectal excision in the operative treatment of carcinoma of the rectum. Journal of American College of Surgeons 1995;181:335-345.

metaidoioplasty sex-change technique

Description
construction of a phallus (phalloplasty) in female-to-male transsexuals; use of anterior vaginal flap rather than groin or abdominal flaps decreases visible scarring

Anatomy
vagina; vaginal wall; vaginal mucosa; urethra; urethral orifice; urethral wall; pars fixa; clitoris; clitoral shaft; glans clitoridis; vestibule; minor labium; labia minora; labia majora; labial spongious corpora; corpora cavernosa; perineum; pars pendulans urethrae

Equipment
standard surgery equipment

Source
Adapted from Hage JJ. Metaidoioplasty: an alternative phalloplasty technique in transsexuals. Plastic and Reconstructive Surgery 1996;97:161-167.

 ## metformin hydrochloride

Brand name
Glucophage

Use
adjunct to diet meant to lower blood glucose in patients with noninsulin-dependent diabetes mellitus (NIDDM), Type II diabetes, whose hyperglycemia cannot be satisfactorily managed on diet alone; may be used concomitantly with a sulfonylurea for adequate glycemic control

Usual dosage:
oral: 500 and 850 mg tablets; usually 1 to 3 g daily in 2 to 3 divided doses

Pharmaceutical company
Bristol-Meyers Squibb Co. Princeton, NJ.

Source
University of Pittsburgh Drug Information and Pharmacoepidemiology Center. Pittsburgh, PA.

 ## methionine/cystine cream

Brand name
Amino acid cream

Use
external treatment of mild cervicitis, postpartum cervical injuries, and cervical wounds associated with some gynecological procedures

Usual dosage
topical: apply once a day

Pharmaceutical company
Hope Pharmaceuticals. Santa Ana, CA.
Source
Stadtlanders Managed Pharmacy Services. Pittsburgh, PA.

 ## methyl salicylate patch

Brand name
TheraPatch

Use
external analgesic for temporary relief of arthritis pain and muscle aches

Usual dosage
topical patches: apply to affected area once a day as needed; available in 2-inch and 3-inch individually wrapped patches

Pharmaceutical company
Del Pharmaceuticals. Plainview, NY.
Source
Stadtlanders Managed Pharmacy Services. Pittsburgh, PA.

 ## metoclopramide

Brand name
Emitasol

Use
topical formulation; an antiemetic administered intranasally for the prevention of emesis associated with cancer chemotherapy

Usual dosage
intranasal: 40 mg 2 hours before chemotherapy, followed by additional doses at 4 and 8 hours after chemotherapy was the dosage studied in clinical trials

Pharmaceutical company
Nastech/Ribogene. Hayward, CA.
Source
Stadtlanders Managed Pharmacy Services. Pittsburgh, PA.

 ## metronidazole/tetracycline, bismuth subsalicylate

Brand name
Helidac

Use
combination therapy for 14 days with bismuth subsalicylate for prevention and eradication of infections caused by *Helicobacter pylori* in patients with peptic ulcer disease

Usual dosage
oral: metronidazole 250 mg three times a day and tetracycline 500 mg four times a day were used concurrently with 5-8 Pepto-Bismol tablets in the clinical trials

Pharmaceutical company
Procter & Gamble. Cincinnati, OH.

Source
University of Pittsburgh Drug Information and Pharmacoepidemiology Center. Pittsburgh, PA.

 ## Miacalcin Nasal Spray

Generic name
see calcitonin (salmon)

 ## mianserin

Brand Name
Athymil

Use
tricyclic antidepressant for use in depressive disorders

Usual Dosage
oral: 30-40 mg daily

Pharmaceutical company
Organon Inc. West Orange, NJ.

Source
University of Pittsburgh Drug Information and Pharmacoepidemiology Center. Pittsburgh, PA.

 ## MIB-1 and PC10 as prognostic markers for esophageal squamous cell carcinoma

Synonyms
none

Indications
esophageal squamous cell carcinoma

Method
representative tissue collection from each tumor and immunohistochemical preparations for MIB-1 and PC10

Normal findings
not applicable

Comments
proliferative activity in esophageal squamous cell carcinoma significantly related to tumor differentiation as defined by MIB-1 immunohistochemical method; potentially valuable as prognostic marker in addition to its use in tumor staging and size; may be good indicator in predicting prognosis in Stage III cancers

Source
Adapted from Lam KY, Law SYK, Som MKP, et al. Prognostic implication of proliferative markers MIB-1 and PC10 in esophageal squamous cell carcinoma. Cancer 1996;77(1):7-13.

 # mibefradil

Brand name
Posicor

Use
calcium channel blocker used for the treatment of hypertension and angina

Usual dosage
oral: doses of 25, 50, or 100 mg once a day were used in clinical trials

Pharmaceutical company
Roche Laboratories. Nutley, NJ.

Source
Stadtlanders Managed Pharmacy Services. Pittsburgh, PA.

 # MicroDigitrapper

Description
MicroDigitrapper-S, MicroDigitrapper-HR, MicroDigitrapper-V, and Digitrapper MkIII series of portable apnea recorders for differential diagnosis of obstructive sleep apnea (OSA) and/or gastroesophageal reflux; records gastric and esophageal pH over a 24-hour period

Source
Synetics Medical product information. Irving, TX.

 # MicroFET2 muscle testing device

Description
ergonomic muscle testing device; shows peak force and test duration

Source
Hoggan Health Industries product information. Draper, UT.

Microgyn II device

Description
patient-controlled stimulation therapy for urinary incontinence; allows increased level of intensity as therapy progresses; probes for vaginal and anal applications

Source
InCare Medical Products of Hollister Inc. product information. Libertyville, IL.

 micrometastases clonogenic assay (MCA)

Synonyms
none

Use
detection of occult tumor cells

Method
soft-agar clonogenic assay

Specimen
bone marrow, peripheral blood stem cell collections

Normal range
no evidence of tumor colonies

Comments
investigational

Source
Blood 1993;82:2605-2610.

 micrometastases detection assay (MDA)

Synonyms
micro-tumor detection

Use
monitoring effectiveness of induction chemotherapy and tumor purging

Method
serial immunocytologic analysis using a panel of tumor-associated mono-clonal antibodies

Specimen
bone marrow

Normal range
no evidence of tumor cell staining

Comments
in active clinical use

Source
Blood 1993;82:2605-2610.

microplate detection of red blood cell antibodies

Synonyms
MMTMATC antibody testing

Use
sensitive and specific detection and identification of red blood cell antibodies

Method
visual detection of antibody bound to immobilized red blood cell monolayers

Specimen
blood

Normal range
no evidence of clinically significant antibodies

Comments
a rapid and low-cost antibody identification method

Source
Adapted from Llopis F, Carbonell-Uberos F, Planelles MD, Montero M, Plasencia I, Carrillo C. A new microplate red blood cell monolayer technique for screening and identifying red blood cell antibodies. Vox Sanguinis 1996;70:152-156.

 Micro Plus spirometer

Description
designed for bedside screening, emergency room use and home patient use; provides digital display of FVC, FEV1, PEF1, FEV1/FVC% and meets accuracy standards; supplied with predicted value calculator

Source
Micro Direct Inc. product information. Auburn, ME.

 Microsampler device

Description
single-step arterial blood sampling with 26-gauge microneedle to provide trauma-free puncture without hematoma; preheparinized capillary syringe provides better sample stability and no ice storage necessary for up to 30 minutes

Source
AVL Scientific Corp. product information. Roswell, GA.

 Microseal ophthalmic handpiece

Description
phacoemulsification surgical instrument for cataract surgery; takes small-incision to micro-incision; offers a more stable intraocular environment; virtually eliminates incision leakage

Source
Storz Ophthalmics product information. St. Louis, MO.

Microsporidia diagnostic procedures

Synonyms
none

Indications
part of differential diagnostic work-up of diarrhea and other *Microsporidia*-associated diseases in immunocompromised patients, particularly AIDS patients; establish diagnosis of microsporidiosis; *Microsporidia* had been demonstrated in immunocompetent persons

Method
staining

Normal findings
none detected

Comments
detection of *Microsporidia* is entirely dependent on adequacy of specimen, staining and preparation of specimen, and experience of person examining specimen

Source
Lexi-Comp Inc. database. Hudson, OH.

 ## microsurgical thoracoscopic vertebrectomy

Description
vertebrectomy and vertebral body reconstruction of anterior thoracic spine; used to treat osteomyelitis, tumors, and compression fractures

Anatomy
intercostal space; vertebral body; spinal cord; pleural cavity; parietal pleura; segmental vessels; rib head; disk; intercostal muscle; neurovascular bundle; azygous vein; hemidiaphragm; thoracic duct; artery of Adamkiewicz; paraspinal tissue; costotransverse ligament; costovertebral ligament; nerve root; neural foramen; pedicle; dura; thecal sac; annulus; cartilaginous endplate; bony endplate

Equipment
double-lumen endotracheal tube; long narrow spine dissection tools; screw plate; methylmethacrylate; bone graft; rigid rod-lens endoscope; lung retractor; chest tube; tissue clamp; blunt-tipped trocar; flexible portal; rigid portal; portal cuff; endoscopic fan retractor; blunt-tipped retractor; fan-shaped retractor; three-dimensional endoscope; video camera; video monitor display system; 30-degree angle endoscope; self-irrigating endoscope; right-angle clamp; Endoshears; fine tissue forceps; ringed tissue forceps; Babcock clamp; drill bit; cutting burr; osteotome; periosteal elevator; bone graft impactor; peanut dissector; Avitene delivery tube; bipolar cautery forceps; monopolar cautery blade; bipolar cautery scissors; monopolar cautery scissors; monopolar tissue forceps; Nuknit; bone wax; sponge stick; Cobb periosteal elevator;

angled Kerrison rongeur; disk rongeur; straight curette; curved curette; Penfield dissector; nerve hook; Midas Rex high-speed air drill; pistol-grip attachment; microscissors; right-angled clamp; disk rongeur; ball-shaped cutting burr; plastic surgical ruler

Source
Adapted from Dickman CA, Rosenthal D, Karahalios DG, Paramore CG, Mican CA, Apostolides PJ, et al. Thoracic vertebrectomy and reconstruction using a microsurgical thoracoscopic approach. Neurosurgery 1996;38:279-293.

 microtiter plate determination of serum total protein

Synonyms
microtiter total protein

Use
determination of total serum protein level in plasmapheresis donors

Method
micro-scale biuret assay with spectrophotometric endpoint

Specimen
serum

Normal range
56.0-73.8 g/liter

Comments
inexpensive and simple assay useful for facilities lacking multichannel chemistry analyzers

Source
Adapted from Mertens G, Muylle L. A microtiter plate method for total protein determination to screen plasma donors. Transfusion 1995;35:968-969.

 MicroVac catheter

Description
microneurosurgical suction and irrigation catheter

Source
Adapted from Johnson JP, Becker DP. A continuous microneurosurgical irrigation and suction system: technical note. Neurosurgery 1996;39:409-411.

 microvascular decompression

Description
microsurgical treatment of glossopharyngeal neuralgia, an uncommon cause of intermittent, lancinating facial pain; T-shaped incision; low lateral retromastoid craniectomy; subarachnoid space opened in the cistern; elevation of flocculus from brain stem; separation of pia-arachnoidal chordae from inferior aspect of the flocculus and cranial nerves

Anatomy

sigmoid and transverse sinuses; posterior fossa; posterior aspect of mastoid eminence; dura; 9th, 10th, and 11th nerves; subarachnoid space; flocculus; pia-arachnoidal chordae

Equipment

standard microvascular surgery equipment; dural tracking suture; microscope; self-retaining retractor; rubber-dam forceps; Cottonoid dissector; Teflon felt

Source

Adapted from Resnik DK, Jannetta PJ, Bissonnette D, Jho HD, Lanzino G. Microvascular decompression for glossopharyngeal neuralgia. Neurosurgery 1995;36:64-69.

 microvascular free flap

Description

microvascular reconstruction of the lower extremity using a mechanical vascular anastomotic device to construct a microvascular free flap graft

Anatomy

anterior tibial artery; venae comitantes; posterior tibial artery; popliteal artery

Equipment

loupe magnification; coupler ring; coupler sizer; 3M microvascular coupling device

Source

Adapted from Denk M, Longaker M, Basner A, Glat P, Karp N, Kasabian A. Microsurgical reconstruction of the lower extremity using the 3M microvascular coupling device in venous anastomoses. Annals of Plastic Surgery 1995;35:601-605.

 Microzide

Generic name

see hydrochlorothiazide

 Micro-Z neuromuscular stimulator

Description

small, lightweight (2 oz) high-volt, neuromuscular stimulator can be worn on the leg, arm, or belt; used in conjunction with Electro-Mesh garment electrodes (gloves, socks, and sleeves); offers nighttime therapy option for treatment; programmable, offering unlimited options up to 24 hours of treatment

Source

PRIZM Medical Inc. product information. Duluth, GA.

Micturin

Generic Name
see terodiline

midodrine

Brand name
ProAmatine

Use
long-acting alpha-adrenergic agonist used for orthostatic hypotension

Usual dosage
oral: 2.5 mg two or three times daily, increasing gradually to a maximum recommended dose of 40 mg daily

Pharmaceutical company
Roberts. Eatontown NJ.

Source
University of Pittsburgh Drug Information and Pharmacoepidemiology Center. Pittsburgh, PA.

midtarsal and tarsometatarsal arthrodesis for primary degenerative osteoarthritis

Description
procedure performed for osteoarthrosis after dislocation with or without a fracture, for primary degenerative osteoarthritis, or for inflammatory arthritis; the extent of the arthrodesis is determined by the degree of the osteoarthrosis

Anatomy
midtarsal joint; tarsometatarsal joint; metatarsocuneiform joints; metatarsocuboid joints; metatarsals; dorsalis pedis artery; deep peroneal nerve

Equipment
standard orthopaedic equipment; Steinmann pins; interfragmentary screws; medial buttress plate

Source
Adapted from Mann RA, Prieskorn D, Sobel M. Midtarsal and tarsometatarsal arthrodesis for primary degenerative osteoarthritis or osteoarthrosis after trauma. The Journal of Bone and Joint Surgery 1996;78:1376-1385.

miglitol

Brand name
Glyset

Use
an alpha-glucosidase inhibitor used to control blood glucose levels in type II diabetes by delaying the intestinal absorption of dietary carbohydrates

Usual dosage
oral: doses of 50 and 100 mg 3 times a day were studied in clinical trials

Pharmaceutical company
Bayer Pharmaceuticals. West Haven, CT.

Source
Stadtlanders Managed Pharmacy Services. Pittsburgh, PA.

 ## Migranal

Generic name
see dihydroergotamine mesylate

 ## Mikamo double-eyelid operation

Description
method produces a second palpebral fold in the Japanese eyelid for aesthetic purposes

Anatomy
upper eyelid; lower eyelid; conjunctiva; tarsus

Equipment
standard oculoplastic instruments

Source
Adapted from Sergile S, Obata K. Mikamo's double-eyelid operation: the advent of Japanese aesthetic surgery. Plastic and Reconstructive Surgery 1997;99:662-667.

 ## MiKasome

Generic name
see amikacin LF

 ## Millenia percutaneous transluminal coronary angioplasty (PTCA) catheter

Description
proprietary 3-D balloon material is unique polymer blend that combines the best characteristics of noncompliant and semi-compliant balloons; rated burst pressure of up to 16 atm (atmosphere); superb tracking; nominal size is attained at a low 6 atm in all diameters; minimizes friction and shear force while transitioning through the target site; designed for improved rewrap characteristics

Source
Medtronic Inc. product information. Minneapolis, MN.

 ## Mill-Rose protected specimen microbiology brushes (PSB)

Description
sealed sterile brushes for collecting specimens in the lower airway

Source
Mill-Rose Laboratories Inc. product information. Mentor, OH.

Mini II and Mini II+ automatic implantable cardioverter defibrillator (AICD)

Description

smaller than previous AICDs; new approved use for larger group of patients to include those at high risk for sudden death from ventricular arrhythmia but with no obvious symptoms

Source

CPI Guidant Corp. product information. St. Paul, MN.

Minidop ES-100VX Pocket Doppler

Description

records velocity waveforms using an electrocardiograph; clinical applications include peripheral vascular procedures, venous compressions, fetal heart rate, blood pressure segmental studies, penile and digit systolic pressures, flow detection in recovery room

Source

Koven Technology Inc. product information. Hazelwood, MO.

Miniguard stress incontinence device

Description

quarter-sized triangular-shaped disposable foam pad with adhesive coating on one side; available by prescription; pad forms a seal over the urethra; can be worn two to five hours and throughout the night with new pad placed after each urination

Source

Advanced Surgical Intervention product information. Dana Point, CA.

minilaparotomy hysterectomy

Description

minisuprapubic incision; continuous repositioning of retractors to expose sections of operative field; alternative to both standard and laparoscopically assisted hysterectomy

Anatomy

subcutaneous fat; abdominal fascia; peritoneum; uterus

Equipment

videolaparoscope; Braun tenaculum; Rochester-Péan forceps; Deaver retractor; self-retaining retractor; electrocoagulating forceps

Source

Adapted from Benedetti-Panici P, Maneschi F, Cutillo G, Scambia G, Congiu M, Mancuso S. Surgery by minilaparotomy in benign gynecologic disease. Obstetrics & Gynecology 1996;87:456-459.

Mini-Motionlogger Actigraph

Description
used in motor activity monitoring to establish sleep length, awakening, and sleep efficiency data

Source
Ambulatory Monitoring Inc. product information. Ardsley, NY.

 MiniOX 1000 and MiniOX 1A oxygen analyzer

Description
oxygen concentration indicator/analyzer ensures an oxygen-enriched atmosphere for patients with lung deficiencies; add-on attachment with interchangeable monitor accurately monitors therapeutic level of oxygen produced by concentrators used in the home; also MiniOX 1A oxygen analyzer

Source
Mine Safety Appliances Co. product information. Pittsburgh, PA.

 miniplate strut

Description
miniplate used as a strut and acrylic is applied using a reinforcement principle

Source
Adapted from Replogle RE, Lanzino G, Francel P, Henson S, Lin K, Jane JA. Acrylic cranioplasty using miniplate struts. Neurosurgery 1996;39:747-749.

 Minulet/Tri-minulet

Generic Name
see gestodene/ethinyl estradiol

 Mirapex

Generic name
see pramipexole

 mirtazapine

Brand name
Remeron

Use
alpha-2 receptor antagonist used in the treatment of depression

Usual dosage
oral: 5 mg to 60 mg daily were studied in the dose-titration trial with the mean final doses usually in the 20-25 mg/day range

Pharmaceutical company
Organon Inc. West Orange, NJ.

Source
University of Pittsburgh Drug Information and Pharmacoepidemiology Center. Pittsburgh, PA.

 ## Mist 14-gauge Eubanks instruments series

Description
surgical instruments include forceps, scissors, probes, needles, and trocars; with a "needlescopic" diameter of 1.7 mm, instruments are capable of being introduced through a 14-gauge (6.5 French) cannula

Source
Mist Inc. product information. Smithfield, NC.

 ## Mitchell penile disassembly for epispadias repair

Description
technique for epispadias repair reported that relies on the unique blood supply of the corpus cavernosum and glans; complete anatomical disassembly is accomplished based on the paired dorsal arteries and neurovascular bundles to each hemiglans, the deep cavernous arteries to the corporeal bodies, and the spongiosum tissue supplying the proximal urethral plate; complete disassembly makes the glans and urethral repair independent

Anatomy
Alcock canal; Buck fascia; corpus cavernosum; coronal sulcus; dorsal arteries; deep cavernous arteries; glans penis; hemicorporeal bodies; internal pudendal artery; meatus; phallus; shaft skin; spongiosum tissue; squamous preputial epithelium; urethral plate; meatus and neomeatus

Equipment
standard urologic surgery equipment; fine-tip electrocautery; methylene blue

Source
Adapted from Mitchell ME, Bagli DJ. Complete penile disassembly for epispadias repair: the Mitchell technique. Journal of Urology 1996;155:300-304.

 ## mitochondrial deoxyribonucleic acid (DNA) analysis

Synonyms
mtDNA analysis; mtDNA typing

Use
detection of mitochondrial DNA mutations in cases of suspected mitochondrial diseases

Method
polymerase chain reaction-based sequencing and amplification of mitochondrial DNA and transfer ribonucleic acid (tRNA)

Specimen
multiple cell or tissue specimens, as appropriate for suspected disorder

Normal range
not applicable

Comments
one of the newest applications of molecular diagnostics

Source
Adapted from Kiechle FL, Kaul KL, Farkas DH. Mitochondrial disorders: methods and specimen selection for diagnostic molecular pathology. Archives of Pathology and Laboratory Medicine 1996;120:597-603.

 mitoguazone

Brand name
Zyrkamine

Use
chemotherapeutic agent for the treatment of relapsed/refractory AIDS-related lymphoma

Usual dosage
intravenous: 600 mg/m^2 on days 1 and 8, then every 2 weeks

Pharmaceutical company
Ilex Oncology. San Antonio, TX.

Source
Stadtlanders Managed Pharmacy Services. Pittsburgh, PA.

▸ *As of June 23, 1997, the FDA Oncologic Drugs Advisory Committee found that there was not substantial evidence that mitoguazone was effective for treatment.*

 Mitolactol

Generic name
see dibromodulcitol (DBD)

 mitral valve reconstruction in sickle cell disease

Description
sickle cell disease has been successfully treated with mitral valve repair undergoing cardiopulmonary bypass; preoperative partial exchange transfusion followed by total exchange transfusion at time of surgery performed to reduce level of hemoglobin S during bypass; other strategies included normothermic bypass with aortic crossclamping, topical hypothermia, and cold crystalloid cardioplegia

Anatomy
anterior and posterior leaflets; interatrial groove; left atrium and ventricle; mitral valve leaflet; pulmonary artery

350

Equipment
Avecor SciMed silicone membrane oxygenator; hard-shell cardiotomy venous reservoir with Medtronic BioMedicus centrifugal pump; Bard arterial line filter; cardiotomy reservoir of Electromedics AT 1000 (autotransfusion) cell-saving device; annuloplasty ring

Source
Adapted from Pagani FD, Polito RJ, Bolling SF. Mitral valve reconstruction in sickle cell disease. Society of Thoracic Surgeons Journal 1996;61:1841-1843.

 ## Mitroflow pericardial heart valve

Description
implantable cardiac device with superior hemodynamics; no anticoagulation required with the implantation of the valve

Source
Mitroflow International Inc. product information. Richmond, BC, Canada.

 ## Mitroflow PeriPatch cylinders

Description
used as a staple line reinforcement; glutaraldehyde-fixed bovine pericardium in a cylindrical configuration designed for use with surgical staplers

Source
Mitroflow International Inc. product information. Richmond BC, Canada

 ## Miyazaki-Bonney test

Synonyms
none

Indications
incontinence

Method
cotton swab tips attached to short Ring forceps simulates the modified Burch procedure by reapproximating the paraurethral fascia and vaginal wall with the lateral pelvic sidewalls

Normal findings
if urine loss is prevented using this test then the patient will benefit from a Burch colpourethropexy

Comments
none

Source
Adapted from Goldman E. Modified Bonney test predicts Burch success. OB.GYN. News 1997;32:23.

Mizuho surgical Doppler

Description
Doppler for the intraoperative evaluation of blood flow; determines patency of parent vessel after aneurysm clipping; locates feeder artery in arteriovenous malformation; confirms patency of major venous sinuses and microvascular anastomoses

Source
Mizuho America Inc. product information. Beverly, MA.

 M4 Kerr Safety Hedstrom instrument

Description
endo instrument with 30-degree oscillation glides along the walls of the canal by mimicking the hand movement most practitioners use in endotherapy; functions without undue torquing

Source
Sybron Dental Specialities Inc. product information. Glendora, CA.

 MMG/O'Neil intermittent catheter system

Description
self-contained pre-lubricated intermittent catheter with removable cover guard over an introducer tip and break-away funnel end for safe and easy urine sampling procedures; catheters come in firm and soft vinyl, plastic, coude tip, and red rubber with smooth polished drainage eyelets and tapered tips for comfort

Source
MMG Healthcare product information. Decatur, GA.

 Moctanin

Generic Name
see monoctanoin

 modified Chrisman-Snook ankle reconstruction

Description
modification of lateral ligament reconstruction, wherein a hole is drilled in the fibula obliquely from proximal to distal, exiting at the tip of the fibula, allowing reconstruction of both the anterior talofibular and calcaneal fibular ligaments; provides a more anatomical repair and addresses the role of the calcaneal fibular ligament in stabilizing subtalar inversion instability

Anatomy
ankle; subtalar joints; anterior talofibular ligament; calcaneal fibular ligament; lateral malleolus; sural nerve; peroneal tendons; fibula; tibiotalar joint

352

Equipment
standard surgery equipment; surgical drill; tendon passer; Jackson-Pratt drain; compressive dressing

Source
Adapted from Smith PA, Miller SJ, Berni AJ. A modified Chrisman-Snook procedure for reconstruction of the lateral ligaments of the ankle: review of 18 cases. Foot & Ankle International 1995;16:259-266.

 modified corncrib (inverted T) procedure

Description
ophthalmic procedure with Quickert suture for repair of involutional entropion; Quickert suture added to re-insert lower eyelid retractors and prevent over-riding of preseptal over pretarsal orbicularis muscle; eyelid margin, tarsal and lower eyelid retractor-conjunctival wound closed vertically; skin and preseptal orbicularis muscle closed horizontally; combined vertical and horizontal wounds create the inverted T

Anatomy
anterior lamella; canthus; cilia; corneoscleral limbus; inferior conjunctival cul-de-sac; orbital rim; preseptal and pretarsal orbicularis oculi muscles; punctum; tarsus

Equipment
15 blade; 5-0 chromic suture; polyglactin suture; Quickert suture; 6-0 silk suture; Westcott scissors

Source
Adapted from Mauriello JA, Abdelsalam A. Modified corncrib (inverted T) procedure with Quickert suture for repair of involutional entropion. Ophthalmology Journal 1997;104:504-507.

 modified Ingelman-Sundberg bladder denervation for urge incontinence

Description
modified Ingelman-Sundberg bladder denervation for urge incontinence; transvaginal local anesthesia to block terminal pelvic nerve branches to bladder

Anatomy
vagina; bladder

Equipment
standard anesthesia equipment

Source
Adapted from Cespedes R, Cross C, McGuire E. Modified Ingleman-Sundberg bladder denervation procedure for intractable urge incontinence. The Journal of Urology 1996;156:1744-1747.

modified Keller resection arthroplasty

Description
modification of traditional technique for management of severe disorders of the first metatarsophalangeal joint; bone is resected from the proximal phalanx, while retaining as much plantar cortex as possible, thus preserving a portion of the attachment of the plantar plate and intrinsic musculature; addresses weakening of first ray and "cock-up" deformity of great toe which may occur after Keller resection arthroplasty

Anatomy
proximal phalanx; phalangeal base; great toe; plantar cortex

Equipment
standard surgery equipment; crescentic saw blade; K-wire stabilization

Source
Adapted from Harper MC. A modified Keller resection arthroplasty. Foot & Ankle International 1995;16:236-237.

 Modulith SL20 device

Description
third-generation extracorporeal shock wave lithotripsy (ESWL) for treatment of urinary calculi in kidney and upper ureter; uses an electromagnetic cylindrical coil system to provide a constant pressure wave source; self-contained unit uses multi-function x-ray as its primary stone localization mechanism

Source
Karl Storz Endoscopy product information. Culver City, CA.

 moexipril hydrochloride

Brand name
Univasc

Use
angiotensin-converting enzyme inhibitor used in the treatment of hypertension

Usual dosage
oral: 3.75, 7.5, and 15 mg daily have been used in clinical trials

Pharmaceutical company
Schwarz Pharma. Milwaukee, WI.

Source
University of Pittsburgh Drug Information and Pharmacoepidemiology Center. Pittsburgh, PA.

moexipril/hydrochlorothiazide

Brand name
Uniretic

Use
combination of ACE inhibitor/diuretic for treatment of hypertension

Usual dosage
oral: one tablet daily. Available in two dosage strengths: 7.5/12.5 mg or 15/25 mg of moexipril/hydrochlorothiazide, respectively

Pharmaceutical company
Schwarz Pharmaceuticals. Mequon, WI.

Source
Stadtlanders Managed Pharmacy Services. Pittsburgh, PA.

 molgramostim

Brand name
Leucomax

Use
human recombinant granulocyte-macrophage colony-stimulating factor used in the treatment of chemotherapy-induced neutropenia

Usual dosage
subcutaneous: adults, 5 to 10 mcg/kg/day for 7 to 10 days after chemotherapy

Pharmaceutical company
Sandoz Pharmaceuticals Corporation. East Hanover, NJ.

Source
University of Pittsburgh Drug Information and Pharmacoepidemiology Center. Pittsburgh, PA.

 mometasone furoate

Brand name
Nasonex

Use
for prevention and treatment of symptoms associated with allergic rhinitis and treatment of perennial rhinitis in patients at least 12 years and older

Usual dosage
topical: one spray in each nostril, once a day

Pharmaceutical company
Schering-Plough Healthcare Product Inc. Liberty Corner, NJ.

Source
Stadtlanders Managed Pharmacy Services. Pittsburgh, PA.

monoctanoin

Brand Name
Moctanin

Use
cholesterol contact solvent used in the dissolution of retained common bile ducts stones or calculi

Usual Dosage
intrabiliary: 3 to 5 ml/hr instilled into the biliary ducts via a T-tube

Pharmaceutical company
Ethitek Pharmaceuticals Company. Skokie, IL.

Source
University of Pittsburgh Drug Information and Pharmacoepidemiology Center. Pittsburgh, PA.

 monocyte monolayer assay (MMA)

Synonyms
none

Use
prediction of clinical significance of red cell antibodies

Method
adherence/phagocytosis assay using serum-sensitized red blood cells

Specimen
serum

Normal range
<4% phagocytosis and/or adherence

Comments
investigational

Source
Adapted from Lown J, Willis J. Monocyte monolayer assay (MMA) reactivity of alloantibodies reacting by the manual polybrene technique but not by an antiglobulin test. Transfusion Medicine 1995;5:281-284.

 Mono-Embolex NM

Generic name
see sandoparin

monospecific anti-human globulin antibody test

Synonyms
monospecific Coombs test, monospecific AHG test

Use
determination of red blood cell compatibility prior to transfusion

Method
serologic reaction of red blood cells, serum, and highly specific anti-human globulin

Specimen
blood

Normal range
no evidence of agglutination

Comments
avoids false-positive interference from clinically insignificant IgM complement-fixing antibodies

Source
American Journal of Clinical Pathology 1995;104:122-125.

 montelukast

Brand name
Singulair

Use
leukotriene antagonist for the treatment of asthma, but not for immediate bronchial relaxation

Usual dosage
oral: 10 mg per day for adults and 5 mg per day for children over age six

Pharmaceutical company
Merck & Co. Inc. West Point, PA.

Source
Stadtlanders Managed Pharmacy Services. Pittsburgh, PA.

 Montgomery laryngeal keel

Description
laryngeal device useful in repair of anterior glottic stenosis (web); can be used with or without vocal cord paralysis; also used following hemilaryngectomy to prevent stenosis

Source
Boston Medical Products Inc. product information. Waltham, MA.

Montgomery speaking valve

Description
device designed to allow tracheostomy patients to vocalize without need for finger occlusion; unique cough release feature eliminates valve blow-out following forceful cough, or excessive airway pressure

Source
Boston Medical Products product information. Waltham, MA.

 ## Montgomery Stomeasure device

Description
special device to allow physician to accurately measure the tracheal stoma for fitting of Montgomery long-term tracheal cannula

Source
Boston Medical Products product information. Waltham, MA.

 ## Monurol

Generic Name
see fosfomycin trometamol

 ## Moonwalker

Description
portable weightbearing system

Source
Lift Aire Inc. product information. Kalamazoo, MI.

 ## Morganstern aspiration/injection system

Description
21F oblique tip sheath for female urethral dilation and examination; allows for accurate, stabilized submucosal needle placement; Panoview II optics for flatter and larger images

Source
Richard Wolf Medical Instruments Corp. product information. Vernon Hill, IL.

Morganstern cystoscope

Description

continuous flow system; for laser-contact tip ablation of prostate, electrohy-draulic lithotripsy, and ultrasound-guided lithotripsy of bladder stones

Source

Richard Wolf Medical Instruments Corp. product information. Vernon Hills, IL.

morphine sulfate

Brand name

Kadian

Use

management of moderate to severe pain where treatment with an opioid analgesic is indicated for more than a few days

Usual dosage

oral: available as extended-release capsule in 20 mg, 50 mg, and 100 mg strength; to be administered 20-50 mg one to two times per day

Pharmaceutical company

Faulding USA. Elizabeth, NJ.

Source

Stadtlanders Managed Pharmacy Services. Pittsburgh, PA.

Mosaic cardiac bioprosthesis

Description

porcine bioprosthesis with zero-pressure fixation designed to preserve leaflet morphology; low-profile stent design; in clinical trials in the U.S., is available in Canada

Source

Medtronic Inc. product information. Minneapolis, MN.

Motilium

Generic Name

see domperidone

Motion Control Limiter (755 MCL)

Description

adjustable plantar flexion range of motion limiter that can be changed to a solid ankle foot orthotic (AFO); varying degrees of plantar flexion are obtained by grinding the stop

Source

Becker Orthopedic product information. Troy, MI.

MouseMitt Keyboarders

Description
fingerless wrist supports constructed of Lycra; keeps wrists warm; reduces strain on finger tendons; promotes circulation; soft pads cushion and support the wrists

Source
MouseMitt International product information. Scotts Valley, CA.

 ## MS Classique balloon dilatation catheter

Description
catheter with large balloon lumen and smaller guide wire lumen; consistent, rapid deflation ensures efficient tracking, maneuverability, and effective vessel dilatation with nominal pressure

Source
Meadox Medicals Inc. product information. Oakland, NJ.

 ## mucin-like carcinoma-associated antigen detection

Synonyms
MCA

Use
monitor therapy and detect metastases and recurrence in patients with breast carcinoma

Method
enzyme immunoassay (EIA)

Specimen
blood

Normal range
less than 11.0 units/ml

Comments
none

Source
Lexi-Comp Inc. database. Hudson, OH.

 ## Mueller Ultralite brace

Description
anterior cruciate ligament (ACL) brace with triaxial hinge; according to manufacturer, the only hinge that can recapture 16 mm of posterior shift of instant center of knee

Source
Mueller Sports Medicine product information. Prairie du Sac, WI.

MULE upper limb exerciser

Description

microcomputer upper limb exerciser (MULE) strengthens upper extremities by playing computer games; develops range of motion (ROM), fine motor control, and eye-hand coordination; assesses upper limb movement capability

Source

Fred Sammons Inc. product information. Western Springs, IL.

 Mullan trigeminal ganglion microcompression set

Description

percutaneous balloon treatment set for trigeminal neuralgia; compression technique offers nonselective treatment affecting the first and second divisions

Source

Cook Inc. product information. Bloomington, IN.

 Multi Axis Ankle

Description

gives natural ankle motion with any bolt-on prosthetic foot; provides smooth roll-over from heel contact to mid-stance as well as inversion/eversion and vertical shock-absorbing characteristics

Source

United States Manufacturing Co. product information. Pasadena, CA.

 Multibite biopsy forceps

Description

multiple sample biopsy forceps designed to obtain multiple specimens in a single pass

Source

Microvasive Boston Scientific Corp. product information. Watertown, MA.

 Multidex dressing

Description

wound filler dressing that attracts white blood cells, macrophages, and fibroblasts to the wound site and stimulates the growth of highly vascularized granulation tissue in as little as 24 hours

Source

DeRoyal Industries Inc. product information. Powell, TN.

multi-directional distractor

Description
surgical device used for craniomaxillofacial callus distraction

Source
KLS Martin LP product information. Jacksonville, FL.

 ## MultiDop XS system

Description
two-channel Doppler unit with flexible probe selection, embolus monitoring and can also be used with endoscopic procedures

Source
DWL Electronic System Inc. product information. Chicago, IL.

 ## MULTIGUIDE mandibular distractor

Description
provides gradual distraction in linear plate and creates angular changes and transverse changes in mandible

Source
Howmedica/Leibinger product information. Dallas, TX.

 ## multiparametric in situ hybridization (ISH) analysis

Synonyms
multiparameter metastasis ISH

Use
prediction of disease recurrence in colon cancer

Method
colorimetric in situ mRNA (messenger ribonucleic acid) hybridization measurement of expression levels for multiple metastasis-related genes

Specimen
biopsy specimen

Normal range
expression levels below threshold

Comments
investigational, but likely to become more widely used

Source
Adapted from Kitadai Y, Ellis LM, Tucker SL et al. Multiparametric in situ mRNA hybridization analysis to predict disease recurrence in patients with colon carcinoma. American Journal of Pathology 1996;149:1541-1551.

Multiple Parameter Telemetry (MPT)

Description
monitoring device to monitor patients while they are moved about the hospital such as from the emergency room to the radiology or coronary care unit; a patient-worn device that constantly and simultaneously records electrocardiogram, digital pulse oximetry, and noninvasive blood pressure using telemetry radiofrequency technique; patient can be ambulatory with this device in place due to digital link radiofrequency receiver

Source
Criticare Systems Inc. product information. Milwaukee, WI.

multiplex polymerase chain reaction (M-PCR)

Synonyms
none

Use
diagnosis of sexually transmitted diseases

Method
polymerase chain reaction with multiple sets of pathogen-specific primer pairs

Specimen
blood

Normal range
negative

Comments
can detect DNA from several bacterial and viral sexually transmitted diseases in a single test

Source
Adapted from Mahony JB. Multiplex polymerase chain reaction for the diagnosis of sexually transmitted diseases. Clinics in Laboratory Medicine 1996;16:61-71.

Multi-Test skin testing

Synonyms
MT skin test

Indications
immediate hypersensitivity skin testing of suspected allergens

Method
semi-automated template administration of candidate allergens to skin

Normal findings
no evidence of reaction

Comments
Multi-Test may be better accepted by children than conventional needle prick testing

Source
Adapted from Rizzo MC, Naspitz CK, Sole D. Comparative performance for immediate hypersensitivity skin testing using two skin prick test devices. Journal of Investigative Allergy and Clinical Immunology 1995;5:354-356.

 MurphyScope neurologic device

Description
endoscope and probe for neuroendoscopy and spinal endoscopy; provides visualization and irrigation to reveal hidden structures and reduce need for wide operative exposure

Source
Clarus Medical Systems Inc. product information. Minneapolis, MN.

 Muse

Generic name
see alprostadil

 mutagenicity assay with in vitro metabolic activating system

Synonyms
none

Use
detection of potentially mutagenic agents

Method
metabolic activation by cultured cells, followed by bioassay for mutations

Specimen
pharmacologic or biologic agent

Normal range
no evidence of mutagenicity

Comments
will likely lead to a a number of cell-line mediated mutation bioassays

Source
Adapted from Rueff J, Chiapella C, Chipman JK et al. Development and validation of alternative metabolic systems for mutagenicity testing in short-term assays. Mutation Research 1996; 353:151-176.

myasthenia gravis evaluation

Use

presence of acetylcholine receptor (AChR) antibodies is 99% specific for myasthenia gravis (MG)

Method

lab testing for autoantibodies to the nicotinic AChR of skeletal muscle in patient's serum

Specimen

serum

Normal range

absence of autoantibodies

Comments

testing has high sensitivity, is cost effective, and extremely low rate of false or unexplained positive results

Source

Specialty Laboratories Inc. database. Santa Monica, CA.

 ***Mycobacterium tuberculosis* detection**

Synonyms

TB test by PCR

Use

detect *Mycobacterium tuberculosis*

Method

polymerase chain reaction (PCR) amplification of conserved gene sequence for the genus *Mycobacterium* sp (13 species); species level identification of screen-reactive samples for typing of *Mycobacterium tuberculosis*

Specimen

sputum; respiratory aspirate

Normal range

uninfected specimen contains no *Mycobacterium tuberculosis*

Comments

Source

Lexi-Comp Inc. database. Hudson, OH.

 ***Mycobacterium tuberculosis* direct test (MTDT)**

Synonyms

Use

rapid diagnosis of infection with *Mycobacterium tuberculosis*

Method

rapid molecular probe reaction

Specimen
sputum or bronchoalveolar lavage

Normal range
negative

Comments
rapid, sensitive and specific; culture remains necessary for drug susceptibility tests, isolation, and identification of non-tuberculous mycobacteria

Source
Adapted from Portaels F, Serruys E, De Beenhouwer H et al. Evaluation of the Gen-Probe amplified *Mycobacterium tuberculosis* direct test for the routine diagnosis of pulmonary tuberculosis. Acta Clinica Belgium 1996;51:144-149.

Mycobacterium tuberculosis hybridization protection drug susceptibility assay

Synonyms
M. tuberculosis hybridization protection assay

Use
detection of drug susceptibility patterns in *M. tuberculosis* isolates

Method
nucleic acid hybridization protection assay

Specimen
clinical isolate

Normal range
susceptible

Comments
may permit more effective, targeted drug therapy

Source
Adapted from Miyamoto J, Koga H, Kohno S, Tashiro T, Hara K. New drug susceptibility test for *Mycobacterium tuberculosis* using the hybridization protection assay. Journal of Clinical Microbiology 1996;34:1323-1326.

mycophenolate mofetil

Brand name
CellCept

Use
maintenance immunosuppressant for the therapy of organ rejection in kidney, heart, and liver transplant patients

Usual dosage
oral: 1 g twice daily up to 3.5 g per day

Pharmaceutical company
Syntex. Palo Alto, CA.

Source
University of Pittsburgh Drug Information and Pharmacoepidemiology Center. Pittsburgh, PA.

myelin-associated glycoprotein antibody detection

Use

two acidic glycolipids are used for detection of myelin-associated glycoprotein (MAG) antibody, namely serum glutamic-pyruvic transaminase (SGPT); presence of antibody to MAG has been associated with sensorimotor neuropathies

Method

enzyme-linked immunosorbent assay (ELISA)

Specimen

blood or cerebrospinal fluid

Normal range

less than 1:400

Comments

approximately 50% of patients with IgM monoclonal gammopathies and associated peripheral neuropathy have detectable MAG antibodies; patients with primarily a sensory neuropathy may have low or no MAG antibody titers but may have elevated titers to sulfatide (a major acidic glycosphingolipid in myelin)

Source

Lexi-Comp Inc. database. Hudson, OH.

 myocardial fractional flow reserve (FFR) measurement

Synonyms

Indications

determination of clinical significance of moderately severe coronary artery stenoses

Method

analysis of pressure measurements made during coronary arteriography

Normal findings

greater than 0.75

Comments

a useful index of the functional severity of stenoses and need for coronary revascularization

Source

Adapted from Pijls NH, De Bruyne B, Peels K et al. Measurement of fractional flow reserve to assess the functional severity of coronary artery stenoses. New England Journal of Medicine 1996;334:1703-1708.

myocardial viability scintigraphy

Synonyms
none

Indications
use when myocardial perfusion scintigraphy indicates regions of poor perfusion using thallium-201 chloride, technetium-99m sestamibi (Cardiolite), or other radiopharmaceuticals and when it is important to determine whether poorly perfused regions are ischemic but still viable and are using anaerobic pathways for energy generation; perform test with view to correct perfusion abnormality with interventional procedure such as coronary artery bypass grafting or percutaneous transluminal coronary angioplasty (PTCA)

Method
fluorine-18 deoxyglucose given intravenously; images generated generally by positron emission tomography (PET) techniques; conventional nuclear imaging techniques such as single photon emission computed tomography (SPECT) gaining use

Normal findings
areas of poor perfusion take up fluorine-18 deoxyglucose if they are viable; if the area of nonperfusion is nonviable no radiopharmaceutical is concentrated, indicating total lack of metabolism and presence of infarction

Comments
none

Source
Nuclear Medicine Consultant. Stedman's Medical Dictionary, 26th edition.

 ## myoglobin assay

Synonyms
serum Mgb assay

Use
early evaluation of suspected myocardial infarction

Method
fluorometric enzyme immunoassay

Specimen
blood

Normal range
less than 70 µg/L

Comments
role in ruling out myocardial infarction currently investigational

Source
American Journal of Clinical Pathology 1995;104:472-476.

Myoscint

Generic name
see imciromab pentetate

 Myotrophin

Generic Name
somatomedin C (IGF-1)

 nalmefene hydrochloride

Brand name
Revex

Use
reversal of opioid drug effects, including postoperative respiratory depression, induced by either natural or synthetic opioids, and for the management of known or suspected opioid overdose

Usual dosage
injectable: dose dependent upon narcotic levels; recommended dose range 0.1 mcg/kg, 0.25 mcg/kg, 0.5 mcg/kg, or 1 mcg/kg primarily as an intravenous bolus, but can be given intramuscularly or subcutaneously if venous access cannot be established

Pharmaceutical company
Ohmeda. Liberty Corner, NJ.

Source
University of Pittsburgh Drug Information and Pharmacoepidemiology Center. Pittsburgh, PA.

 Naprelan

Generic name
see naproxen

 naproxen

Brand name
Naprelan

Use
nonsteroidal anti-inflammatory for relief of mild to moderate pain

Usual dosage
oral: over the counter product; controlled-release tablet formulation; available in 375 mg naproxen (412.5 mg naproxen sodium) and 500 mg naproxen (550 naproxen sodium); to be administered in doses of 750 mg to 1000 mg as single daily dose

Pharmaceutical company
Wyeth-Ayerst Laboratories. Philadelphia, PA.
Source
Stadtlanders Managed Pharmacy Services. Pittsburgh, PA.

 Naraghi-DeCoster reduction clamp

Description
orthopaedic instrument designed for reduction of femoral shaft fractures prior to passing the guide pin during intramedullary fixation
Source
Innomed Inc. product information. Savannah, GA.

 naratriptan

Brand name
Amerge
Use
treatment of migraines that offers less recurrences and a better safety profile over sumatriptan
Usual dosage
oral: 1, 2.5, 5, 7.5, and 10 mg doses have been used in clinical trials to alleviate migraine
Pharmaceutical company
GlaxoWellcome Inc. Research Triangle Park, NC.
Source
Stadtlanders Managed Pharmacy Services. Pittsburgh, PA.

 Naropin

Generic name
see ropivacaine

 NarrowFlex catheter

Description
intra-aortic flexible balloon catheter; features a wire-reinforced outer gas lumen with an inner central lumen made from nitinol
Source
Arrow International Inc. product information. Reading, PA.

nasal cilia beat-frequency analysis

Synonyms
nasal cilia biopsy test

Use
evaluation of cilia beat frequency for diagnosis of abnormal cilia

Method
computer-enhanced transmitted phase-contrast photometry

Specimen
nasal cilia tissue biopsy

Normal range
5 to 8 Hz at 77 F

Comments
abnormal cilia beat frequency requires electron microscopy to determine structural abnormality

Source
University of Minnesota Department of Laboratory Medicine and Pathology. Minneapolis, MN.

 Nasarel

Generic name
see flunisolide

 Nasonex

Generic name
see mometasone furoate

 natural killer cell activation

Synonyms
NK cell activation; NK effector cell therapy; ex vivo activated killer cells

Use
natural killer (NK) cell activation provides patients who have poorly treatable cancers with activated cells having tumor-killing ability

Method
cytapheresis is performed to collect peripheral blood lymphocytes from a patient, cells are grown in culture with interleukin-2, causing natural killer cell activation, and the cells are reinfused

Specimen
peripheral blood cytapheresis product

Normal range
investigational use

Comments
currently limited to patients with advanced breast cancer or lymphoma

Source
University of Minnesota Department of Laboratory Medicine and Pathology. Minneapolis, MN.

Natural Profile abutment system

Description
dental anatomic abutment and abutment body that are identically contoured, simulating the form of a natural tooth; used for tooth replacement; restores natural function

Source
Impla-Med Implant Group product information. Sunrise, FL.

Navelbine

Generic name
see vinorelbine

Navoban

Generic name
see tropisetron

n-docosanol

Brand name
Lidakol

Use
topical cream to reduce size and pigmentation of cutaneous lesions caused by Kaposi sarcoma in patients with HIV-1 infection

Usual dosage
topical: applied as a 10% cream to active lesions

Pharmaceutical company
Lidak Pharmaceuticals. La Jolla, CA.

Source
Stadtlanders Managed Pharmacy Services. Pittsburgh, PA.

Neckcare pillow

Description
hot/cold pillow for relief of headache and neck pain

Source
FlagHouse Rehab product information. Mt Vernon, NY.

 ## Necktrac

Description
portable neck traction device

Source
Lossing Orthopedic Inc. product information. Minneapolis, MN.

 ## nefazodone hydrochloride

Brand name
Serzone

Use
serotonin and norepinephrine reuptake inhibitor used in the treatment of depression

Usual dosage
oral: starting dose 200 mg daily administered in two divided doses; effective dosage range 300 to 600 mg daily

Pharmaceutical company
Bristol-Meyers Squibb Co. Princeton, NJ.

Source
University of Pittsburgh Drug Information and Pharmacoepidemiology Center. Pittsburgh, PA.

 ## nelfinavir

Brand name
Viracept

Use
protease inhibitor for use in treatment of HIV infection

Usual dosage
oral: 500 mg to 750 mg three times a day studied in clinical trials

Pharmaceutical company
Agouron Pharmaceuticals. San Diego, CA.

Source
Stadtlanders Managed Pharmacy Services. Pittsburgh, PA.

Nellcor Symphony N-3000 pulse oximeter

Description
incorporates Oxismart; advanced signal processing and alarm management in high-motion or low-perfusion patient environments; designed to identify and reject artifacts attributed to motion and electronic or optical noise interference; maintains good saturated partial pressure of oxygen (SpO$_2$) signal in the critical care or step-down/intermediate care unit, transport unit, and/or general care unit; also has a blood pressure monitor attachment

Source
Nellcor Puritan-Bennett product information. Pleasanton, CA.

G5 Neocussor percussor

Description
provides soothing, precise treatment to help loosen and mobilize secretion build-up in neonates; 3 different-shaped disposable applicators help prevent cross-contamination

Source
General Physiotherapy Inc. product information. St. Louis, MO.

NeoDerm dressing

Description
secures epidural catheters; designed for small-framed and pediatric patients who require catheter stabilization; the rectangular shape and adhesive foam border anchors the catheter in place

Source
ConMed Corp. product information. Utica, NY.

neodynium:yttrium-lithium-fluoride (Nd:YLF) laser segmentation

Description
used for retinal traction associated with proliferative diabetic retinopathy; picosecond pulse photodisruptive laser Food and Drug Administration-approved for phase I; indications for treatment were: distortion and shallow elevation of the macula caused by adherent posterior hyaloid interface, traction retinal detachment involving fovea, and fovea-threatened traction retinal detachment; traction release accomplished by laser segmentation of detached hyaloid interface and proliferative tissue; Nd:YLF low pulse energy

Anatomy
central macular region; choroid; fovea; fundus; hyaloid interface; macula; pars plana; retina; vitreous

Equipment
Nd: YLF laser

Source
Adapted from Cohen BZ, Wald KJ, Toyama K. Neodymium: YLF picosecond laser segmentation for retinal traction associated with diabetic retinopathy. American Journal of Ophthalmology 1997;123:515-522.

 Neonatal Y TrachCare

Description
sidestream catheter combines closed suction with high frequency oscillators, high frequency jet-ventilators, volume, and physiologic monitors; fits all neonates, even very low birth weight; has a single lavage port, numbered and color-coded catheter for precise depth of suction control; detachable catheter for convenient catheter changes; portal for accessories accomodates 5 French (5-Fr), 6 French (6-Fr), and 8 French (8-Fr) sizes with multiple Y adapter sizes for specific endotracheal tube size

Source
Ballard Medical Products product information. Draper, UT.

 Neoprobe 1000 radioisotope detection system

Description
device designed for invasive and noninvasive procedures; detects a wide range of radionuclides; features sound-guided localization of targeted tissues; continuous display of gamma counts

Source
Neoprobe Corp. product information. Dublin, OH.

 Neoral

Generic name
see cyclosporine microemulsion

 NeoVO₂R volume control resuscitator

Description
ensures uniform ventilation; eliminates hypoinflation and hyperinflation, eliminates hypoventilation and hyperventilation, and reduces risk of pneumothorax; delivers up to 100% O₂ or a specific fraction of inspired oxygen (FiO₂) at selected volume and rates without atmospheric air dilution; secondary port allows installation of normal saline or surfactant, bronchial lavage, or suctioning while ventilating; connector can accommodate endotracheal tube or face mask

Source
NeoMed Corp. product information. London, Ontario, Canada.

Nerve Fiber Analyzer laser ophthalmoscope

Description
laser beam instrument that measures thickness of retinal nerve fiber layer (RNFL) rather than surface topography; sensitive test for detecting early glaucomatous damage

Source
Laser Diagnostics Technologies Inc. product information. San Diego, CA.

 # Nerve Integrity Monitor 2 (NIM2)

Description
facial nerve monitor; sensitive detector of minute responses; minimizes possibility of trigeminal nerve stimulation producing false-positive facial responses

Source
Xomed product information. Jacksonville, FL.

 # Neuhann cystotome

Description
ophthalmic irrigating surgical instrument; provides stability to penetrate anterior capsule without bending while providing sufficient irrigation to maintain positive pressure

Source
Visitec Co. product information. Sarasota, FL.

 # Neumega

Generic Name
see recombinant human interleukin 11

 # neu-metoclopramide

Brand name
Neu-Sensamide

Use
formulation of metoclopramide used as a radiation and chemotherapy sensitizing agent

Usual dosage
intravenous or intramuscular: 1.8 mg/kg in clinical trials

Pharmaceutical company
Oxigene. New York, NY.

Source
Stadtlanders Managed Pharmacy Services. Pittsburgh, PA.

Neuprex

Generic name
see recombinant bactericidal/permeability-increasing protein (rBPI$_{21}$)

 neural crest tumor localization study

Synonyms
pheochromocytoma and neuroblastoma localization study; adrenergic tumor localization study

Indications
localize primary and metastatic adrenergic tumors including pheochromocytoma, neuroblastoma, carcinoid, and nonfunctioning paragangliomas, all of which have avidity for the compound

Method
intravenous injection of iodine-131 metaiodobenzylguanidine (MIBG or Iobenguane sulfate) is given after doses of iodide (as with Lugol solution) are administered to block thyroid gland; sequential imaging performed over several days

Normal findings
no uptake unless tumor is present

Comments
a similar radiopharmaceutical iodine-123 MIBG with better imaging properties and lower radiation dose is under development and evaluation

Source
Nuclear Medicine Consultant. Stedman's Medical Dictionary, 26th edition.

 Neurelan

Generic name
see fampridine

 NeuroAvitene applicator

Description
Avitene preloaded syringe for neurosurgical applications; 100% microfibrillar topical collagen hemostat potentiates natural clotting without swelling

Source
MedChem Products Inc. product information. Woburn, MA.

 neuroendocrine tumor localization study

Synonyms
tumor localization study; indium-111 octreotide scintigraphy; OctreoScan

Indication
indium-111 pentetreotide is an agent for the scintigraphic localization of primary and metastatic neuroendocrine tumors bearing somatostatin receptors

Method
administer indium-111 intravenously to well-hydrated patients followed by sequential whole body and regional scintigraphic imaging for up to 72 hours after administration

Normal findings
no localization of the radioactive compound other than at sites of normal elimination; abnormalities include, but are not limited to, carcinoids, gastrinomas, insulinomas, neuroblastomas, pituitary adenomas, pheochromocytomas, and medullary thyroid carcinomas demonstrate localization of the radiopharmaceutical

Comments
indium-111 octreotide scintigraphy is also useful for detecting oat cell lung carcinomas, lymphomas, and granulomas

Source
Nuclear Medicine Consultant. Stedman's Medical Dictionary, 26th edition.

Neuroguard transcranial Doppler

Description
blood flow monitoring for real-time observation of cerebral circulation during carotid endarterectomy, coronary artery bypass graft surgery, and orthopaedic procedures using transcranial Doppler (TCD) technology.

Source
Medasonics Inc. product information. Mountain View, CA.

Neuromeet nerve approximator

Description
neurologic surgical instrument that simplifies approximation; very fine surgical hooks are positioned for easy nerve attachment and precise alignment along a flexible runner

Source
Accurate Surgical & Scientific Instruments Corp. product information. Westbury, NY.

Neuropedic mattress

Description
patented mattress with four sections of polyurethane foam; each section has a specific density and firmness; conforms to and supports the weight of the entire body

Source
Neuropedic product information. White Plains, NY.

neurovascular infrahyoid island flap for tongue reconstruction

Description
fasciomuscular flap formed from the sternothyroid, sternohyoid, and upper part of the omohyoid muscles used for total reconstruction of the tongue or large defects of the tongue base

Anatomy
sternothyroid muscle; sternohyoid muscle; omohyoid muscle; lymph nodes; tongue; larynx; carotid artery; jugular vein; superior thyroid artery and vein; ansa cervicalis of the hypoglossal nerve

Equipment
retractor; dissector; scalpel

Source
Adapted from Remmert S, Sommer K, Majocco A, et al. The neurovascular infrahyoid muscle flap. Plastic and Reconstructive Surgery 1997;99:613-618.

 ## Neuroview neuroendoscope

Description
semirigid biopsy forceps can be passed through brain parenchyma to extract a 0.8-cc sample; alligator tooth design on the grasping forceps ensures effective tissue manipulation for minimally invasive neurosurgery; indicated for biopsies, third ventriculoscopy, shunt placement, and cyst fenestration; Neuro-Navigational and Neuroview System Model 100 neuroendoscope models

Source
Neuro Navigational product information. Costa Mesa, CA.

 ## Neu-Sensamide

Generic name
see neu-metoclopramide

 ## nevirapine

Brand name
Viramune

Use
non-nucleoside reverse transcriptase inhibitor (NNRTI); used in combination with nucleoside analogues in the treatment of HIV/AIDS infection

Usual dosage
oral: available in 200 mg tablets; to be administered 200 mg once a day for the first 14 days, then 200 mg twice a day, thereafter with nucleoside analogues

Pharmaceutical company
Boehringer Ingelheim Pharmaceuticals Inc. Ridgefield, CT.
Source
Stadtlanders Managed Pharmacy Services. Pittsburgh, PA.

New Beginnings topical gel sheeting

Description
clear silicone gel sheeting used in treatment for keloid and hypertrophic scars
Source
PMT Corporation product information. Chanhassen, MN.

Nexerciser Plus

Description
neck muscle exercise and testing system for neck rehabilitation
Source
Nexerciser Plus product information. Bedford, NH.

Niamtu Video Imaging System

Description
portable computer video miniaturization imaging system compatible with Windows 3.1 or Windows 95; enables physician to perform surgical imaging and digital photography in minutes; compatible with S-video endoscopes and intraoral cameras
Source
Niamtu Video Imaging System product information. Richmond, VA.

NicCheck-I

Synonyms
none
Use
determines nicotine level
Method
test strip is dipped into urine specimen; color change determines amount of nicotine
Specimen
urine

Normal range
low reading

Comments
test can be done in a doctor's office or other outpatient setting; results available in 15 minutes; easy to use

Source
Adapted from MDDI Reports - The Gray Sheet 1997;23:I&W2-I&W3.

 # nicergoline

Brand name
Sermion

Use
a cerebral vasodilator for treatment of Alzheimer disease

Usual dosage
oral: 30 mg twice a day

Pharmaceutical company
Pharmacia and Upjohn Co. Kalamazoo, MI.

Source
Stadtlanders Managed Pharmacy Services. Pittsburgh, PA.

 # Nicolet Compass EMG instrument

Description
computerized instrument for electromyography (EMG) and nerve conduction studies; includes motor and sensory nerve conductions, F-waves, H-reflexes, neuromuscular junction test, and needle electromyography (free run, rastered and triggered)

Source
Nicolet Biomedical Inc. product information. Madison, WI.

 # nicorandil

Brand name
Icorel

Use
vascular smooth muscle relaxant used in the treatment of angina pectoris

Usual dosage
oral: 5 to 20 mg doses given twice daily have been used in clinical studies

Pharmaceutical company
Rhone-Poulenc Rorer Pharmaceuticals Inc. Collegeville, PA.

Source
University of Pittsburgh Drug Information and Pharmacoepidemiology Center. Pittsburgh, PA.

nicotine nasal spray

Brand name
Nicotrol NS

Use
aid in smoking cessation for the relief of nicotine withdrawal symptoms

Usual dosage
nasal spray: one dose or spray in each nostril administers 1 mg of nicotine (0.5 mg/spray); patients are recommended to start with one or two doses per hour but not exceeding 40 mg (80 sprays) per day

Pharmaceutical company
McNeil Pharmaceutical. Raritan, NJ.

Source
University of Pittsburgh Drug Information and Pharmacoepidemiology Center. Pittsburgh, PA.

 Nicotrol NS

Generic name
see nicotine nasal spray

 nifedipine

Brand name
Geomatrix

Use
used for the treatment of hypertension

Usual dosage
oral: 30 to 60 mg once a day, not to exceed 120 mg a day

Pharmaceutical company
Gensia Laboratories LTD. Irvine, CA.

Source
Stadtlanders Managed Pharmacy Services. Pittsburgh, PA.

 Nilandron

Generic name
see nilutamide

 nilutamide

Brand name
Nilandron

Use
nonsteroidal androgen blocker used in the treatment of metastatic prostate cancer in combination with surgical castration

Usual dosage
oral: dosages of 150 mg/day and 300 mg/day (in three divided doses) have been used in clinical trials

Pharmaceutical company
Roussel. Somerville, NJ.

Source
University of Pittsburgh Drug Information and Pharmacoepidemiology Center. Pittsburgh, PA.

 Nimbex

Generic Name
see cisatracurium

 Niplette

Description
noninvasive over-the-counter device to correct flat or inverted nipples; tissue expansion achieved through long-term suction

Source
Avent America product information. Addison, IL.

 nisoldipine

Brand name
Sular

Use
extended release calcium channel blocker used in the treatment of hypertension

Usual dosage
oral: 20 mg daily and the dose can be increased by 10-mg increments

Pharmaceutical company
Zeneca Pharmaceuticals Group. Wilmington, DE.

Source
University of Pittsburgh Drug Information and Pharmacoepidemiology Center. Pittsburgh, PA.

 nitrendipine

Brand name
Baypress

Use
calcium channel blocker for the treatment of mild to moderate hypertension

Usual dosage
oral: 10 mg daily titrated to a maximum of 40 mg daily

Pharmaceutical company
Miles Inc. Elkhart, IN.

Source
University of Pittsburgh Drug Information and Pharmacoepidemiology Center. Pittsburgh, PA.

Nordan-Ruiz trapezoidal marker

Description
ophthalmologic surgery incision marker

Source
ASSI product information. Westbury, NY.

norethindrone acetate and ethinyl estradiol

Brand name
Estrostep

Use
oral contraceptive in new class called Estrophasic oral contraceptives; provides low, gradually increasing amounts of estrogen with low, constant dose of progestin

Usual dosage
28-day pill pack with 20, 30, 35 µg ethinyl estradiol and 1 mg norethindrone acetate; contains 7 inactive tablets to help women maintain their regimen

Pharmaceutical company
Warner-Lambert Co. Morris Plains, NJ.

Source
Warner-Lambert Co. press release on Internet.

Norfolk intrauterine catheter set

Description
delivery catheter used for introduction of washed spermatozoa into the uterine cavity; translucent catheter designed to fit coaxially through the introducing cannula

Source
Cook OB/GYN product information. Spencer, IN.

norgestimate/ethinyl estradiol

Brand name
Ortho TriCyclen

Use
oral contraceptive approved as a treatment for moderate acne vulgaris

384

Usual dosage
oral: 1 tablet a day in 28-tablet pill package; 21 out of 28 tablets contain 35 g ethinyl estradiol and increasing doses of norgestimate (0.18 mg in 7 tablets, 0.215 mg in 7 tablets, and 0.25 mg in 7 tablets); the last 7 of the 28 tablets contain inert chemical

Pharmaceutical company
Ortho Pharmaceuticals Corp. Raritan, NJ.

Source
Stadtlanders Managed Pharmacy Services. Pittsburgh, PA.

Normix

Generic name
see rifaximin

Norvir

Generic name
see ritonavir

"no-touch" technique, coronary artery bypass graft

Description
internal mammary artery (IMA) and the great saphenous vein (SV) are grafts of choice for coronary artery bypass graft (CABG) surgery; during harvesting of the SV a protracted spasm occurs; a technique has been developed in which a cushion of surrounding tissue is left around the vein to prevent spasm; studies are being performed to evaluate this new technique

Anatomy
arterial pedicle; arterial and venous tributaries; connective perivascular tissue; lumen; lymphatic drainage system; media and intima of IMA; saphenous vein bed; vasa vasorum

Equipment
standard CABG surgical equipment

Source
Adapted from Souza D. A new no-touch preparation technique. Scandinavian Journal of Thoracic Cardiovascular Surgery 1996;30:41-44.

Novagold

Description
PVP (polyvinylpyrrolidone)-hydrogel-filled single-lumen mammary implant that feels natural and is highly radiolucent

Source
NOVAMEDICAL Products product information. Mannheim, Germany.

Novascan scanning headpiece

Description
lightweight laser ideal for performing cosmetic skin resurfacing procedures over broad areas resulting in minimal necrosis and limited thermal damage; provides controllable depth ablation

Source
Luxar Corp. product information. Bothell, WA.

 ## Novastan

Generic name
see argatroban

 ## Novatec LightBlade

Description
investigational, surgical work station with solid state surface PRK laser which performs vision correction for myopia, hyperopia, astigmatism, and therapeutic uses

Source
Novatec Laser Systems product information. Carlsbad, CA.

 ## novel plasminogen activator or lanoteplase

Brand name
nPA

Use
thrombotic (anti-clotting) agent, a naturally occurring protein, which dissolves clots and restores blood flow to the heart in patients with acute myocardial infarction; presently in clinical trials

Usual dosage
one-time, weight-adjusted bolus administered by single injection

Pharmaceutical company
Bristol-Myers Squibb. Princeton, NJ.

Source
Bristol-Myers Squibb press release on the Internet.

 ## nPA

Generic name
see novel plasminogen activator or lanoteplase

Nugent criteria

Synonyms
vaginal Gram stain

Use
method for detection of bacterial vaginosis

Method
vaginal swab

Specimen
secretions high in the posterior vaginal fornix

Normal range
no evidence of bacterial infection

Source
Adapted from Schwebke JR, Hillier SL, Sobel JD, McGregor JA, Sweet RL. Validity of the vaginal Gram stain for the diagnosis of bacterial vaginosis. Obstetrics and Gynecology 1996;88:573-576.

Nu-Hope skin barrier strip

Description
flexible, solid-strip sticks used to build up areas around ostomy pouch openings; fills in any creases or dips; provides tight seal application

Source
Nu-Hope Laboratories product information. Pacoima, CA.

NuStep body recumbent stepper

Description
low-impact all-in-one aerobic strengthening exerciser; adjustable, total body exerciser for individuals with physical limitations such as cardiac problems, diabetes, lower back injuries, and orthopaedic conditions

Source
LifePlus Inc. product information. Ann Arbor, MI.

Nu-Trake Weiss emergency airway system

Description
AE-1300 Nu-Trake cricothyrotomy device with syringe, stylet, needle and housing unit; 4.5-mm, 6-mm, and 7.2-mm airway diameters with obturator and tie; also AA-925 Nu-Trake and AE-1310 Pedia-Trake

Source
Armstrong Medical Industries Inc. product information. Lincolnshire, IL and San Diego, CA.

Nu-Vois artificial larynx

Description
produces a voice with artificial larynx or with intraoral adapter to be used as a mouth-type artificial larynx; operates with standard alkaline or rechargeable 9 volt batteries

Source
Bivona Medical Technologies product information. Gary, IN.

Nuwave transcutaneous electrical nerve stimulator

Description
transcutaneous electrical nerve stimulator (TENS) device; reusable "lo-back" electrodes offer evenly distributed stimulation; biphasic symmetrical waveforms

Source
Staodyn Inc. product information. Longmont, CO.

Nyotran

Generic name
see nystatin

Nystar Plus ENG

Description
electronystagmogram (ENG) instrument conducts a battery of standard and advanced tests; standard tests include caloric, smooth pursuit, optokinetic, positional, saccade, fistula, positioning, spontaneous, gaze, and rotation

Source
Nicolet Biomedical Inc. product information. Madison, WI.

nystatin

Brand name
Nyotran

Use
lipid based formulation of nystatin for the treatment of fungal infections

Usual dosage
intravenous: 0.25 mg/kg, 0.5 mg/kg, 0.75 mg/kg, or 1 mg/kg in phase I dose-ranging studies

Pharmaceutical company
Aronex Pharmaceuticals Inc. Woodlands, TX.

Source
Stadtlanders Managed Pharmacy Services. Pittsburgh, PA.

Obagi Blue Peel

Description

Blue Peel chemical peel treatment; markedly improved skin laxity, corrects wrinkles, melasma, scars, laxity, large pores and nonfacial skin conditions

Source

Worldwide Products Inc. product information. Glendora, CA.

Oberto mouth prop

Description

a specialized product for use in electroconvulsive therapy (ECT) and epileptic spasm; latex with central air vent

Source

Rusch Inc. product information. Duluth, GA.

oblique osteotomy for tibial deformity

Description

correction of tibial shaft malunion in deformities of less than 2.5 cm using one cut in the bone; single bone cut preserves bone and speeds healing; technique involves oblique osteotomy with placement of lag screw and neutralization plate; fibular osteotomy and Achilles tendon lengthening performed as indicated

Anatomy

tibia; fibula; Achilles tendon; knee; lower extremity; proximal and distal tibial metaphysis; tibial plafond

Equipment

standard surgery equipment; tourniquet; somatosensory evoked potential monitoring; Schanz pins; Hohmann retractors; Synthes femoral distractor; Synthes angled blade plate instrument set; surgical saw; bone reduction forceps; Synthes dynamic compression plate; Robert Jones dressing

Source

Adapted from Sanders R, Anglen JO, Mark JB. Oblique osteotomy for the correction of tibial malunion. The Journal of Bone and Joint Surgery 1995;77-A:240-246.

O₂Boot

Description

lightweight, portable, disposable topical hyperbaric oxygen wound treatment; accommodates wounds of various sizes and locations; delivers oxygen topically to the wound at pressures slightly above atmospheric pressure; enhances wound healing by establishing favorable tissue oxygenation; promotes growth of new blood vessels; produces less recidivism

Source

GWR Medical LLP product information. Chadds Ford, PA.

Ocoee scalp cleansing unit

Description
automatic scalp cleansing machine mounted in cabinet; wets, debrides, cleanses and rinses scalp, applies shampoo or disinfectant; removes postsurgical residue from scalp and hair follicles in six minutes; minimizes infection

Source
Ocoee Inc. product information. Nashville, TN.

octreotide and fluorodeoxyglucose thyroid scintigraphy

Synonyms
none

Use
detection of thyroid cancer metastases

Method
imaging scintigraphy

Normal findings
no evidence of localized uptake

Comments
particularly useful when the initial radioiodine scan is negative

Source
Adapted from Reinhardt MJ, Moser E. An update on diagnostic methods in the investigation of diseases of the thyroid. European Journal of Nuclear Medicine 1996;23:587-594.

Ogden Anchor soft tissue device

Description
reattachment device for anchoring soft tissue to bone; used for soft tissue reattachment in rotator cuff repairs; recently cleared by the Food and Drug Administration (FDA; Feb. 1995) for expanded shoulder, multiple soft tissues, and orthopaedic attachment applications in lower extremity

Source
American Medical Electronics Inc. product information. Richardson, TX.

olanzapine

Brand Name
Zyprexa

Use
treatment of schizophrenia

Usual Dosage
oral: 7.5 to 17.5 mg/day have been used in clinical trials

Pharmaceutical company
Eli Lilly and Company. Indianapolis, IN.

Source
University of Pittsburgh Drug Information and Pharmacoepidemiology Center. Pittsburgh, PA.

 olopatadine

Brand name
Patanol

Use
ophthalmic antihistamine for the relief of itching eye symptoms caused by allergic conjunctivitis

Usual dosage
topical: 1 to 2 drops into eye(s) twice a day, every 5 to 8 hours

Pharmaceutical company
Alcon Laboratories. Fort Worth, TX.

Source
Stadtlanders Managed Pharmacy Services. Pittsburgh, PA.

 Olympus CYF-3 OES cystofibroscope

Description
cystofibroscope with 5.4-mm outer diameter, 2.2-mm instrument channel, 210-degree up, and 90-degree down angulation, 120-degree angle of view, and insertion measurement markers

Source
Olympus America Inc. product information. Lake Success, NY.

 Olympus EUS-20 endoscopic ultrasound

Description
instrument that provides view of all five layers of gastrointestinal tract; uneclipsed 360-degree view of cross-sectional anatomy of superficial mucosa, deep mucosa, submucosa, muscularis propria, and serosa

Source
Olympus America Inc. product information. Lake Success, NY.

 OmegaPort access port

Description
only access port with no-sludge warranty, according to manufacturer; sludge is thrombosed blood and drug residuals that accumulate in reservoirs of conventional access ports

Source
Norfolk Medical product information. Skokie, IL.

omentectomy for leiomyosarcoma of colon

Description
leiomyosarcoma of the colon is extremely rare, comprising less than 0.1 percent of colonic malignancy; rectal involvement occurs 2 to 3 times more frequently than involvement of the rest of the colon; tumors grow in various ways, including intracolonic (invading into the bowel), exoclonic (growing away from the lumen), and intramural; pain, burning, cramping, changes in bowel habits, bleeding, fever, and chills are predominant symptoms; abdominal mass is not common symptom; surgical treatment omentectomy for leiomyosarcoma of colon (continued)

Anatomy
descending colon; bowel lumen; mesenteric nodes

Equipment
standard surgery equipment

Source
Adapted from Fallahzadeh H. Leiomyosarcoma of colon: report of two cases. American Surgeon 1995;61:294-296.

Omnicef

Generic name
see cefdinir

Omni-LapoTract support system

Description
surgical multidirectional device designed for minimally invasive procedures; holds either the scope (camera) or a grasper, giving the surgeon an extra pair of hands

Source
Omni-Tract Surgical product information. Minneapolis, MN.

Omni Pulse-MAX holmium laser

Description
can fragment urinary tract stones including cystine or calcium oxalate monohydrate; minimizes intraluminal trauma

Source
Trimedyne Inc. product information. Irvine, CA.

Omni-Sal/ImmunoComb II HIV-1 and HIV-2 assay

Synonyms
salivary HIV antibody assay

Use
laboratory diagnosis of HIV infection

Method
oral fluid collection device linked to microimmunoassay

Specimen
saliva

Normal range
no evidence of antibody reactivity

Comments
rapid, sensitive, highly accurate assay, and does not require blood specimen

Source
Adapted from Saville RD, Constantine NT, Holm-Hansen C, Wisnom C, DePaola L, Falkler WA Jr. Evaluation of two novel immunoassays designed to detect HIV antibodies in oral fluids. Journal of Clinical Laboratory Analysis 1997;11:63-68.

 Oncaspar

Generic name
see pegaspargase

 Oncolym

Generic name
see Lym-1 monoclonal antibody with radioisotope iodine-131

 Ontosein

Generic Name
see orgotein

 OnTrak rapid urine latex agglutination immunoassay

Synonyms
cocaine AIA test

Use
rapid screening for cocaine use

Method
card-based latex agglutination immunoassay for the cocaine metabolite benzoylecgonine

Specimen
urine

Normal range
negative

Comments
permits rapid, accurate screening for cocaine use in an emergency department setting

Source
Adapted from Westdorp EJ, Salomone JA III, Roberts DK, McIntyre MK, Watson WA. Validation of a rapid urine screening assay for cocaine use among pregnant emergency patients. Academic Emergency Medicine 1995;2:795-798.

 Onyx

Description
self-contained finger pulse oximeter

Source
Nonin Medical Inc. product information. Plymouth, MN.

 "open" exit foramen: new sign of unilateral interfacetal dislocation or subluxation (UID/S) in lower cervical spine

Synonyms
facet dislocation

Indications
injury resembling facet subluxation, to perching or frank dislocation (jumped or locked facets), interfacetal joint malalignment

Method
radiological clinical assessment and quantitative measurements

Normal findings
not applicable

Comments
additional radiologic sign to detect such injuries can be identified on axial CT or MR; unilateral enlargement of injured exit foramen compared to uninvolved contralateral foramen occurs on axial images; "open" exit foramen sign; classical descriptions of these injuries include: rotation of spinous processes toward side of injury at levels above injury, malalignment of uncovertebral joints, enterolisthesis, bare facet signs

Source
Adapted from McConnell Jr CT, Wippold II FJ, West OC, Angtuaro ECE, Gado MH. The "open" exit foramen: a new sign of unilateral interfacetal dislocation or subluxation in the lower cervical spine. Emergency Radiology 1995;2:296-302.

 OperaSTAR resectoscope system

Description
specialized tissue-aspirating resectoscope allows physicians to remove tissues causing abnormal uterine bleeding by ablation

Source
FemRx product information. Sunnyvale, CA.

Operating Arm stereotactic navigator

Description
advanced image-guided neurosurgical instrument surgery system for frame-less stereotactic navigation

Source
Radionics product information. Burlington, MA.

ophthalmic vitreous surgical techniques

Description
techniques for sulcus fixation of posteriorly dislocated or secondarily implanted posterior chamber intraocular lens, repair of iridodialysis, and management of decentered intraocular lens during vitreous surgery using 25 gauge forceps; forceps have a curved shaft, tip with distal platform to grasp suture, and proximal groove to grip haptic; insert through grooved scleral incision into the plane of the ciliary sulcus; forceps designed for anterior segment applications during vitreous surgery

Anatomy
choroid; ciliary sulcus; cortical vitreous; corneoscleral limbus; capsular diaphragm; crystalline lens; iris diaphragm; iris root; iris stroma; periretinal membrane; peripheral iris; pars plana; retina; sclera; scleral groove; sulcus

Equipment
standard ophthalmic surgery equipment; crescent knife; curved needle; end-gripping forceps; fixation suture; fenestrated needle; hand-held cautery; 25 gauge intraocular forceps; intraocular lens haptic; nylon suture; polypropylene suture; polymethyl methacrylate optic; polypropylene haptic; slip knot

Source
Adapted from Chang S, Coll EC. Surgical techniques for repositioning a dislocated intraocular lens, repair of iridodialysis, and secondary intraocular lens implantation using innovative 25 gauge forceps. American Journal of Ophthalmology 1995;119:165-174.

OPOL

Generic name
see live oral polio vaccine

Oppociser exercise device

Description
device especially designed to assist in strengthening the opponens muscle; features adjustable tension provided by rubber bands in two sizes

Source
Sammons Inc. product information. Western Springs, IL.

opportunistic laparoscopic strategy

Description
three guidelines to make vaginal phase of laparoscopy as easy and nonmorbid as possible

Anatomy
cervix; vagina; uterine arteries; uterine fundus; corpus

Equipment
bipolar forceps; unipolar cutting needle

Source
Adapted from Pelosi MA, Pelosi MA III. A comprehensive approach to morcellation of the large uterus. Contemporary OB/GYN 1997;42:106-125.

 ## Optelec Passport magnifier

Description
portable video magnifying instrument operates on battery or any power source; magnifies print up to 40 times for people who are vision impaired

Source
Optelec product information. Westford, MA.

 ## Optetrak total knee replacement system

Description
orthopaedic knee prosthesis with superior motion and stability; requires less bone removal; solves problems of articular stress and patellofemoral malfunction seen with other knee prostheses

Source
Exactech Inc. product information. Gainesville, FL.

 ## optical coherence tomography (OCT)

Synonyms
none

Indications
assess plaque morphology at micron scale

Method
low coherent infrared light or ultrashort laser pulses used to generate tomographic images

Normal findings
not applicable

Comments

OCT represents promising new diagnostic technology for intracoronary imaging, which could permit in vivo evaluation of critical vascular pathology

Source

Adapted from Brezinski ME, Tearney GJ, Bouma BE, et al. Imaging of coronary artery microstructure (in vitro) with optical coherence tomography. American Journal of Cardiology 1996;77:92-93.

 Optima diamond knife

Description

KOI-130 and KOI-130T with 45 degree cutting edges, 1-mm width and 0.15-mm thicknesses

Source

KOI Western Medical Products Inc. product information. San Diego, CA.

 Option Orthotic Series

Description

this series features two premolded orthotic bases including the Lite Option and the Pro Option; the Lite Option is a red UCOlite base that provides cushioning with accommodative support; the Pro Option is a white PRO XP II base that provides control and balance in a mid-range device; each Option base fits easily in most shoes and may be reshaped with heat to create a custom fit

Source

UCO Inc. product information. Prospect Heights, IL.

 OPTP Slant

Description

positioning for stretching gastrocnemius soleus complex; important for prevention and treatment of many common lower leg and foot problems; assists with general stretching and weightbearing; can promote more stable gait

Source

OPTP product information. Minneapolis, MN.

 Orapette/SalivaCard HIV-1/HIV-2 assay

Synonyms

salivary HIV antibody assay

Use

laboratory diagnosis of HIV infection

Method

oral fluid collection device linked to card-based immunoassay

Specimen
saliva

Normal range
no evidence of antibody reactivity

Comments
rapid, sensitive, highly accurate assay, and does not require blood specimen

Source
Adapted from Saville RD, Constantine NT, Holm-Hansen C, Wisnom C, DePaola L, Falkler WA Jr. Evaluation of two novel immunoassays designed to detect HIV antibodies in oral fluids. Journal of Clinical Laboratory Analysis 1997;11:63-68.

 Orascoptic acuity system

Description
Dimension-3 magnifying telescopes with fiberoptic or halogen lighting systems to reduce neck, back, and eye fatigue during lengthy procedures; replaces need for fiberoptic handpieces in dentistry and greatly enhances overhead lighting in operating room; works with any vision or safety system including laser goggles, safety goggles, and prescription lenses

Source
Orascoptic Research Inc. product information. Madison, WI.

 OraSure HIV-1 collection device

Description
collection device used in collection of oral fluid specimens for human immunodeficiency virus type 1 (HIV-1) antibody testing in subjects 13 years of age and older; used with the oral fluid Vironostika HIV-1 Micro-ELISA System screening test

Source
Epitope Inc. product information. Beaverton, OR.

 Orbis-Sigma valve

Description
variable resistance valve which automatically controls cerebrospinal fluid drainage in patients with hydrocephalus

Source
Cordis Corporation product information. Miami, FL.

Orbital shoulder stabilizer brace

Description
Orbital shoulder stabilizer (OSS) strengthens unstable shoulder by developing stability in the proximal shoulder, chest, and back muscles; provides feedback and may be used in multiple positions and rotations

Source
Charles Group Inc. product information. Park City, UT.

 ## orbit blade

Description
rotatable curved blade with unique cutting window that can be rotated within the field of view without removing it mid-procedure to bend and change its configuration

Source
Smith & Nephew Dyonics Inc. product information. Andover, MA.

 ## Orca surgical blade

Description
cataract surgical blade available in stab, inserter, spoon, and crescent styles

Source
Mentor Ophthalmics product information. Mentor, OH.

 ## Orgaran

see danaparoid sodium

 ## orgotein

Brand Name
Ontosein

Use
bovine-derived superoxide dimutase (bSOD)/anti-inflammatory agent used in the treatment of osteoarthritis of the knee

Usual Dosage
intra-articularly: in clinical trials 4 mg or 8 mg initially then on days 7 and 14. If necessary, may repeat on day 28

Pharmaceutical company
DDI Pharmaceuticals Inc. Mountain View, CA.

Source
University of Pittsburgh Drug Information and Pharmacoepidemiology Center. Pittsburgh, PA.

orlistat

Brand name
Xenical

Use
lipase inhibitor that blocks approximately 30% of fat eaten in food; first of new class of non-central nervous system, nonsystemic drugs for treatment of obesity

Usual dosage
not given

Pharmaceutical company
Roche Laboratories. Nutley, NJ.

Source
Food and Drug Administration Internet site.

 Orthex Relievers shoe inserts

Description
featuring Viscolas, a shock-absorbent viscoelastic polymer from E-A-R Specialty Composites; have been shown to reduce the back, leg and foot pain associated with standing or walking for long periods, particularly in occupational applications; the full-cushion insole features a hypoallergenic viscoelastic polymer layer, with a breathable Cambrelle cover that will not rot or support fungal growth

Source
Viscolas Inc. product information. Chattanooga, TN.

 OrthoBone pillow

Description
uniquely shaped design combines proper neck support with head support of a traditional bed pillow, washable, comes with cover

Source
Products Unlimited Inc. product information. Omaha, NE.

 orthognathic occlusal relator

Description
microadjustable surgical device ensures accuracy in orthognathic presurgical splint construction

Source
Gnathodontic Services Inc. product information. Owensboro, KY.

Orthomedics Stretch and Heel splint

Description
a splint for alleviating plantar fasciitis, Achilles tendinitis and other lower extremity overuse injuries; comes in two sizes with optional liner and derotation bar available

Source
Orthomedics Inc. product information. Pasadena, CA.

 Ortho TriCyclen

Generic name
see norgestimate/ethinyl estradiol

 Orthovisc

Generic Name
see hyaluronic acid

 OrthoVise orthopaedic instrument

Description
surgical instrument with slap hammer; designed with the option of using a slap hammer on three locations on the OrthoVise for better adaptability; can be attached to the end or on either side

Source
Innomed Inc. product information. Savannah, GA.

 OrthoWedge healing shoe

Description
protects forefoot by removing most pressure from the metatarsal heads and digits after forefoot surgery or in treatment of diabetic ulcerations

Source
Darco International Inc. product information. Huntington, WV.

 Osher gonio/posterior pole lens

Description
ocular lens provides surgeon with clear view of angle and posterior pole simultaneously; view through two mirrors confirms critical anatomical landmarks that involve intraocular lens haptics

Source
Ocular Instruments Inc. product information. Bellevue, WA.

Osher keratometer

Description
ophthalmic surgical instrument designed for intraoperative identification and confirmation of steep meridian when performing a stigmatic keratotomy at time of cataract surgery

Source
Ocular Instruments product information. Bellevue, WA.

 ## OsmoCyte pillow wound dressing

Description
wound care dressing with controlled moisture absorption; unique hydropolymer beads incorporate exudate into molecular structure; locks in moisture providing an optimal wound healing environment; does not macerate; comes out intact, leaving no residue minimizing patient discomfort and damage to newly formed tissue

Source
ProCyte Corp. product information. Kirkland, WA.

 ## OSSEOTITE implant

Description
dental implant with a microtextured surface and increased surface area that allows for increased bone apposition

Source
3i Implant Innovations product information. Palm Beach Gardens, FL.

 ## osseous coagulum trap (OCT)

Description
surgical device offers improved method for collecting osseous material for bone grafting; osseous material is collected in filter basket for quick retrieval

Source
Quality Aspirators product information. Duncanville, TX.

 ## osteoblast proliferation fluorometric assay

Synonyms
AlamarBlue osteoblast proliferation assay

Use
studies of osteoblast cell growth, particularly in diseases of bone formation

Method
fluorometric measurement of oxidation-reduction indicator AlamarBlue in response to metabolic activity

Specimen
cultured osteoblasts

Normal range
investigational

Comments
may facilitate testing of bone growth-promoting agents

Source
Adapted from Jonsson KB, Frost A, Larsson R, Ljunghall S, Ljunggren O. A new fluorometric assay for determination of osteoblastic proliferation: effects of glucocorticoids and insulin-like growth factor-I. Calcified Tissue International 1997;60:30-36.

 osteochondral autograft transfer system (OATS)

Description
offers a comprehensive surgical treatment for most full-thickness femoral condyle defects of the knee; the OATS technique incorporates a series of thin-walled cutting tubes to harvest autogenous plugs of bone capped with healthy hyaline cartilage that will be transferred to the damaged area; these osteochondral core autografts are then press fit into one or more sockets created in the condylar defect; may be carried out arthroscopically or as an open procedure

Anatomy
intra-articular notch; lateral femoral condyle; sulcus terminalis; subchondral bone

Equipment
arthroscope; set of sizer/tamps with Delrin heads of 5-10 cm diameters; OATS single-use tube harvesters; tube harvester driver/extractor; pin calibrator; OATS alignment stick

Source
Arthrex Inc. product information. Naples, FL.

 OsteoGraf/D

Description
bone grafting material with rounded particles that minimizes tissue trauma; vial-syringe interconnect system with three style syringes

Source
Ultimatics Inc. product information. Springdale, AR.

·Osteo Implant

Description
dental implant with a 3.00-mm minor diameter and 3.75-mm major diameter; has self-tapping feature with a standard external hex drive
Source
Osteo Implant Corp. product information. New Castle, PA.

 OSTEOMIN

Description
demineralized freeze-dried bone available in syringes; advantages are osteoinduction and no second surgery needed for removal
Source
Park Dental Research Corp. product information. New York, NY.

 Osteoplate implant

Description
osseointegration blade implant used in cases that have insufficient bone for endosteal implants; highly resorbed into alveolar bone
Source
Tronicsoral product information. Bremen, Germany.

 osteotomy analysis simulation software (OASIS)

Description
uses AP x-ray of leg to identify bony landmarks, contours, and joint contacts; computer analysis of axial alignment joint force, ligament force, pressure distribution; displays color line drawings; allows interactive simulation to show projected results of various types of osteotomies
Source
Zona Medical Technologies U.S.A. Inc. product information. Sausalito, CA.

 Otocap myringotomy blade

Description
safety cap designed for myringotomy scalpels; according to the manufacturer, only myringotomy blade in the world to offer the safety cap
Source
ScalpelTEC product information. Memphis, TN.

404

 ## Otto Bock Greissinger Plus foot

Description
model IA30 is a prosthesis that utilizes a joint that emulates the multi-axial movement of the human foot making uneven surfaces easier to negotiate; the source of the flexibility is a rocking rubber that completely encircles the ankle axis; available in three durometers

Source
Otto Bock Orthopaedic Industry Inc. product information. Minneapolis, MN.

 ## Otto Bock modular rotary hydraulic knee

Description
model 3R80 is a knee joint for amputees; features a 135-degree flexion angle that is an advantage for bicycling, entering a car, kneeling or sitting; recommended for patients with moderate to higher activity levels and weighing up to 220 pounds

Source
Otto Bock Orthopaedic Industry Inc. product information. Minneapolis, MN.

 ## Otto Bock system electric hands

Description
myoelectric upper limb prosthesis with microchip control circuitry; dynamic mode control has 2 independent systems that proportionally control both grip force and speed; strength of muscle signal directly controls grip speed and force which immediately adapts to signal changes; finger speed ranges from 15-130 mm per second providing amputee with well-controlled physiological grasp

Source
Otto-Bock Orthopedic Industry Inc. product information. Minneapolis, MN.

 ## oxcarbazepine

Brand name
Trileptal

Use
for the treatment of patients with refractory seizures

Usual dosage
oral: 600-1200 mg

Pharmaceutical company
Novartis Pharmaceuticals. East Hanover, NJ.

Source
Stadtlanders Managed Pharmacy Services. Pittsburgh, PA.

OxiLink

Description
disposable oximetry probe cover; polyurethane film functions as a barrier between the probe and the patient's skin while ensuring adhesion to the finger

Source
BCI International product information. Waukesha, WI.

 OxiScan pulse oximeter

Description
device providing a complete system to conduct, interpret, and retrieve overnight oximetry studies of adults and newborns

Source
AirSep Corp. product information. Buffalo, NY.

 oxycodone hydrochloride

Brand name
OxyContin

Use
extended release tablet formulation of opioid analgesic for moderate to severe pain

Usual dosage
oral: available as 10, 20, 40 mg oxycodone hydrochloride; 1 tablet every 8 to 12 hours as needed for pain

Pharmaceutical company
The Purdue Frederick Co. Norwalk, CT.

Source
Stadtlanders Managed Pharmacy Services. Pittsburgh, PA.

 OxyContin

Generic name
see oxycodone hydrochloride

 Oxydome

Description
body-enclosing oxygen therapy system for premature neonates

Source
Nascor product information. Crows Nest, Australia.

406

 Oxy-Holter

Description
evaluates oxygen therapy patients for desaturation while monitoring arrhythmias in 1 overnight recording; overnight pulse oximetry with full disclosure 3-lead ECG recordings

Source
Synectics Medical product information. Irving, TX.

 Oxypleth pulse oximeter

Description
provides measurement and display of arterial oxygen saturation of blood and pulse rate; internal 4-hour battery provides ability to monitor patients during transport and/or power failures

Source
Novametrix Medical Systems Inc. product information. Wallingford, CT.

 Oxypod

Description
oxygen hood for newborns

Source
Nascor product information. Crows Nest, Australia.

 OxyTemp

Description
integrated model 3301T hand-held pulse oximeter with infrared thermometry temperature sensing for spot-checking pulse rate, SpO_2, and temperature

Source
BCI International product information. Waukesha, WI.

 OxyTip sensors

Description
neonatal/toddler pulse oximeter sensors and adult/pediatric pulse oximeter sensors provide reliable readings and reduced falsealarms; re-usable OxyLead interconnect cables compatible with Ohmeda oximetry equipment

Source
Ohmeda Medical Systems product information. Madison, WI.

Oxy-Ultra-Lite ambulatory oxygen systems

Description
provides a 1 L/min oxygen-requiring patient with 7 hours of ambulation; some models are supplied with carrying pouches to be used during exercise, gardening, shopping, etc.

Source
Chad Therapeutics Inc. product information. Chatsworth, CA.

 Pacesetter Tendril DX steroid-eluting active-fixation pacing lead

Description
pacing lead tip secretes a small amount of steroid minimizing tissue inflammation at the lead implant site; manufactured by St. Jude Medical

Source
Internet news sources.

 p53 allelotyping

Synonyms
p53 tumor suppressor gene analysis

Use
colorectal cancer patients having tumors with deletion of the p53 (chromosome 17p) gene are far more likely to show tumor recurrence and have shorter disease-free survival than patients with tumors retaining both copies of the gene; recent data indicate allelotype analysis may have greater prognostic significance than deoxyribonucleic acid (DNA) ploidy analysis

Method
southern blot hybridization

Specimen
solid tumor and whole blood; solid tumor and normal colonic mucosa

Normal range
investigational use

Comments
performance characteristics have not been established

Source
Lexi-Comp Inc. database. Hudson, OH.

PalmCups

Description
manual percussors for assisting in the performance of chest physiotherapy; soft vinyl cups are easily used by a clinician or a family member who may be providing therapy at home

Source
Diemolding Healthcare Division product information. Canastota, NY.

 PalmVue ECGstat

Description
12-lead communication system; first pocket-size wireless system; enables palmtop computer to display and store 12-lead ECG waveforms, test messages and computerized ECG interpretations; built-in paging system, error detection and security features

Source
Hewlett-Packard product information. Andover, MA.

 PAL pump for air mattress overlay

Description
powered air loss (PAL) pump for mattress overlay provides continuous pressure relieving performance; alternating pressure systems generally provide pressure relief less frequently

Source
Gaymar Industries Inc. product information. Orchard Park, NY.

 Paluther

Generic name
see artemether

 PAM2 and PAM3 monitors

Description
evaluates and monitors body movements; applications include sleep/wake studies, circadian rhythms, insomnia, restless leg syndrome, Parkinson tremor, hyperactivity, ergonomics; recorder is worn on the wrist, arm, waist, or leg; data is generated by movement, totaled and time stamped at intervals, and then downloaded through an interface adapter for presentation and analysis

Source
IM Systems product information. Baltimore, MD.

Panasol II home phototherapy system

Description
freestanding electrically operated unit that utilizes ultraviolet B (UVB) light;
physician-prescribed treatment for unsightly patches and scales associated
with psoriasis

Source
National Biological Corp. product information. Twinsburg, OH.

pancreatic juice antidiuretic hormone (ADH) assay

Synonyms
pancreatic ADH level

Use
detection of ectopic ADH production in tumor diagnosis

Method
ADH-specific immunoassay

Specimen
pancreatic juice aspirate

Normal range
not yet established, but likely less than 1 picogram (pg)/ml

Comments
useful in evaluation of patients with unexplained syndrome of increased
ADH (SIADH)

Source
Adapted from Nagashima Y, Iino K, Oki Y et al. A rare case of ectopic antidiuretic hormone-producing pancreatic
adenocarcinoma: new diagnostic approach. Internal Medicine 1996;35:280-284.

pancreatic oncofetal antigen detection

Synonyms
POA

Use
may be useful in the diagnosis and management of pancreatic cancer and
other cancers

Method
rocket immunoelectrophoresis (Laurell method)

Specimen
blood

Normal range
less than 15 pancreatic oncofetal antigen (POA) units/ml

Comments
sensitivity of the assay is 0.7 POA units/ml

Source
Lexi-Comp Inc. database, Hudson, OH.

Pandel

Generic name
see hydrocortisone buteprate

 "pants" vein jump graft in liver transplantation

Description
portal vein thrombosis has been a surgical challenge in orthotopic hepatic transplantation; the technique of the venous "jump" graft from the superior mesenteric vein has been standardized; one of the limiting factors of the technique is the lack of a sufficient segment of the superior mesenteric vein (SMV) from which the venous vein can be anastomosed; the technique of anastomosing two iliac venous allografts separately to two jejunal branches of the SMV to reconstitute portal vein flow to the allograft has been utilized

Anatomy
confluence of superior mesenteric and portal vein; iliac veins; jejunal branches; liver; mesenteric root; retropancreatic segment of SMV; supramesocolic area; transverse colon

Equipment
standard surgical equipment

Source
Pinna AD, Lim JW, Sugitani AD, Starzl TE, Fung JJ. "Pants" vein jump graft for portal vein and superior mesenteric vein thrombosis in transplantation of the liver. Journal of American College of Surgeons 1996;183:527-528.

 Papercuff blood pressure cuff

Description
disposable blood pressure cuff; outer layer does not stretch so that inflated pressure is transferred to patient's arm; inner layer does stretch so that there are no gaps between cuff and arm; minimizes contact with blood or body fluids that can contaminate fabric of standard cuff; accuracy comparable to standard cuff

Source
CAS Medical Systems Inc. product information. Branford, CT.

 Parachute stone retrieval device

Description
urologic stone retrieval basket with "O" tip, or filiform tip

Source
Microvasive Boston Scientific Corp. product information. Natick, MA.

paraffin section immunophenotyping

Synonyms
none

Use
immunohistological evaluation of acute leukemia specimens

Method
paraffin-embedded tissue including bone marrow clot and trephine needle biopsy specimens are evaluated for immunohistochemistry

Specimen
bone marrow

Normal range
not applicable

Comments
in the past this was limited by inability to detect many lineage-related antigens in paraffin sections; improvement in immunohistochemical methods and introduction of new antibodies has reduced that limitation

Source
Adapted from Arber DA, Jenkins KA. Paraffin section immunophenotyping of acute leukemias in bone marrow specimens. American Journal of Clinical Pathology 1996;106:462-468.

 Paragon laser

Description
carbon dioxide (CO_2) surgical laser system; five ClearPulse char-free tissue effects at every watt; built-in laparoscopic smoke evacuator

Source
Heraeus Surgical Inc. product information. Milpitas, CA.

 Paragon single-stage dental implant system

Description
single-stage implant manufactured with an internal or external hex configuration; packaged with a healing collar that functions as a fixture mount during implant placement and as a healing collar during the nonsubmerged healing period

Source
DENTSPLY Implant product information. York, PA.

paraPRO needle

Description
paracentesis needle with a two-part trocar that provides a visual indicator of entry while extending a blunt tip to help prevent accidental organ injury

Source
Denver Biomaterials Inc. product information. Golden, CO.

 Parascan scanning device

Description
designed to provide swift and gradual vaporization of delicate tissue while reducing treatment time of aesthetic laser surgery

Source
Heraeus Surgical Inc. product information. Milpitas, CA.

 parathyroid hormone-related protein (PTHrP)

Synonyms
none

Use
test for evaluation of hypercalcemic syndromes; overproduction is indicative of certain malignancies and activates parathyroid hormone (PTH)/PTHrP receptors in bone and kidney

Method
immunoradiometric assay (IRMA) and radioimmunoassay (RIA)

Specimen
none

Normal findings
38-64 pg/mL

Comments
none

Source
Adapted from Bruns D, Brunes E. Parathyroid hormone-related protein in benign lesions. American Journal of Clinical Pathology 1996;105:377-379.

 parathyroid tumor localization study

Synonyms
parathyroid adenoma localization study

Indications
localize parathyroid tumors before the first operation or after parathyroid exploration with persistent hyperparathyroidism to localize ectopic parathyroid lesions for surgical removal

Method

inject intravenously with technetium-99m sestamibi (Cardiolite) followed by sequential visualization; thyroid tissue tends to have decreased localization with time whereas parathyroid tissue has relatively increased concentration; alternatively, dual radiopharmaceutical study may be done with technetium-99m sestamibi and technetium-99m pertechnetate (latter goes to the thyroid, the former to both thyroid and parathyroid); subtraction of the pertechnetate image from the sestamibi image reveals the location of the parathyroid tumor

Normal findings

no parathyroid tumor localization

Comments

thyroid tumors also localize the radiopharmaceutical

Source

Nuclear Medicine Consultant. Stedman's Medical Dictionary, 26th edition.

 Park-O-Tron drill system

Description

dual motor drill system; microelectric drill system for implants and use in oral surgery

Source

Park Dental Research Group product information. New York, NY.

 pars plana Baerveldt tube insertion with vitrectomy

Description

treatment of glaucoma associated with pseudophakia and aphakia is often difficult; technique of combined pars plana vitrectomy and pars plana insertion of Baerveldt tube provides intraocular pressure control in eyes with shallow anterior chamber or vitreous prolapse and glaucoma associated with pseudophakia or aphakia; Baerveldt glaucoma implant is a nonvalved, single-plate drainage device usually placed on the superotemporal aspect of the globe because of ease of insertion at this site

Anatomy

anterior chamber; corneal endothelium; corneoscleral limbus; conjunctiva; choroid; episclera; iris; inferior fornix; lateral rectus muscle; superotemporal aspect of globe; pars plana; retina; sclera; superior oblique and superior rectus muscles; Tenon capsule; vitreous

Equipment

standard ophthalmic surgery equipment; Baerveldt implant; calipers; ophthalmoscope; infusion cannula; microvitreoretinal blade; muscle hook; vitreous cutter

Source

Adapted from Varma T, Heuer DK, Lundy DC, Baerveldt G, Lee P, Minckler DS. Pars plana Baerveldt tube insertion with vitrectomy in glaucomas associated with pseudophakia and aphakia. American Journal of Ophthalmology 1995;119:401-407.

414

 passive hemagglutination (PHA) test

Synonyms
passive HA reaction

Use
rapid measurement of circulating tetanus, diphtheria, or hepatitis antibodies to determine immunity or exposure

Method
passive hemagglutination reaction using highly purified antigens covalently coupled to turkey red blood cells

Specimen
blood

Normal range
not applicable – antibody reactivity may be normal or abnormal depending on the disease and whether the individual has been immunized deliberately

Comments
circulating antibodies can be assessed in 20 minutes using one drop of blood

Source
Adapted from Relyveld EH, Huet M, Lery L. Passive hemagglutination tests using purified antigens covalently coupled to turkey erythrocytes. Developmental Biology Standards 1996;86:225-241.

 Patanol

Generic name
see olopatadine

 Patellar Band knee protector

Description
light-weight protection for the knee during sports activities; for prevention of sports injury, for patellofemoral disorders, and/or preservative treatment; prevents outward rotation of patella

Source
Nakamura Brace Co. Ltd. product information. Oda, Japan.

 Pautler infusion cannula

Description
ophthalmic instrument designed to provide continuous irrigation during complicated posterior segment surgery; angled flange that allows it to be sutured to the sclera, while cannula enters anterior segment through the cornea

Source
Visitec Co. product information. Sarasota, FL.

PB-FOxS pediatric femoral sensor kit

Description
femoral sensor kit for use with PB3300 intra-arterial blood gas (IABG) monitoring system; enables clinicians to use continuous IABG monitoring in pediatric patients

Source
Puritan-Bennett Corp. product information. Carlsbad, CA.

 PC Performer knee prosthesis

Description
fully programmable centroid, full range adjustable flexion stability, ultra-light composite prosthesis

Source
Daw Industries product information. San Diego, CA.

 Peacekeeper cannula

Description
ophthalmic surgical instrument that combines Wet-Field hemostasis for controlled retinotomy and targeted coagulation with an extrudable cannula to achieve controlled subretinal drainage

Source
Mentor O&O Inc. product information. Norwell, MA.

 Peak gait module

Description
motion measurement system; provides accurate 3-dimensional analysis of joint dynamics of human gait; computes orientation of the body's lower segments as well as the forces at work within the hip, knee, and ankle joints

Source
Peak Performance Technologies Inc. product information. Englewood, CO.

 PEARL (physiologic endometrial ablation/resection loop) technology

Description
provides ability to perform resection and ablation procedures using isotonic irrigation solutions such as normal saline; eliminates possible complications of non-isotonic solution tissue absorption; part of the OPERA (outpatient endometrial resection/ablation) system

Source
FemRx Inc. product information. Sunnyvale, CA.

pediatric pressure relief ankle foot orthosis (PRAFO) attachment

Description
a brace that is most useful for the spina bifida and cerebral palsy population; it allows continual stretch of the Achilles tendon during sleep time

Source
Anatomical Concepts Inc. product information. Boardman, OH.

 Pedi-Cushions

Description
over-the-counter foot pads and cushions

Source
Pedifix Inc. product information. Mt. Kisco, NY.

 pegaspargase

Brand name
Oncaspar

Use
therapeutic use in a broad range of cancers

Usual dosage
intramuscular (preferred): 2500 IU/m2 every 14 days; intravenous: 2500 IU/m2 every 14 days

Pharmaceutical company
Enzon Inc. Piscataway, NJ.

Source
University of Pittsburgh Drug Information and Pharmacoepidemiology Center. Pittsburgh, PA.

 pegorgotein

Brand name
Dismutec

Use
treatment of severe head injury

Usual dosage
intravenous: 10,000 units/kg or 20,000 units/kg within 8 hours of injury in clinical trials

Pharmaceutical company
Enzon Inc. Piscataway, NJ.

Source
Stadtlanders Managed Pharmacy Services. Pittsburgh, PA.

Pelosi fibrotome

Description
knife designed specifically for morcellation techniques

Source
Adapted from Pelosi MA, Pelosi MA III. A comprehensive approach to morcellation of the large uterus. Contemporary OB/GYN 1997;42:106-125.

 ## penciclovir

Brand name
Denavir

Use
treatment of recurrent herpes labialis (cold sores) on face and lips

Usual dosage
topical: 1% cream; apply to cold sores every 2 hours during waking hours for a period of 4 days

Pharmaceutical company
SmithKline Beecham Pharmaceuticals. Pittsburgh, PA.

Source
Stadtlanders Managed Pharmacy Services. Pittsburgh, PA.

 ## pentostan polysulfate sodium

Brand Name
Elmiron

Use
semi-synthetic glycosaminoglycan-like substance; anti-inflammatory used in the treatment of interstitial cystitis

Usual Dosage
oral: 200-400 mg/day

Pharmaceutical company
IVAX Corporation. Miami, FL.

Source
University of Pittsburgh Drug Information and Pharmacoepidemiology Center. Pittsburgh, PA.

 ## Percu-Stay catheter fastener

Description
percutaneous drainage catheter fastener minimizes chance of catheter working its way out, comfortable yet sticks securely

Source
Percu-Stay product information. *(Editor note: Unable to verify company address)*

percutaneous bladder neck stabilization (PBNS)

Description

procedure for correcting stress urinary incontinence; also called Vesica procedure; this technique uses sutures affixed to the pubic bone to suspend the bladder neck; a bone locator serves as a stabilizer for the suture anchorsystem; physician ensures that there is equal tension on the suspending sutures; use of the suture anchor system provides consistent elevation on both sides of the urethra; procedure takes about 25 minutes to perform versus an hour for traditional strategies and it shortens recovery time for some women; one side-effect is the potential for a punctured bladder which can be easily identified through cystoscopy

Anatomy

urethra; bladder; vagina

Equipment

standard surgical equipment

Source

Adapted from Mark A. Newman, staff writer. New Incontinence Therapy May Be Safer, Easier. Ob.Gyn.News March 1996.

 percutaneous endoscopic gastrojejunostomy

Description

percutaneous endoscopic gastrojejunostomy (PEG-J) increasingly used to maintain long-term enteral nutrition; precise placement defined as placement of the jejunostomy tube beyond the ligament of Treitz; Glidewire is advantageous for placement due to its resistance to forming kinks and a wet hydrophilic coating that makes the wire slippery and easily steerable, facilitating maneuverability of the angles of the upper intestine

Anatomy

ampulla of Vater, duodenum, ligament of Treitz, pylorus

Equipment

standard endoscopic surgery equipment; endoscope; rubber-tipped Olympus forceps; hydropolymer-coated Glidewire; 28F Super percutaneous endoscopic gastrostomy (PEG) tube; 12F polyurethane jejunostomy tube; 12F straight biliary catheter with stiffening cannula; torque device

Source

Adapted from Parasher VK, Abramowicz CJ, Bell C, Delledonne AM, Wright A. Successful placement of percutaneous gastrojejunostomy using steerable Glidewire - a modified controlled push technique. Gastrointestinal Endoscopy 1995;41:52-54.

percutaneous transluminal endomyocardial revascularization (PTER)

Description
catheter-based minimally invasive procedure for treatment of coronary artery disease by creating channels in oxygen-starved areas of the heart muscle

Anatomy
not given

Equipment
can be performed without general anesthesia

Source
CorMedica and CR Bard distributor press release on Internet.

 ## perendoscopic injection of botulinum toxin

Description
intrasphincteric injection of botulinum toxin for the treatment of achalasic patients who failed previous therapy with myotomy or pneumatic dilation

Anatomy
lower esophageal segment (LES) region

Equipment
sclerotherapy needle; Arndorfer catheter; Sensor Medics pump

Source
Adapted from Annesse V, Basciani M, Lombardi G et al. Perendoscopic injection of botulinum toxin is effective in achalasia after failure of myotomy or pneumatic dilation. Gastrointestinal Endoscopy 1996;44(4):461-464.

 ## perflubron

Brand name
LiquiVent

Use
oxygen-carrying liquid, also known as liquid oxygen, is delivered intratracheally to patients on mechanical ventilation to improve oxygen delivery to the lungs

Usual dosage
intratracheal: enough LiquiVent is administered to replace the lung's functional residual capacity; dose of LiquiVent will vary with individual needs; patients typically receive it for a few hours to a few days; when no longer needed it is allowed to evaporate

Pharmaceutical company
Hoechst Marion Roussel Pharmaceuticals Inc. Somerville, NJ.

Source
Stadtlanders Managed Pharmacy Services. Pittsburgh, PA.

Perf-Plate cranial plate

Description
cranial plate that offers alternative to traditional cranial flap suturing techniques

Source
Zimmer Inc. product information. Warsaw, IN.

pericardioplasty in pectus excavatum repair

Description
pectus excavatum involves redundant pericardial sac, levocardia, and an empty space in the mediastinum into which the sternum is pulled; pericardioplasty repositions the heart; use transverse submammary curved (lazy-3) incision or vertical median incision from manubrium to xiphoid; subperichondrial resection of deformed cartilage occurs; incise pericardial sac vertically to develop flap; suture to right costal border to reposition the heart; bony wedge stabilizes the sternum

Anatomy
sternum; sternal body; retrosternal space; manubrium; xiphoid process; rib; chest wall; pectoralis muscle; costal border; costal and costochondral cartilage; intercostal space; perichondrium; perichondrial bed; periosteum; angle of Louis; mediastinum; pericardium; pericardial sac; stem of pulmonary artery; diaphragm; aponeurosis

Equipment
standard surgery equipment; Gigli saw; wire suture

Source
Adapted from Teixeira JP, Teixeira-Filho J. Operative correction of pectus excavatum using the right ventricle as a sternal support. Journal of the American College of Surgeons 1995;180:346-348.

PERI-COMFORT cushion

Description
seating cushion is an auto-inflating air seating cushion with foam core; fits most chairs, wheelchairs, and seating situations

Source
Chi'Am International product information. Circle Pines, MN.

Periotest

Synonyms
none

Indications
assesses buccolingual, mesiodistal, and rotational mobility of dental implant; endosseous dental implants require assessment of osseointegration in order to prevent infection

Method
at 3-, 6-, 9-, and 12-month intervals assessment made of inflammation, gingival hyperplasia, gingival recession, plaque index, gingival index, and width of keratinized gingiva

Normal findings
no abnormal findings

Comments
none

Source
Adapted from Barber HD, Seckinger RJ, Silverstein K, et al. Comparison of soft tissue healing and osseointegration of IMZ implants placed in one-stage and two-stage techniques: a pilot study. Implant Dentistry 1996;5:11-14.

 Peri-Strips staple line reinforcement

Description
strips of bovine pericardium sutured to a backing material; used for lung volume reductions, segmentectomies, lobectomies, wedge resections, bronchial resections, pneumonectomies and other soft tissue repairs

Source
Bio-Vascular Inc. product information. St. Paul, MN.

 peritoneal tethering

Description
prevention of colostomy prolapse by peritoneal tethering; prolapse defined as protrusion of colostomy for more than 4 cm beyond the skin surface; the technique of anchoring the colon loop to a length of peritoneum three times the width of the stoma offers the potential for prevention of prolapse, provided the whole anchorage remains intact during the colostomy period

Anatomy
abdominal wall; distal loop of colon; hepatic flexure; lumen of bowel; parietal peritoneum; seromuscular coat; subfascial area

Equipment
standard surgical equipment; absorbable sutures

Source
Adapted from Ng WT, Book KS, Wong MK, Cheng PW, Cheung CH. Prevention of colostomy prolapse by peritoneal tethering. Journal of American College of Surgeons 1997;184:313-315.

422

 peritoneovenous shunt

Description
placement of peritoneovenous shunt as palliative treatment for ascites secondary to gynecologic malignancy; replaces painful and inconvenient intermittent abdominal paracentesis for patients in final stages of illness

Anatomy
ovary; peritoneum; endometrium; fallopian tubes; abdomen Equipment standard surgery equipment; B.G. Medical Leveen or Denver shunt

Source
Adapted from Faught W, Kirkpatrick JR, Krepart GV, Heywood MS, Lotocki RJ. Peritoneovenous shunt for palliation of gynecologic malignant ascites. Journal of the American College of Surgeons 1995;180:472-474.

 Permark pigment colors and Enhancer III

Description
presterilized iron oxide base colors with alcohol and glycerol that can be used with pigmenting units; uses include for nipple-areola after reconstruction; replacing pigment loss to scars, burns or laser hypopigmentation; cosmetic applications such as lip or eye liners

Source
Micropigmentation Devices Inc. product information. Edison, NJ.

 Perma Sharp suture and needle

Description
finely honed surgical stainless steel needle that cuts easily through the suture site; suture material is laser-drilled and provides smoother, more uniform attachment, resulting in less tissue disruption

Source
Hu-Friedy Manufacturing Company Inc. product information. Chicago, IL.

 peroral insertion technique of self-expanding metal stent

Description
a reliable insertion technique for malignant gastric outlet and duodenal stenoses

Anatomy
duodenum; greater curvature of the stomach; ampulla; descending duodenum

Equipment

Gianturco Z-stent; Teflon delivery sheath; extra-stiff guidewire; balloon dilator; biliary self-expanding metal stent

Source

Adapted from Maetani I, Inoue H, Sato M, Ohashi S, Igarashi Y, Sakai Y. Peroral insertion techniques of self-expanding metal stents for malignant gastric outlet and duodenal stenoses. Gastrointestinal Endoscopy 1996;44(4):468-471.

 ## P-glycoprotein (Pgp) assay for tumor cell multidrug resistance

Synonyms

Pgp assay

Use

evaluation of drug resistance in adult acute leukemic disorders

Method

flow cytometric detection of Pgp-expressing cells, and flow cytometric measurement of fluorescent-labeled drug accumulation

Specimen

blood or bone marrow

Normal range

investigational

Comments

clinical trials of Pgp modulation can be expected in the near future

Source

Adapted from Broxterman HJ, Sonneveld P, Feller N, Ossenkoppele GJ, Währer DCR, Eekman CA, Schoester M, Lankelma J, Pinedo HM, Löwenberg B, Schuurhuis GJ. Quality control of multidrug resistance assays in adult acute leukemia: correlation between assays for P-glycoprotein expression and activity. Blood 1996;87:4809-4816.

 ## Phaco-4 diamond knife

Description

ophthalmic surgical instrument with keratome-shaped blade; features four double-beveled cutting edges for smooth clear cataract incisions

Source

Katena Products Inc. product information. Denville, NJ.

 ## pharmacoradiologic disimpaction of esophageal foreign bodies

Synonyms

Indications

impaction of foreign body; possibility of perforation

Method

use of glucagon and diazepam; use of glucagon, an effervescent agent and water; or use of glucagon only

Normal findings
not applicable

Comments
relatively safe and inexpensive method of cure

Source
Adapted from Maglinte DDJ, Chernish SM, Kelvin FM, Lappas JC. Pharmacoradiologic disimpaction of esophageal foreign bodies: review and recommendation. Emergency Radiology 1995;2:151-157.

 Pharmorubicin

Generic name
see epirubicin

 phentolamine

Brand name
Vasomax

Use
an oral agent for the treatment of male erectile dysfunction

Usual dosage
oral: 50 mg taken 1.5 hours before coitus in clinical trials

Pharmaceutical company
Zonagen. The Woodlands, TX.

Source
Stadtlanders Managed Pharmacy Services. Pittsburgh, PA.

 PhosphorImager system

Description
filmless autoradiography computer program system used for fast, accurate quantitation of radioactive gels, blots, and samples, and as detector in x-ray crystallography

Source
Molecular Dynamics product information. Sunnyvale, CA.

 photochemical inactivation of transfusion-transmissible hepatitis B virus

Synonyms
photoinactivation; blood product sterilization; blood product decontamination

Use
pretransfusion inactivation of hepatitis B virus in platelet concentrates

Method
photochemical decontamination using 8-methoxypsoralen and ultraviolet A light

Specimen
platelet concentrate

Normal range
not applicable

Comments
investigational, but likely to evolve into a standard clinical practice

Source
Adapted from Eble BE, Corash L. Photochemical inactivation of duck hepatitis B virus in human platelet concentrates: a model of surrogate human hepatitis B virus infectivity. Transfusion 1996;36:406-418.

 PhotoDerm PL

Description
noninvasive pulsed light device used in treating pigmented lesions and tattoos. *(Editor note: also there is PhotoDerm VL)*

Source
ESC Medical Systems Ltd. product information. Yokneam, Israel.

 PhotoFix alpha pericardial bioprosthesis

Description
prosthesis for aortic valve replacement; leaflets constructed from bovine pericardium and treated with a fixation process that uses photo-oxidation to create stable collagen crosslinks; currently in clinical trials

Source
CarboMedics Inc. product information. Austin, TX.

 Photofrin

Generic name
see porfimer sodium

 PhotoGenica laser system

Description
pulsed dye laser system for treating vascular or pigmented lesions; PhotoGenica-P destroys only melanin containing cells; PhotoGenica-V targets microvasculature and controls coagulation

Source
Cynosure Inc. product information. Bedford, MA.

PhotoGenica T laser system

Description
PhotoGenica T is a Q-switched alexandrite laser; safely removes multi-colored tattoos and pigmented lesions; PhotoGenica P removes benign pigmented lesions such as café au lait birthmarks, sun spots, liver spots, freckles and brown pigmented lesions (cells that contain melanin); PhotoGenica V improves or eliminates port wine birthmarks and stretch marks, telangiectasias, warts and hypertrophic scars (microvascular areas and coagulation control) (Editor note: PhotoGenica P and V are in Word Watcher Vol. 1, issue 1; due to the sound similiarity in the names specific details of each is presented in this issue)

Source
Cynosure Inc. product information. Bedford, MA.

photopheresis

Synonyms
extracorporeal photochemotherapy

Use
treatment of known or suspected immune-mediated diseases

Method
cytapheresis is performed to collect peripheral blood lymphocytes from a patient, cells are treated with a drug, which is then activated by exposure to ultraviolet light, and the cells are reinfused, where they modulate the patient's immune system

Specimen
peripheral blood cytapheresis product

Comments
currently in use or under investigation for cutaneous T-cell lymphoma, scleroderma, and organ transplant rejection

Source
University of Minnesota Department of Laboratory Medicine and Pathology. Minneapolis, MN.

Pinwheel System

Description
dermatome testing instrument

Source
Cronin Pinwheel System product information. Whitefish, MT.

PIP/DIP strap

Description
finger flexion hook-and-loop strap increases and holds proximal interphalangeal (PIP) and distal interphalangeal (DIP) joints in flexion with constant force

Source
Fred Sammons Inc. product information. Western Springs, IL.

 Pixykine

Generic name
see interleukin-3/granulocyte macrophage-colony stimulating factor fusion protein

 Plak-Vac oral suction brush

Description
dental tool attached to suction to evacuate bacteria, dental plaque, saliva, fluids and food debris; reduces bacterial infection, chronic halitosis, and the potential hazards of aspiration; reduces risk of systemic infection when patient is "at risk" due to suppressed host defenses

Source
Trademark Medical product information. Fenton, MO.

 plantar fasciitis night splint

Description
splint device stabilizes the forefoot in 10 to 20 degrees of dorsiflexion while stretching the plantar fascia; lessens contractures and muscle tightening and minimizes painful steps the following morning; 3 universal sizes fit left or right extremity

Source
Orthomerica Products Inc. product information. Newport Beach, CA.

 plastic endosurgical system (P.E.S.)

Description
plastic surgery precision instruments designed for advanced endoscopic techniques; digital camera and video accessories

Source
Storz Instrument Co. product information. St. Louis, MO.

platelet antigen system genotyping by polymerase chain reaction (PCR) and ligation-based typing

Synonyms
HPA 1-5 genotyping

Use
rapid platelet genotyping of platelet donors, screening for critical antigens in pregnant women

Method
multiplex PCR-based amplification combined with ligation-based typing; visualized by enzyme-linked immunoabsorbent assay

Specimen
blood

Normal range
not applicable

Comments
more readily automated than other platelet typing methods

Source
Adapted from Legler TJ, Kohler M, Mayr WR, Panzer S, Ohto H, Fischer GF. Genotyping of the human platelet antigen systems 1 through 5 by multiplex polymerase chain reaction and ligation-based typing. Transfusion 1996;36:426-431.

 plateletpheresis product white blood cell count

Synonyms
apheresis platelet WBC; single-donor platelet WBC

Use
determination of white blood cell contamination of apheresis platelet products

Method
ultraviolet microscopy of fluorochrome-stained cells dispensed into micro-wells by repeating microsyringe

Specimen
plateletpheresis product

Normal range
<5 x 10^6 WBC

Comments
simpler and more precise than conventional high-sensitivity methods

Source
Adapted from Borzini P, Riva M, Dassi M, et al. A very simple method for counting white cells in platelet units collected by apheresis. Transfusion 1995;35:884-885.

Platypus diagnostic software

Synonyms
none

Indications
identification of fetal abnormalities seen on ultrasound

Method
database of over 360 fetal anomalies; updated regularly by world experts; real-time ultrasound images with motion control; text with differential diagnoses, sonographic features, associated syndromes, reference list

Normal findings
no fetal abnormalities

Comments
diagnostic and training aid

Source
Toi Kinnoir Inc. product information. Ottawa, Canada.

 Plavix

Generic name
see clopidogrel

 PLI-100 pico-injector pipette system

Description
microinjection device that enables independent control of an injection pipette by gathering, retaining, and delivering a single sperm while a second holding pipette retains an oocyte

Source
Medical Systems Corp. product information. Greenvale, NY.

 PlumeSafe Whisper 602 smoke evacuation system

Description
noiseless solution to smoke evacuation during laser and electrosurgical procedures

Source
Buffalo Filter/Medtek Devices Inc. product information. Buffalo, NY.

Plyoball

Description
medicine ball with no oscillation, no bounce

Source
OPTP product information. Minneapolis, MN.

 p53 mutation analysis in mantle cell lymphoma (MCL)

Synonyms
p53 testing; p53 MCL mutation detection

Use
prognostic evaluation of patients with mantle cell lymphoma

Method
polymerase chain reaction DNA amplification screened by denaturing gradient gel electrophoresis

Specimen
tissue biopsy

Normal range
no evidence of p53 mutation amplification product

Comments
investigational but likely to evolve into a standard clinical test

Source
Adapted from Greiner TC, Moynihan MJ, Chan WC, Lytle DM, Pedersen A, Anderson JR, Weisenburger DD. p53 mutations in mantle cell lymphoma are associated with variant cytology and predict a poor prognosis. Blood 1996;87:4302-4310.

 Pneu-trac cervical collar

Description
patient-controlled cervical orthosis allows patient to inflate or release the bulb/valve for static or intermittent cervical stretch

Source
Zinco Industries Inc. product information. Pasadena, CA.

 pocked erythrocyte count

Synonyms
PE count; RE system testing

Use
evaluation of splenic reticuloendothelial (RE) function in patient with suspected hyposplenia or asplenia

Method
examination of glutaldehyde-treated blood smear using interference contrast microscopy with Nomarski optics

Specimen
EDTA (ethylenediaminetetraacetic acid)-anticoagulated blood

Normal range
<3% pocked erythrocytes

Comments
considered a "gold standard" test for several years, but requires specialized microscopy

Source
Adapted from Tham KT, Teague MW, Howard CA, Chen SY. A simple splenic reticuloendothelial function test. American Journal of Clinical Pathology 1996;105:548-552.

 ## Pocket-Dop 3 monitor

Description
compact obstetrical Doppler with a digital fetal heart rate display; has auto-correlation like full-sized antepartum and intrapartum monitors; wall-mounted or counter top recharging system; interchangeable probes such as 2 MHz obstetrical probe or 3 MHz obstetrical probe; a Pocket-Dop 2 system with 5 MHz vascular probe and 8 MHz vascular probe is also available

Source
Imex Medical Systems product information. Golden, CO.

 ## Pocketpeak peak flow meter

Description
portable peak flow meter with ergonomic design making monitoring peak flow throughout the day convenient and practical for all ages of patients; Steel-Flex operating mechanism provides user with appropriate readings to establish their normal baseline or peak expiratory flow rate (PEFR); includes diary and easy to read instructions

Source
Hudson RCI product information. Temecula, CA.

 ## PodoSpray nail drill system

Description
nail drill system for dustless and painless removal of onychomycotic nails; continuously coats nail with a fine aerosol mist that entraps dust on the surface of the nail before it can become airborne; eliminates friction burns by constantly cooling the burr

Source
Darco product information. Huntington, WV.

432

 point-of-care assay for C-reactive protein

Synonyms
CRP office laboratory assay

Use
monitoring disease activity in multiple disorders

Method
automated immunoassay

Specimen
blood

Normal range
0.8 mg/dl

Comments
can be expected to become commonly used in primary care settings

Source
Adapted from Hobbs FD, Kenkre JE, Carter YH, Thorpe GH, Holder RL. Reliability and feasibility of a near patient test for C-reactive protein in primary care. British Journal of General Practice 1996;46:395-400.

 polymerase chain reaction (PCR) assay for Lyme disease

Synonyms
Lyme disease PCR; *Borrelia burgdorferi* PCR

Use
diagnosis of Lyme disease

Method
nested PCR rapid cycle amplification assay specific for *Borrelia burgdorferi* outer surface protein A DNA

Specimen
serum or synovial fluid

Normal range
negative

Comments
particularly valuable in seronegative patients with early, partially treated, or chronic disease

Source
Adapted from Mouritsen CL, Wittwer CT, Litwin CM, Yang L, Weis JJ, Martins TB, Jaskowski TD, Hill HR. Polymerase chain reaction detection of Lyme disease. American Journal of Clinical Pathology 1996;105:647-654.

 polymerase chain reaction (PCR)-based detection of hepatitis G virus (HGV)

Synonyms
HGV detection

Use
diagnosis of HGV infection; blood product screening

Method
polymerase chain reaction with hepatitis G-specific primers

Specimen
blood

Normal range
HGV-specific PCR product not detected

Comments
HGV is a newly identified virus, but is transfusion-transmissible; clinical HGV testing is expected to become standard

Source
Adapted from Linnen J, Wages J Jr, Zhang-Keck Z-Y, et al. Molecular cloning and disease association of hepatitis G virus: a transfusion-transmissible agent. Science 1996;271:505-508.

 ### polymerase chain reaction (PCR)-based diagnosis of Kaposi sarcoma

Synonyms
detection of Kaposi sarcoma-associated herpesvirus (KSHV)-like DNA sequence; KSHV DNA polymerase chain reaction (PCR)

Use
diagnosis of Kaposi sarcoma

Method
PCR using primer pairs for Kaposi sarcoma-associated herpesvirus-like DNA sequence (KSHV DNA)

Specimen
biopsy specimen

Normal range
KSHV-specific PCR product not detected

Comments
investigational

Source
Adapted from Jin Y-T, Tsai S-T, Yan J-J, Hsaio J-H, Lee Y-Y, Su I-J. Detection of Kaposi sarcoma-associated herpesvirus-like DNA sequence in vascular lesions: a reliable diagnostic marker for Kaposi's sarcoma. American Journal of Clinical Pathology 1996;105:360-363.

 ### polymerase chain reaction (PCR)-based K-ras codon 12 mutation detection

Synonyms
K-ras codon 12 mutation PCR

Use
diagnosis of pancreatic carcinoma

Method
PCR with wild-type and mutated primer pair

Specimen
cytology smear

Normal range
K-ras codon 12 mutation-specific PCR product not detected

Comments
complements, but does not replace cytologic analysis

Source
Adapted from Apple SK, Hecht JR, Novak JM, Nieberg RK, Rosenthal DL, Grody WW. Polymerase chain reaction-based K-ras mutation detection of pancreatic adenocarcinoma in routine cytology smears. American Journal of Clinical Pathology 1996;105:321-326.

 polymerase chain reaction (PCR) detection of *bcl*-1 rearrangement in mantle cell lymphoma

Synonyms
bcl-1 PCR; t(11;14) PCR

Use
diagnosis and prognostic evaluation of mantle cell lymphoma

Method
polymerase chain reaction with Southern blot detection

Specimen
frozen and paraffin-embedded tissue biopsy

Normal range
no amplified product detected

Comments
highly sensitive, specific detection of a translocation characteristic of mantle cell lymphoma

Source
Adapted from Pinyol M, Campo E, Nadal A, Terol MP, Jares P, Nayach I, Fernandez PL, Piris MA, Montserrat E, Cardesa A. Detection of the *bcl*-1 rearrangement at the major translocation center in frozen and paraffin-embedded tissues of mantle cell lymphomas by polymerase chain reaction. American Journal of Clinical Pathology 1996;105:532-537.

 polymerase chain reaction (PCR) detection of *Mycoplasma pneumoniae*

Synonyms
Mycoplasma pneumoniae PCR; *M. pneumoniae* PCR

Use
diagnosis of *Mycoplasma pneumoniae* infection

Method
polymerase chain reaction using *Mycoplasma pneumoniae*-specific primers

Specimen
throat swab specimen

Normal range
no reaction products detectable

Comments
PCR appears significantly superior to standard serological tests for *Mycoplasma pneumoniae*, particularly in adult patients

Source
Adapted from Blackmore TK, Reznikov M, Gordon DL. Clinical utility of the polymerase chain reaction to diagnose *Mycoplasma pneumoniae* infection. Pathology 1995;27:177-181.

 polymerase chain reaction (PCR) single-strand conformation polymorphism (SSCP) platelet antigen typing

Synonyms
PCR-SSCP human platelet antigen (HPA) genotyping; PCR-SSCP HPA typing

Use
diagnosis of thrombocytopenia; platelet donor selection

Method
PCR followed by single-strand non-denaturing polyacrylamide gel electrophoresis

Specimen
blood

Normal range
not applicable

Comments
detects previously identified and novel polymorphisms

Source
Adapted from Fujiwara K, Tokunaga K, Isa K, et al. DNA-based typing of human platelet antigen systems by polymerase chain reaction-single-strand conformation polymorphism method. Vox Sanguinis 1995;69:347-351.

 Polytec PI LaseAway

Description
ruby laser technology for removing tattoos and pigmented lesions; beam shaping and rapid pulse repetition reduces treatment time; up to 4-mm spot size; 10 J/cm2 treatment fluences

Source
Polytec PI product information. Costa Mesa, CA.

 polytetrafluoroethylene membrane graft

Description
extraction of fractured central incisors in maxillary anterior region for treatment of osseous defects; microporous hydroxyapatite graft placed in extraction sites to preserve ridge form; graft material packed to overfill sockets; excess material removed; high-density polytetrafluoroethylene (PTFE) membrane cut and shaped to conform to ridge; clear acrylic resin temporary splint fabricated with denture teeth serves as temporary prosthesis

Anatomy
central incisor sockets; gingival papilla; mesial root space; mucoperiosteal flap; barrier membrane; alveolar mucosa; anterior maxillary ridge

Equipment
standard oral surgery equipment; polytetrafluoroethylene microporous hydroxyapatite graft; acrylic resin splint; tissue forceps

Source
Adapted from Bartee BK. The use of high-density polytetrafluoroethylene membrane to treat osseous defects. Implant Dentistry 1995;4:21-26.

POMS 20/50 oxygen conservation device

Description
pulsed-dose oxygen management system (POMS) conservation device for oxygen containers; ensures delivery of prescribed amount of oxygen during exercise and rest; POMS 20 for liquid oxygen; POMS 50 for gas

Source
Pulsair product information. Fort Pierce, FL.

porfimer sodium

Brand name
Photofrin

Use
photosensitizing agent used as a component of photodynamic therapy for the treatment of localized superficial or solid malignant tumors

Usual dosage
intravenous bolus: usually 2 mg/kg followed in 24 to 72 hours by application of light to the tumor; optimal doses remain to be established

Pharmaceutical company
Lederle Laboratories. Wayne, NJ.

Source
University of Pittsburgh Drug Information and Pharmacoepidemiology Center. Pittsburgh, PA.

PortaFlo urine collection system

Description
urine collection system with adjustable funnel to provide ease of use, comfort and movement for patients with incontinence; features a valve between the funnel and urine collection bag that eliminates the risk of bag reflux, leakage and odor

Source
MMG Healthcare product information. Atlanta, GA.

portal vein embolization prior to hepatic resection

Description
when resection is feasible but not practical because of the amount of functional reserve in the remaining liver, preoperative left hepatic hypertrophy induced by right portal vein embolization has been reported to have promising results; the portal vein is entered percutaneously through a transhepatic route; using ultrasonic guidance the left portal branch is accessed with a Chiba needle and portal blood is aspirated; the portal trunk is catheterized using Seldinger technique; embolization of the portal vein and necessary branches is performed under fluoroscopic control

Anatomy
hepatic capsule; hepatic parenchyma; iliac vein; liver; lobe; parenchymal space; pulmonary circulation; portal branch; portal vein; sectorial branches

Equipment
catheter; Chiba needle; fibrin glue (Tissucol); fluoroscopic imaging apparatus; n-butyl-2-cyanoacrylate (Histoacryl); Lipiodol; ultrasound equipment

Source
Adapted from Azoulay D, Raccuia JS, Castaing D, Bismuth H. Right portal vein embolization in preparation for major hepatic resection. Journal of American College of Surgeons 1995;181:267-269.

 portal vein reconstruction

Description
use of left renal vein graft for reconstruction of portal vein at the hepatic hilus due to carcinoma invasion of great vessels; the left renal vein is well-suited for this procedure due to its length and collateral branches, and its diameter matches well with the portal vein branch at the hepatic hilar bifurcation

Anatomy
hepatic hilus; portal vein; hepatic artery; abdomen; left renal vein; right renal vein; gonadal vein; renal-azygous and splenorenal communications; portal trunk

Equipment
standard vascular surgery equipment

Source
Adapted from Miyazaki M, Itoh H, Kaiho T, Ambiru S, Togawa A, et al. Portal vein reconstruction at the hepatic hilus using a left renal vein graft. Journal of the American College of Surgeons 1995;180:497-498.

438

 Porta-Resp monitor

Description
noninvasive and portable monitor displays digital maximum respiratory pressure readings; peak inspiratory and expiratory pressure to assess thoracic strength; measures positive or negative gas pressure

Source
S&M Instrument Co. Inc. product information. Doylestown, PA.

 Portex Per-fit tracheostomy kit

Description
percutaneous bedside tracheostomy kit with beveled tip and low-profile cuff; 7, 8, and 9 mm tracheostomy tube

Source
SIMS product information. Keene, NH.

 PortSaver PercLoop device

Description
ligating loop, which may be introduced percutaneously; saves a "port," allowing surgeon flexibility of introduction of instrument; designed for single-handed minimally invasive surgery

Source
Advanced Surgical Inc. product information. Princeton, NJ.

 Posicor

Generic name
see mibefradil

 posteroventral pallidotomy (PVP)

Description
treatment for intractable tremor, dyskinesia, and rigidity of Parkinson disease; combined with standard stereotactic thalamotomy for maximum therapeutic effect; burr hole created; radiofrequency probe used to create serial lesions in ventro-oralis posterior (VOp) and ventralis intermedius (Vim) nuclei

Anatomy
VOp nuclei; Vim nuclei; thalamus; anterior commissure (AC); posterior commissure (PC); AC-PC line; AC-PC plane; mammillary body; floor of third ventricle; foramen of Monro; internal capsule; globus pallidus; ansa lenticularis

Equipment
Unified Parkinson Disease Rating Scale (UPDRS); standard surgery equipment; CRW ring; phantom base; ventriculostomy catheter; Radionics thermocouple radiofrequency probe

Source
Adapted from Iacono RP, Henderson JM, Lonser RR. Combined stereotactic thalamotomy and posteroventral pallidotomy for Parkinson disease. Journal of Image-Guided Surgery 1995;1:133-140.

 Posture S'port

Description
posture support that pulls shoulders, spine, and lower back into neutral position to decrease pain

Source
The Saunders Group Inc. product information. Chaska, MN.

 potassium bicarbonate

Brand name
Xosten

Use
for prevention and treatment of osteoporosis in postmenopausal women

Usual dosage
oral: 60-120 mmol has been used in the clinical trial

Pharmaceutical company
Proctor & Gamble Pharmaceuticals. Cincinnati, OH.

Source
Stadtlanders Managed Pharmacy Services. Pittsburgh, PA.

 Potocky needle

Description
long needle (27 gauge) used with syringe; developed for cervical application of local anesthesia

Source
CooperSurgical product information. Shelton, CT.

 power Doppler ultrasound

Synonyms
color Doppler energy; CDE; ultrasound angiography

Indications
supplements standard color Doppler imaging; improves assessment of ovarian pathology, musculoskeletal inflammation, scrotal disease, transplant ischemia, and carotid artery stenosis

Method
signal processing technique modifies Doppler signal received from a standard hand-held ultrasound transducer producing greater sensitivity to vascular blood flow

Normal findings
improved visualization of small vessels and vessels with slow flow

Comments
increases sensitivity of standard color Doppler imaging

Source
University of Maryland Department of Diagnostic Radiology. Baltimore, MD.

 ## PowerProxi Sonic Interdental Toothbrush system

Description
battery-operated dental hygiene system designed for patients concerned about tooth decalcification, decay, and permanent staining

Source
Dentist Preferred Inc. product information. Yardley, PA.

 ## Powervision ultrasound system

Description
directional color angiography

Source
Toshiba America Medical Systems product information. Tustin, CA.

 ## pramipexole

Brand name
Mirapex

Use
dopamine (D_2) receptor agonist; used for the treatment of early Parkinson disease

Usual dosage
oral: maximum dose up to 4.5 mg/day was used in clinical trials

Pharmaceutical company
Upjohn Co. Kalamazoo, MI.

Source
Stadtlanders Managed Pharmacy Services. Pittsburgh, PA.

pramlintide

Brand name
not yet available

Use
used to control hyperglycemia in types I & II diabetes

Usual dosage
subcutaneous: 30-300 µg, 30 minutes before meals has been studied in clinical trials

Pharmaceutical company
Amylin/Lifescan. Milpitas, CA.

Source
Stadtlanders Managed Pharmacy Services. Pittsburgh, PA.

 pranlukast

Brand name
Ultair

Use
leukotriene antagonist used in the treatment of asthma

Usual dosage
oral: 225-450 mg twice daily in clinical trials

Pharmaceutical company
SmithKline Beecham. Philadelphia, PA.

Source
Stadtlanders Managed Pharmacy Services. Pittsburgh, PA.

 prasterone

Brand name
DHEA (dehydroepiandrosterone)

Use
as a supplement for patients with DHEA deficiency; should be used only in men above 30 to 40 years of age

Usual dosage
oral: 50 mg a day for DHEA deficient patients

Pharmaceutical company
Elan Corp. Atlanta, GA.

Source
Stadtlanders Managed Pharmacy Services. Pittsburgh, PA.

precise lesion measuring (PLM) device

Description
clear plastic instrument used to obtain precise measurements of scars, excisions, grafts, lesions, and tracking wound repairs

Source
MEDPRO INTL product information. Elk Grove, IL.

 Preclude peritoneal membrane

Description
permanent peritoneal implant; provides safe, effective, and inert barrier for use in peritoneal reconstruction of adhesiolysis sites, myomectomy incisions, and ablation sites

Source
WL Gore & Associates Inc. product information. Flagstaff, AZ.

 Precose

Generic name
see acarbose

 pregnancy-associated plasma protein A

Synonyms
PAPP-A

Use
prenatal screening for trisomy 21 and neural tube defect in first trimester of pregnancy

Method
immunoassay

Specimen
serum

Normal range
investigational

Comments
may permit detection of trisomy 21 and neural tube defects earlier in pregnancy than possible with currently used markers

Source
Adapted from Prenatal Screening Program, British Columbia Children's Hospital. Medscape, 1996.

Premphase

Generic name
see conjugated estrogens/medroxyprogesterone acetate

 Prempro

Generic name
see conjugated estrogens/medroxyprogesterone acetate

 Prep-IM

Description
precementing total hip bone preparation kit with tools and implants to facilitate cleaning the osteotomized femur and plugging the medullary canal; enhances improved interstitial penetration of bone cement; kit contains femoral canal brush, Buck cement restrictors, and a disposable inserter tool

Source
Smith & Nephew Richards product information. Memphis, TN.

 pressure relief ankle foot orthosis (PRAFO)
knee-ankle-foot orthosis (KAFO)

Description
also known as PKA PRAFO KAFO; PKA 650 (adult) and PKA 550 (pediatric) address complications associated with the ankle/foot while providing suspension and rotation control

Source
Anatomical Concepts Inc. product information. Boardman, OH.

 Presto and/or Presto-Flash spirometry system

Description
Presto is a stand-alone spirometry system that provides easy-to-understand prompts to perform forced vital capacity (FVC), flow/volume loop, slow vital capacity (SVC), and maximal ventilatory volume (MVV) testing with numeric and graphic results within 30 seconds; Presto-Flash is portable, performs all standard tests including inhalation challenge and trend analysis

Source
Burdick Inc. product information. Milton, WI.

Preston overhead pulleys

Description
chrome-plated steel, heat-adjustable overhead pulley system consisting of wall-mounted pulley arm, 2 swivel pulleys, 2 handles with rope, weight pan, and assorted weights up to 8.8 pounds
Source
J.A. Preston Corp. product information. Jackson, MI.

 Prevacid

Generic name
see lansoprazole

 preVent Pneumotach

Description
exercise testing flowmeter accurately measures exercise ventilation
Source
MedGraphics product information. St. Paul, MN.

 Price corneal transplant system

Description
ophthalmic surgical instruments consisting of donor cornea punch and set of three radial markers; provides accurate means of cutting donor cornea, and matching tissue to recipient cornea
Source
American Surgical Instruments Corp. product information. Westmont, IL.

 Prima Series specula

Description
loop electrical excision procedure (LEEP) polymer specula that are lighter, smoother, highly resistant to temperature change; non-stick material makes placement and removal easier after electrosurgery and eliminates the possibility of electrical shock; incorporates an innovative "Vu-More" design providing 25% increase of instrument access over standard specula
Source
Cooper Surgical product information. Shelton, CT.

Primer modified Unna boot

Description
bandage of 100% cotton gauze impregnated with a nonhardening zinc oxide paste; provides comfortable, moist environment for management of leg ulcers; Primer is packaged with Medi-Rip in Unna-Pak

Source
Glenwood Inc. product information. Tenafly, NJ.

 ## PRISM automated transfusion microbiology screening system

Synonyms
none

Use
automated infectious disease screening by blood donation testing laboratories

Method
automated immunoassay

Specimen
blood

Normal range
nonreactive

Comments
represents an improvement in process control for large-volume blood centers

Source
Adapted from Reeves I, Wenham D, Perry K, Williamson L, Allain JP. An evaluation of the Abbott PRISM transfusion microbiology screening system. Transfusion Science 1996;12:5.

 ## Prizm Electro-Mesh Z-Stim-II stimulator

Description
portable pulsed galvanic stimulator for treatment of the diabetic foot, postoperative care, and reflex sympathetic dystrophy; stops pain, increases blood circulation and range of motion, prevents venous thrombosis, and retards disuse atrophy; electrodes fit onto the Prizm Electro-Mesh sock

Source
Prizm Medical Inc. product information. Norcross, GA.

ProAdvantage knee

Description
high-quality prosthetic knee; series includes PK-1600, PK-1000-4PA, PK-1078

Source
Cascade Orthopaedic Supply product information. Plano, TX.

 ## Pro-Air

Generic name
see procaterol

 ## ProAmatine

Generic name
see midodrine

 ## Pro-Bal protected balloon-tipped catheter

Description
specimen collection catheter designed for use with bronchoscopes

Source
Mill-Rose Laboratories Inc. product information. Mentor, OH.

 ## procaterol

Brand name
Pro-Air

Use
beta-adrenergic agonist used in the treatment of bronchial asthma

Usual dosage
oral: 0.05-0.1 mg twice daily
inhalation: 0.01-0.02 mg inhaled 3 times daily

Pharmaceutical company
Parke-Davis. Morris Plains, NJ.

Source
University of Pittsburgh Drug Information and Pharmacoepidemiology Center. Pittsburgh PA.

ProCyte transparent dressing

Description
moisture vapor permeable, thin sheet dressing that may be used as a primary or secondary dressing

Source
ProCyte Corp. product information. Kirkland, WA.

 ## Proderm topical spray

Description
topical spray that stimulates capillary beds to help promote the healing process

Source
Dow Hickam Pharmaceuticals product information. Sugarland, TX.

 ## product-enhanced reverse transcriptase (PERT) assay

Synonyms
none

Use
detection and quantitation of viral load in HIV-1-infected patients

Method
modified reverse transcriptase polymerase chain reaction assay

Specimen
blood or plasma

Normal range
no evidence of particle-associated reverse transcriptase product

Comments
may come to be used as a staging assay in treating patients infected with HIV-1

Source
Adapted from Boni J, Pyra H, Schupbach J. Sensitive detection and quantification of particle-associated reverse transcriptase in plasma of HIV-1-infected individuals by the product-enhanced reverse transcriptase (PERT) assay. Journal of Medical Virology 1996;49:23-28.

 ## ProDynamic monitor

Description
urodynamic monitoring system for outpatient setting testing of bladder and sphincter activity

Source
Browne Medical Systems product information. White Bear Lake, MN.

Profile VS (valve system)

Description
valve device designed to minimize overdrainage of cerebrospinal fluid and maintain intraventricular pressure within physiologic range; components include occluder, reservoir chamber, needle guard, valve seat and anti-siphon membrane

Source
Heyer-Schulte NeuroCare product information. Pleasant Prairie, WI.

Profix total knee replacement system

Description
orthopaedic knee prosthesis reduces operative time with simpler, more accurate fitting; design reduces wear and prolongs life of prosthesis

Source
Smith & Nephew Richards Inc. product information. Memphis, TN.

Profore Four-Layer bandage system

Description
unique four-layer bandage system specifically designed for management of venous leg ulcers; provides consistent compression; easily adapted to any size or shape of leg; provides clean environment for healing

Source
Smith & Nephew Inc. product information. Largo, FL.

ProForma cannula

Description
precurved cannula for biliary endoscopy

Source
Bard International Products Division product information. Billerica, MA.

ProForma papillotome

Description
papillotome for biliary endoscopy; guaranteed orientation between 11 o'clock and 1 o'clock for common bile duct entry

Source
Bard International Products Division product information. Billerica, MA.

progenitor assay

Synonyms
colony-forming assay; stem cell assay; colony-forming unit assay

Use
colony-forming unit assay (CFU) detects and enumerates functional blood progenitor and stem cells in bone marrow, peripheral blood stem cell cytapheresis products, and umbilical cord blood

Method
culture in semi-solid media with growth factors, followed by morphological identification of colonies as colony-forming unit-granulocyte/macrophage (CFU-GM), burst-forming unit-erythroid (BFU-e), or colony-forming unit-granulocyte/erythrocyte/megakaryocyte/macrophage (CFU-GEMM)

Specimen
bone marrow; peripheral blood stem cell cytapheresis product; umbilical cord blood

Normal range
investigational use, but generally 2 x 105 CFU-GM/kg recipient body weight

Comments
semi-quantitative assay, but the principal measure of progenitor cell function

Source
University of Minnesota Department of Laboratory Medicine and Pathology. Minneapolis, MN.

 progesterone (micronized)

Brand name
Prometrium

Use
oral progesterone for secondary amenorrhea and abnormal uterine bleeding due to hormonal imbalance in postmenopausal women

Usual dosage
oral: 200 mg/day of micronized progesterone on days 1-12 of the month with 0.625 mg/day of conjugated estrogen therapy in 28-day month cycles

Pharmaceutical company
Schering-Plough Corp. Kenilworth, NJ.

Source
Stadtlanders Managed Pharmacy Services. Pittsburgh, PA.

progesterone (natural)

Brand name
Crinone

Use
treatment of severe amenorrhea and prevention of endometrial cancer in postmenopausal women who are receiving hormone replacement therapy

Usual dosage
topical: sustained-release bioadhesive delivery in doses of 45 mg to 90 mg have been used in the studies

Pharmaceutical company
Wyeth-Ayerst Laboratories. Philadelphia, PA.

Source
Stadtlanders Managed Pharmacy Services. Pittsburgh, PA.

proglumide

Brand name
Gastronol

Use
an inhibitor of gastric acid secretion to prevent or treat patients with peptic ulcer or other gastrointestinal disorders

Usual dosage
oral: in doses of 0.8 g to 1.6 g daily before meals

Pharmaceutical company
Barrows Research Group Inc. Valley Stream, NY.

Source
Stadtlanders Managed Pharmacy Services. Pittsburgh, PA.

Prograf

Generic name
see tacrolimus

ProLine endoscopic instruments

Description
reusable hand instruments with tip configurations to perform current laparoscopic procedures; scissors, dissectors, needle holders, and graspers that utilize jaws with striations instead of teeth

Source
Smith & Nephew Dyonics Inc. product information. Andover, MA.

PROloop

Description
electrosurgical tool for transurethral resection of prostate using electro-surgery

Source
ENDOcare Inc. product information. Irvine, CA.

Prometrium

Generic name
see progesterone (micronized)

pronation spring control device

Description
pronation spring control (PSC) device is an ankle-foot orthosis for support and control; assists lifting function and neutral alignment positioning; for plantar fasciitis, shin splints, heel spurs, and stress fractures in the metatarsal area

Source
Fabri-foam Products product information. Exton, PA.

Propaq Encore vital signs monitor

Description
monitoring device for patients of all ages; gives information on 3- or 5-lead electrocardiogram, noninvasive and invasive blood pressure, Nellcor pulse oximetry, mainstream capnography, impedance respiration, apnea and temperature

Source
Protocol Systems Inc. product information. Beaverton, OR.

Propecia

Generic name
see finasteride

propiram

Brand name
Dirame

Use
opioid analgesic used for moderate to severe pain following gynecologic and surgical procedures

Usual dosage
oral: 50 to 100 mg every 4-6 hours as needed

Pharmaceutical company
Roberts Pharmaceutical Corp. Eatontown, NJ.

Source
University of Pittsburgh Drug Information and Pharmacoepidemiology Center. Pittsburgh, PA.

 Pro-Post System

Description
acid-etched posts to facilitate creation of a bond between dentinal tubule and the metal post, 8 custom-sized post drills and 4 appropriate-sized verifiers to aid in seating the post

Source
Tulsa Dental Products product information. Tulsa, OK.

 ProstaScint Kit (Capromab Pendetide)

Description
imaging study and kit containing nonradioactive imaging agent (Indium-111 ProstaScint) for additional diagnostic analysis of patients with suspected metastatic prostate cancer

Source
Cytogen Corp. product information. Princeton, NJ.

 prostate-specific antigen testing by bispecific immunoprobe

Synonyms
rapid bispecific immunoprobe PSA assay

Use
screening and follow-up of prostate cancer patients

Method
immunoassay using bispecific monoclonal antibody (immunoprobe)

Specimen
blood

Normal range
investigational

Comments
immunoprobe will facilitate development of improved clinical laboratory assays, as well as physician office laboratory screening tests

Source
Adapted from Kreutz FT, Suresh MR. Novel bispecific immunoprobe for rapid and sensitive detection of prostate-specific antigen. Clinical Chemistry 1997;43:649-656.

 Prosynap

Generic name
see lubeluzole

 ProSys Urihesive System LA and System NL

Description
ProSys leg bag system for people with urinary incontinence; may be used with male external catheters or indwelling catheters; anti-reflux valve at the intake port protects against backflow of urine and possible infection

Source
VonvaTec product information. Princeton, NJ.

 Protara

Generic name
see acadesine

 Protec

Generic name
see lisofylline (LSF)

 prothelen sets

Description
drilling templates, sockets, and container/frames for below-the-knee and above-the-knee amputations; thermo-moldable; also called prothelen blue

Source
IPOS Orthopedics Industry product information. Niagara Falls, NY.

Prothiaden

Generic Name
see dothiepin

 ProTouch resectoscope

Description
gynecologic surgical instrument designed specifically for operative hysteroscopy; maximal high continuous flow rate for clearer operative field; large outflow holes for bubble and tissue removal

Source
CooperSurgical Inc. product information. Shelton, CT.

 Protovir

Generic name
see sevirumab

 Proxiderm wound closure system

Description
nonsurgical treatment of nonhealing diabetic or pressure ulcers and nonhealing wounds; tissue hooks inserted into healthy skin at wound margin; gentle constant traction from Proxiderm device stretches healthy skin over wound; new skin growth through tissue expansion and angiogenesis; provides full-thickness skin coverage

Source
Progressive Surgical Products product information. Westbury, NY.

 Proxi-Floss interproximal cleaner

Description
disposable interproximal cleaning appliance specifically designed for orthodontic, periodontal, and implant applications; cleans bridgework and implant abutments effectively

Source
Advanced Implant Technologies Inc. product information. Beverly Hills, CA.

proximal balloon occlusion

Description
treatment of dissecting vertebral artery aneurysms accompanied by subarachnoid hemorrhage (SAH); dissecting aneurysms diagnosed on basis of
angiographic findings including "pearl and string" sign; endovascular proximal balloon occlusion performed in extracranial portion of vertebral artery
after successful balloon Mata test to confirm safety of permanent occlusion
and after period of cerebral vasospasm

Anatomy
vertebral artery; femoral artery; thyrocervical trunk

Equipment
standard neurosurgery equipment; guiding catheter; double-lumen wedge
pressure catheter; detachable latex valve balloon; coaxial catheter

Source
Adapted from Tsukahara T, Wada H, Satake K, Yaoita H, Takahashi A. Proximal balloon occlusion for dissecting
vertebral aneurysms accompanied by subarachnoid hemorrhage. Neurosurgery 1995;36:914-920.

Pryor anterior wedge morcellation technique

Description
technique for removing enlarged uterus vaginally utilizing a predetermined
symmetrical pattern in a coronal plane

Anatomy
cervix; vagina; uterine arteries; bladder; cornua; adnexa

Equipment
knife or heavy scissors; retractors

Source
Adapted from Pelosi MA, Pelosi MA III. A comprehensive approach to morcellation of the large uterus.
Contemporary OB/GYN 1997;42:106-125.

pubovaginal sling

Description
procedure for treatment of women with Type III stress urinary incontinence;
modification of traditional Goebell-Stoeckel-Frangenheim procedure;
addresses complications of urinary retention and detrusor instability caused
by excessive tension on the sling at surgery; cystoscopy-assisted technique
adjusts tension

Anatomy
urethra; vesical neck; detrusor; urethral sphincter; vagina; rectus fascia; bladder; vaginal epithelium; endopelvic fascia; pubis

Equipment
standard surgery equipment; Foley catheter; Metzenbaum scissors; DeBakey clamp; nonabsorbable sutures; Allis clamps; trocar 12F suprapubic tube; cystoscope; vaginal pack

Source
Adapted from Blaivas JG. Keys to successful pubovaginal sling surgery. Contemporary OB/GYN 1995;40:46-61.

Pucci pediatrics hand orthoses

Description
patented air inflation system to apply stretch therapy

Source
D'Mannco Inc. product information. High Springs, FL.

pull-through gynecomastia reduction

Description
liposuction treatment of fatty glandular gynecomastia in male; clamp used to pull additional breast parenchymal tissue through liposuction cannula incision

Anatomy
breast; anterior axillary pillar; mammary sulcus; areola; subareolar area; glandular tissue; pectoral fascia; parenchyma

Equipment
scalpel; liposuction cannula; clamp; electrocautery; suction drain

Source
Adapted from Morselli PG. Pull-through: a new technique for breast reduction in gynecomastia. Plastic and Reconstructive Surgery 1996;97:450-454.

pulmonary surfactant

Brand name
Curosurf

Use
porcine pulmonary surfactant; used for the treatment and prevention of respiratory distress syndrome in premature infants

Usual dosage
intratracheal: doses of 100 mg/kg-200 mg/kg were used in clinical trials

Pharmaceutical company
Chiesi Pharmaceuticals Inc. Ridgefield, CT.

Source
Stadtlanders Managed Pharmacy Services. Pittsburgh, PA.

Pulmosonic ultrasonic nebulizer

Description
portable nebulizer device that allows for deep, penetrating therapy without noise and lengthy treatment times of compressor nebulizers

Source
DeVilbiss Sunrise Medical product information. Somerset, PA.

 ## Pulsair.5 oxygen portable unit

Description
compact liquid oxygen tank weighs just over 6 pounds when full; features PulseDose oxygen delivery technology (Editor note: pronounced "pulse-air point five")

Source
DeVilbiss Health Care Inc. product information. Somerset, PA.

 ## pulsed galvanic stimulator

Description
GV 350 2-channel device provides alternating and/or continuous coordination between stimulation output

Source
BioMedical Life Systems Inc. product information. Vista, CA.

 ## PulseDose portable compressed oxygen systems

Description
Hideaway and Walkabout portable compressed oxygen systems feature unit technology to deliver a consistent, measured dose of oxygen at the leading edge of inspiration, which is critical for maintaining optimum oxygen levels; features 11 selectable flow rates from 5 to 6 lpm (liters per minute); audible and visual inspiratory delay indicator reassures patient of sufficient battery power; PulseDose indicator offers visual confirmation of pulse response; toggle switch to continuous flow backup to set standard flow rate at 2 lpm

Source
DeVilbiss Health Care Inc. product information. Somerset, PA.

 ## Pump-It-Up pneumatic socket

Description
customized fabricated prosthesis with pneumatic socket volume management mechanism (inner socket and air bladder unit); allows control over volumetric fit; provides improved proprioception

Source
Knit-Rite Inc. product information. Kansas City, MO.

PumpPals

Description

comfort insoles for women's shoes; alternative to customized orthotics; temporary or long-term use

Source

Pedifix product information. Mount Kisko, NY.

 Puritan-Bennett 7250 metabolic monitor

Description

instrument used with Ventilator 7200 that measures body oxygen consumption and carbon dioxide production; measurements are used to calculate several metabolic parameters that help determine ventilatory, metabolic, and nutritional requirements

Source

Puritan-Bennett Corp. product information. Carlsbad, CA.

 P-wave electrical detection of sick sinus syndrome

Synonyms

Indications

sick sinus syndrome

Method

signal averaged P-wave electrocardiograms were recorded through bandpass filter of 40-300 Hz with P-wave triggering technique; voltage and duration were measured

Normal findings

not applicable

Comments

long, low amplitude signals early in filtered P wave on signal-averaged ECGs are characteristic of sick sinus syndrome (Editor note: P wave is hyphenated when used as an adjective but not when it stands alone)

Source

Adapted from Yamada T, Fukunami M, Kumagai K et al. Detection of patients with sick sinus syndrome by use of low amplitude potentials early in filtered P wave. Cardiology 1996;28:738-750.

pylorus-preserving pancreatoduodenectomy (PPPD)

Description
gastroduodenal artery preservation in PPPD for periampullary cancer with pancreatic remnant maintaining a normal function is evaluated; the preservation also included the right gastroepiploic artery, division of the anterior superior pancreaticoduodenal artery, and division of the posterior superior pancreaticoduodenal artery; distal pancreas reconstructed with anastomosis to posterior wall of stomach; surgery also performed for distal bile duct, ampullary, and islet cell cancers

Anatomy
arteries: common hepatic, gastroduodenal, proper hepatic, posterior superior pancreaticoduodenal, and right gastroepiploic; ampulla of Vater; distal common bile duct; head and tail of pancreas; islet cell; pancreatic duct; pancreas; parenchyma; pyloric ring; pylorus

Equipment
standard surgery equipment

Source
Adapted from Nagai H, Ohki J, Kondo Y, Yasudo T, et al. Pancreatoduodenectomy with preservation of the pylorus and gastroduodenal artery. Annals of Surgery 1996;223:194-198.

 Pyrilinks-D urine assay

Synonyms
deoxypyridinoline crosslinks urine assay

Indications
identification and monitoring of patient at risk for bone loss

Method
measures deoxypyridinoline (Dpd), a crosslink of type 1 collagen in bone; marker for bone resorption; excreted unmetabolized in urine; results unaffected by diet; elevated levels indicate excessive bone resorption and loss of bone mass

Normal findings
normal levels of Dpd

Comments
none

Source
Metra Biosystems Inc. product information. Mountain View, CA.

Q-Tee cleaning swab

Description
fiber-free, polyspun cleaning swab on a break-resistant wand for all cleaning applications in reprocessing medical devices; specifically useful for cleaning the flexible endoscope valve openings and buttons

Source
Chris Lutz Medical product information. Languana Hills, CA.

QuadPolar electrode

Description
latest in intra-aortic balloon pump technology and critical-care catheterization products; maintains flexibility and torqueability at body temperature

Source
Arrow/Kontron Instruments product information. Everett, MA.

Quadramet

Generic name
see samarium-EDTMP

quadrantic sclerectomies with internal drainage

Description
surgical management of idiopathic uveal effusion syndrome; internal drainage of subretinal fluid performed with quadrantic partial-thickness sclerectomies used as treatment of secondary retinal detachment in uveal effusion syndrome; pars plana vitrectomy also done in conjunction with above and fluid-gas exchange; procedure hastens reattachment of neurosensory retina

Anatomy
choroid; ciliochoroid; epithelium; ora serrata; pars plana; peripheral fundus; retina; subretinal space; suprachoroidal space; uvea; vitreous cavity

Equipment
standard ophthalmic surgical equipment

Source
Adapted from Schneiderman TE, Johnson MW. A new approach to the surgical management of idiopathic uveal effusion syndrome. American Journal of Ophthalmology 1997;123:262-263.

quantitative immunoassay for urine myoglobin

Synonyms
urine myoglobin immunoassay

Use
prediction of renal dysfunction following rhabdomyolysis

Method
automated Stratus II myoglobin immunoassay

Specimen
urine

Normal range
<20,000 mg/liter

Comments
a modification of the serum myoglobin assay

Source
Adapted from Loun B, Astles R, Copeland KR, Sedor FA. Adaptation of a quantitative immunoassay for urine myoglobin. American Journal of Clinical Pathology 1996;105:479-486.

Quantrex Sweep 650 (QS650) ultrasonic cleansing system

Description
cleans blood, debris, and bioburden from surgical instruments; provides proper asepsis; handles volume cleaning, yet is compact

Source
L & R Manufacturing Co. product information. Kearny, NJ.

Quantum enhancement knife

Description
ophthalmic surgical instrument without footplates; provides safety and precision in extending keratotomy incisions; safety stop minimizes inadvertent overextension; allows for precise astigmatic incision extension

Source
Storz Ophthalmics product information. St. Louis, MO.

Quartzo device

Description

device that delivers manually or electrically powered stimulators that cause the brain to produce natural pain relieving substances; used to reduce patient dependence on analgesics and anti-inflammatory drugs; a 2-minute application produces up to 3 hours of pain relief from lumbago, chronic neck pain, and rheumatic pain; device is applied to area of joint pain, muscle pain, tendon pain, etc. and then to the lower back or neck as directed

Source

French Technology product information. Chicago, IL.

quetiapine

Brand name

Seroquel

Use

a serotonin and dopamine (D2-linked) receptor antagonist used in the treatment of schizophrenia

Usual dosage

oral: up to 750 mg/day was used in clinical trials

Pharmaceutical company

Zeneca Pharmaceuticals Group. Wilmington, DE.

Source

University of Pittsburgh Drug Information and Pharmacoepidemiology Center. Pittsburgh, PA.

Quick-Sil starter kits

Description

a faster, more cost-effective way to use silicone modifications in everything from distal-end pads to body jackets; the five-minute silicone now available in a 330-ml cartridge suitable for use in prosthetic labs and the 50-ml cartridge that works well for modifications

Source

UCO Inc. product information. Prospect Heights, IL.

Quickswitch irrigation/aspiration ophthalmic system

Description

hand-held device with irrigation and aspiration (I/A) tips for cataract surgery; interchangeable tips for clean-up and removal, and aspiration of infusions and solutions

Source

Katena Products Inc. product information. Denville, NJ.

QuickVue *Chlamydia* rapid test

Description
one-step predictor technology provides rapid test results

Source
Quidel Corp. product information. San Diego, CA.

 ## QuickVue human chorionic gonadotropin (hCG) pregnancy tests

Description
one-step predictor technology includes QuickVue hCG, QuickVue hCG Combo cards, QS hCG

Source
Quidel Corp. product information. San Diego, CA.

 ## Quinton PermCath catheter

Description
chronic hemodialysis catheter with oval pull-apart introducer for percutaneous insertion

Source
Quinton Instrument Co. product information. Seattle, WA.

 ## quinupristin/dalfopristin

Brand Name
Synercid

Use
anti-infective used in the treatment of vancomycin resistant enterococus (VRE) infection

Usual Dosage
intravenous: 5 or 7.5 mg/kg infused over 1 hour at every 8 hours interval for 5 to 14 days

Pharmaceutical company
Rhone-Poulenc Rorer Pharmaceuticals Inc. Collegeville, PA.

Source
University of Pittsburgh Drug Information and Pharmacoepidemiology Center. Pittsburgh, PA.

464

 radial artery forearm free flap urethral reconstruction

Description
reconstruction of scarred urethra due to multiple surgical procedures for hypospadias or trauma; full-thickness skin graft is excised and sutured into tube shape; with attached radial artery is sutured to inferior epigastric artery in groin and tunneled subcutaneously and sutured in place to correct urethral defect

Anatomy
forearm; radial artery; groin; inguinal ligament; external oblique muscle; conjoined tendon; lateral margin of rectus abdominis muscle; urethra

Equipment
standard surgery equipment

Source
Adapted from Morrison WA, Webster HR, Kumta S. Urethreral reconstruction using the radial artery forearm free flap: conventional and prefabricated. Plastic and Reconstructive Surgery 1996;97:413-416.

 radial artery graft

Description
treatment for hemangiopericytoma involving the torcular herophili is total resection; affected sinuses removed and successfully reconstructed with radial artery interposition graft between straight and right transverse sinus; complete removal of tumor

Anatomy
dural, transverse, and superior sagittal sinuses; torcular Herophili; cerebellar tentorium; intima of straight sinus; radial artery; right occipital lobe

Equipment
standard surgery equipment; ultrasonic aspirator; Doppler flowmeter; Sugita long-blade clips; nylon sutures

Source
Adapted from Nagashima H, Kobayashi S, Takayama T, Tunica Y. Total resection of torcular herophili hemangiopericytoma with radial artery graft: case report. Neurosurgery 1995;36:1024-1027.

 radical cystectomy using endoscopic stapling devices

Description
radical cystectomy followed by urinary reconstruction is a lengthy procedure; various techniques have been tried to minimize blood loss; hemostasis of the deep dorsal vein complex has been accomplished with the endoscopic stapler to ligate and divide the bladder and prostatic lateral ligaments that contain abundant vessels

Anatomy
bladder; deep dorsal vein complex; Denonvilliers space; endopelvic fascia; neurovascular bundle; prostatic apex; prostatic lateral ligaments; puboprostatic ligaments; vas deferens; venous plexus; urethra

Equipment
Multifire Endo TA 30-3.5 stapler; Multifire Endo GIA 30-3.5 stapler; titanium staples

Source
Adapted from Yamashita T, Muraishi O, Umeda S, Matsushita T. Radical cystectomy using endoscopic stapling devices: preliminary experience with a simple and reliable technique. Journal of Urology 1997;157:263-265.

 radiofrequency catheter ablation

Description
management of recurrent ventricular tachycardia (VT) following failure of antitachycardia pacing and implantation of first generation implantable cardioverter defibrillator (ICD); early ventricular activity localized in midposterior septum; radiofrequency ablation delivered with successful termination of ventricular tachycardia

Anatomy
left ventricle; right ventricle; midposterior septum

Equipment
standard cardiovascular surgery equipment; electrophysiologic catheters; hexapolar catheter; quadripolar catheter; radiofrequency pulse generator

Source
Adapted from Porterfield JG, Porterfield LM, Fiallo LA. Management of ventricular tachycardia with ablation therapy in a patient with a previously implanted cardioverter defibrillator. The Journal of Invasive Cardiology 1995;7:53-56.

 radiographic spherical endotracheal tube cuff signals tracheal injury

Synonyms
none

Indications
tracheobronchial injury; signs of breathing difficulty

Method
esophagoscopy

Normal findings
not applicable

Comments
tracheobronchial injury is uncommon manifestation of trauma; mechanism of injury is usually severe, high-velocity deceleration-type of injury as would result from motor vehicle accident, airplane crash or fall; failure to make early diagnosis can lead to disastrous acute/delayed complications

Source
Adapted from Rao P, Novelline R, Dobins J. The spherical endotracheal tube cuff: a plain radiographic sign of tracheal injury. Emergency Radiology 1996;3:87-90.

RadioVisioGraphy (RVG)

Description
filmless digital intraoral x-ray imaging system

Source
Trophy Radiology Inc. product information. Marietta, GA.

 Railguard bed rail

Description
inflatable/deflatable accessory for standard hospital bed offers safety, comfort, and protection from hard metal bed railing; provides optimal tissue safe environment for wound healing

Source
Bazooka Portable Specialty Bed. University Hospital Service product information. Bloomington, MN.

 raloxifene

Brand name
Evista

Use
anti-estrogen used in the prevention and treatment of osteoporosis in post-menopausal women

Usual dosage
oral: 200 mg daily was used in clinical trials

Pharmaceutical company
Eli Lilly and Co. Indianapolis, IN.

Source
University of Pittsburgh Drug Information and Pharmacoepidemiology Center. Pittsburgh, PA.

 ranitidine bismuth citrate

Brand name
Tritec

Use
prophylaxis of *Helicobacter pylori*-induced peptic ulcer disease

Usual dosage
each 400 mg tablet contains 150 mg ranitidine base and 240 mg bismuth citrate: one tablet twice a day for 4 weeks in combination with clarithromycin (Biaxin 500 mg 3 times a day) for treatment of *H. pylori*-induced ulcers

Pharmaceutical company
Glaxo Wellcome Research. Triangle Park, NC.

Source
University of Pittsburgh Drug Information and Pharmacoepidemiology Center. Pittsburgh, PA.

Rapamune

Generic name
see sirolimus

Rapide wound suture

Description
Vicryl coated suture for short-term wound support; sutures begin to fall off within 7 to 10 days
Source
Ethicon Inc. (Johnson & Johnson) product information. Piscataway, NJ.

rapid exchange (RX) Elipse catheter

Description
dilatation balloon catheter with Microglide coating; Dynacross shaft and low-friction tapered tip
Source
Advanced Cardiovascular Sys. Inc. product information. Santa Clara, CA.

rapid exchange (RX) Flowtrack catheter

Description
dilatation balloon catheter with radiopaque markers, patented peel-away shaft, 10 proximal and 4 distal perfusion holes, and tapered tip
Source
Advanced Cardiovascular Sys. Inc. product information. Santa Clara, CA.

rapid Rh D genotyping

Synonyms
Rh D PCR
Use
alternative to traditional serologic Rh typing
Method
polymerase chain reaction (PCR) to amplify DNA to detect the presence of Rh D DNA
Specimen
blood
Normal range
Rh D positive or negative

Comments
investigational use

Source
Blood 1995:85:2975-2980.

 Rapid Vue human chorionic gonadotropin (hCG) rapid pregnancy test

Description
one-step predictor technology provides accurate in-office screening

Source
Quidel Corp. product information. San Diego, CA.

 Rappazzo intraocular manipulator

Description
used for manipulation of nucleus during cataract surgery; special finger-like extrusions provide grasping ability

Source
Storz Ophthalmics product information. St. Louis, MO.

 Rath treatment table

Description
mechanical physical therapy treatment table designed for use with the McKenzie method; newly developed lateral-shift belt ratchet system allows patient to exercise with no assistance from therapist

Source
Hill Laboratories Co. product information. Malvern, PA.

 Raxar

Generic name
see grepafloxacin

 Reactine

Generic name
see cetirizine

 Real-EaSE neck and shoulder relaxer

Description
advanced cervical neck support system that cradles the neck and base of the skull; muscle comfort can be appreciated within 30 seconds

Source
Kenshin Trading Corp. product information. Torrance, CA.

real-time, low-intensity x-ray (RTLX)

Description
dental imaging equipment where a full-motion digital image appears instantly on a video monitor with no film or processing required; produced at radiation levels that are substantially below levels emitted by conventional x-rays

Source
Panoramic Corp. product information. Fort Wayne, IN.

 recombinant bactericidal/permeability-increasing protein (rBPI$_{21}$)

Brand name
Neuprex

Use
used in the treatment of meningococcemia for its ability to increase the permeability of bacterial cells; also being studied for use in hemorrhagic trauma and with antibiotics in intra-abdominal infections

Usual dosage
intravenous: an initial bolus dose of 0.5 mg/kg over 30 minutes, then an infusion dose up to 2 mg/kg given over 24 hours for meningococcemia; 1, 2, and 4 mg/kg/day for 3 days in clinical trials for intra-abdominal infections

Pharmaceutical company
Xoma Corp. Berkley, CA.

Source
Stadtlanders Managed Pharmacy Services. Pittsburgh, PA.

 recombinant human interleukin 11 (IL-11)

Brand Name
Neumega

Use
recombinant hematopoietic growth factor with stimulatory effects on multiple hematopoietic progenitor cells

Usual Dosage
continuous intravenous infusion: 10,000-320,000 Cetus units/m2/day for 14 days, post transplantation was used in phase-1 clinical trials

Pharmaceutical company
Cetus. Emeryville, CA.

Source
University of Pittsburgh Drug Information and Pharmacoepidemiology Center. Pittsburgh, PA.

recombinant human tumor necrosis factor receptor fixed chain fusion protein (rhTNFR:Fc)

Brand name
Enbrel

Use
a tumor necrosis factor inhibitor used to reduce the inflammation associated with rheumatoid arthritis

Usual dosage
injectable: doses of 2 or 16 mg/m^2 subcutaneously administered twice weekly are being studied in clinical trials

Pharmaceutical company
Immunex Co. Seattle, WA.

Source
Stadtlanders Managed Pharmacy Services. Pittsburgh, PA.

 recombinant thyroid stimulating hormone

Brand name
Thyrogen

Use
boosts bloodstream levels of thyroid stimulating hormone (TSH) prior to annual or biannual screening for recurrence of thyroid cancer without causing symptoms of hypothyroidism

Usual dosage
oral: 0.9 mg a day for 2 days or 0.9 mg every 72 hours for one week were doses used in clinical trials prior to thyroid examination

Pharmaceutical company
Genzyme Corp. Cambridge, MA.

Source
Stadtlanders Managed Pharmacy Services. Pittsburgh, PA.

 Redux

Generic name
see dexfenfluramine hydrochloride
► As of September 15, 1997, Redux has been withdrawn from the market.

 Re-Entry Malecot catheter set

Description
nephrostomy catheter set consisting of C-Flex Re-Entry catheter, flexible stylets, and drainage bag connecting tube

Source
Microvasive Boston Scientific Corp. product information. Natick, MA.

Reflection I, V, and FSO acetabular cups

Description
prosthetic cups for hip fractures with MicroStable liner locking mechanism; minimizes polyethylene surface abrasion and reduces motion-induced debris; Reflection I has one hole in the center for a screw, Reflection V has five holes for pegs, screws or both, and Reflection FSO (for screws only)

Source
Smith & Nephew Richards Inc. product information. Memphis, TN.

Reflex articulating endoscopic cutter (AEC)

Description
surgical instrument combining 360-degree rotation and 45-degree bilateral articulation provides the surgeon with maneuverability, access and control

Source
Richard-Allan product information. Richland, MI.

REGENTEX GBR-200

Description
second-generation, high density, microporous membrane that is soft and easy to custom contour to the defect

Source
Advanced Surgical Technologies product information. Sacramento, CA.

regional cerebral blood flow scintigraphy

Synonyms
brain perfusion study; rCBF

Indications
detect and localize recurrent brain tumor; diagnose Alzheimer disease and other dementias; localize seizure foci; evaluate brain injury and location, size, and prognosis of cerebral ischemia; diagnose brain death

Method
single photon emission computed tomography (SPECT): inject technetium-99m HMPAO (Ceretec) or technetium-99m ECD (Neurolite) intravenously; patient in supine position with head secured; acquire images by a rotating gamma camera and reconstruct for interpretation
positron emission tomography (PET): inject oxygen-15 water intravenously, follow SPECT method using a PET detector

Normal findings
normal distribution of brain perfusion

Comments
patient must remain still during acquisition; Diamox (acetazolamide) may
be administered to elicit abnormalities

Source
Lexi-Comp Inc. database. Hudson, OH.
Nuclear Medicine Consultant. Stedman's Medical Dictionary, 26th edition.

Regranex

Generic name
see becaplermin

2+2 Rehab Collar

Description
stabilizer collar with elastic component for exercise with a pouch for hot or
cold pack inserts; enables patient to perform isometric and isokinetic exercises

Source
Ortho-Care Inc. product information. Raytown, MO.

ReJuveness scar treatment

Description
soft, pliable silicone sheet that is applied over a scar for a few hours a day;
softens, smooths, and flattens scars and restores skin to its normal texture
and color

Source
RichMark International Corp. product information. Everett, MA.

relaxin H2

Brand name
ConXn

Use
recombinant human relaxin hormone; used to decrease collagen synthesis in
patients with scleroderma

Usual dosage
injectable: 1-100 ng/ml were used in human fibroblast cell lines in preclinical trials

Pharmaceutical company
Genentech Inc. South San Francisco, CA.

Source
Stadtlanders Managed Pharmacy Services. Pittsburgh, PA.

release of the flexor hallucis longus tendon

Description
operative release of the flexor hallucis longus for the treatment of isolated stenosing tenosynovitis at the level of the ankle joint after nonoperative therapy has failed; used in patients who place high demands on the foot and ankle

Anatomy
ipsilateral thigh; medial malleolus; subtalar joint; medial retinaculum; neurovascular bundle; flexor hallucis longus tendon; sustentaculum tali

Equipment
standard orthopaedic equipment

Source
Adapted from Kolettis GJ, Micheli LJ, Klein JD. Release of the flexor hallucis longus tendon in ballet dancers. The Journal of Bone and Joint Surgery 1996;78:1386-1390.

 release of traction for hypotony and vitreoretinopathy

Description
early surgery to release traction over the anterior retina and uveal tissue in eyes with chronic hypotony and anterior proliferative vitreoretinopathy can increase intraocular pressure and stabilize visual acuity; removal of the anterior proliferative tissue releases traction on the iris, pars plicata, and vitreous base, and reattaches the anterior retina; this increases the intraocular pressure; vitreoretinopathy is graded according to Lewis and Aaberg classification

Anatomy
anterior hyaloid tissue; ciliary epithelium; pars plana; pars plicata; posterior chamber intraocular lens; retinal pigment epithelium; vitreous gel

Equipment
standard ophthalmic surgical equipment; vitreoretinal pick

Source
Adapted from Lewis H, Verdaguer JI. Surgical treatment for chronic hypotony and anterior proliferative vitreoretinopathy. American Journal of Ophthalmology 1996;122:228-235.

 Reliance device

Description
urinary control insert for women; balloon-tipped, single-use device for stress urinary incontinence

Source
UroMed Corp. production information. Watertown, NY.

Relief Band device

Description
non-drug device for treatment of gastric distress, nausea, vomiting, and motion sickness; transcutaneous electrical nerve stimulation (TENS) on the underside of a wrist band blocks gastric distress signals to the brain

Source
Maven Laboratories product information. Yuba City, CA.

 Remeron

Generic name
see mirtazapine

 remifentanil

Brand name
Ultiva

Use
short-acting µ-opioid analgesic during induction and maintenance of general anesthesia

Usual dosage
injectable: 1 µg/kg as bolus followed by an infusion of 0.0125-1.0 µg/kg/min were used as a component of nitrous oxide-opioid-relaxant anesthesia in a dose-ranging pilot study; continuous infusion of remifentanil in doses of 0.1 mg/kg/min is currently under investigation for analgesia effect

Pharmaceutical company
Glaxo Wellcome Inc. Research Triangle Park, NC.

Source
Stadtlanders Managed Pharmacy Services. Pittsburgh, PA.

 Reminyl

Generic name
see sabeluzole

 Remisar

Generic name
see bropirimine

Remune

Generic name
see AIDS vaccine glycoprotein 120 (gp 120)

 Renaissance spirometry system

Description
patient-friendly assessment of lung condition demonstrates effects of smoking on lung function before other symptoms appear; diagnostic information includes forced vital capacity, flow volume loops, predicted values, and a suggested interpretation; portable

Source
Puritan-Bennett product information. Wilmington, MA.

 renal lesion superselective catheterization/embolization

Description
embolization of renal vascular lesions with platinum microcoils delivered through microcatheter system; conserves most of renal parenchyma when lesions are too peripheral to be catheterized in standard angiographic fashion; coaxial variable stiffness catheter system facilitates precise super selective catheterization

Anatomy
kidneys; vascular system; peripheral renal artery; renal parenchyma

Equipment
Tracker-18 microcatheter; platinum microcoils; variable stiffness catheter; 5F cobra catheter; sidewinder catheter; steerable guidewire; rotating hemostatic valve; torque device; coil pusher; N-butyl-cyanoacrylate glue; iodized oil; color Doppler flow sonograph

Source
Adapted from Beaujeux R, Saussine C, Al-Fakir A, et al. Superselective endovascular treatment of renal vascular lesions. Journal of Urology 1995;153:14-17.

 Renormax

Generic name
see spirapril hydrochloride

 Renova

Generic Name
see tretinoin cream

ReoPro

Generic name
see abciximab

 repair of alveolar ridge defect

Description
the repair of severe ridge defects presents a challenge for tooth replacement with dental implants; staged technique of implants following bone regeneration pose the advantages of larger osseous surface contributing to bone formation, allows improved implant alignment which permits better initial stability, and increased maturation of the new bone with probable improved apposition to implant surface

Anatomy
alveolar ridge; anterior mandible; anterior nasal spine; cortical bone; crestal bone; canine fossa regions; central incisors; inferior and lateral rim of nasal cavity; mandibular symphysis; maxillary arch; maxillofacial region; mucogingival junction; mucosa; nasal floor; osseous tissue; osteogenic cells; premaxilla; periapical region; periosteum; vestibule (vestibulum oris)

Equipment
standard dental implant surgery equipment; demineralized freeze-dried bone; resorbable hydroxyapatite; tissue scissors; scalpel blade; surgical template fabricated from a diagnostic "wax up"; titanium alloy screws

Source
Adapted from Misch CM, Misch CE. The repair of localized severe ridge defects for implant placement using mandibular bone grafts. Implant Dentistry Winter 1995;4:261-265.

 Repel bioresorbable barrier film

Description
for prevention and reduction of postoperative adhesions; expected to be available in US in 1999

Source
Life Medical Sciences Inc. product information. Edison, NJ.

 Replace implant system

Description
implant system that facilitates placement between adjacent teeth with converging roots; reduces off axis loading

Source
Steri-Oss product information. Yorba Linda, CA.

replication-competent retrovirus (RCR) assay

Synonyms
RCR testing

Use
detection of replication-competent retrovirus in genetically-engineered cell specimens

Method
cell culture-based assay

Specimen
retrovirally-transduced cell suspension

Normal range
no evidence of replication-competent retrovirus

Comments
investigational, but required for all retrovirus-based genetic engineering

Source
University of Minnesota Department of Laboratory Medicine and Pathology. Minneapolis, MN.

 Requip

Generic name
see ropinirole

 Rescriptor

Generic name
see delavirdine mesylate

 resection of dumbbell and paraspinal tumors

Description
most tumors of the thoracic and lumbar spine are accessible through standard spinal exposures; adequate surgical exposure is difficult for large dumbbell and other paraspinal tumors so lateral extracavitary approach is useful in these situations; the single-stage approach provides exposure of intradural structures, as well as access to the paraspinal region, ventral spinal canal, and vertebral body; one of the big advantages is that both the anterior and posterior portion of the procedure can be performed through one incision

Anatomy
anterior paraspinal region; ascending lumbar vein; autonomic rami; disc space; dorsal root ganglion; dorsal segmental and foraminal branches from intercostal or lumbar vessels; epidural structure; intradural space; intervertebral foramen; nerve root sleeve; perineural venous rete; psoas muscle; sensory fascicles; spinal canal; transverse process

Equipment
standard neurosurgery equipment; curette; cautery; Cotrel-Dubousset rods; Gelfoam; high-speed drill; Kerrison rongeurs; osteotome; reverse angle curette

Source
Adapted from McCormick PC. Surgical management of dumbbell and paraspinal tumors of the thoracic and lumbar spine. Journal of Neurosurgery 1996;38:67-75.

 ## resection of pituitary tumor, transfacial approach

Description
surgical resection by traditional approaches of giant invasive pituitary adenomas are reportedly impossible; they are rare tumors that have extensively involved the cranial base, as well as other intra- and extracranial structures; tumors were resected via a transfacial approach which incorporated an osteoplastic maxillotomy with palatal division and posterior pharyngeal incision, providing exposure from the suprasellar region to C2; the tumor was resected using standard techniques; the transfacial approach allows a safe exposure for maximal surgical resection

Anatomy
buccal mucosa; carotid arteries; cavernous sinus; clivus; dura; ethmoid sinus; foramen magnum; hypothalamus; maxillary sinus; nasal septum; nasopharyngeal soft tissue; optic chiasm; palatal mucosa; parasellar region; pituitary gland; pterygoid process; retropharyngeal space; sella turcica; sphenoid sinus; soft palate/hard palate junction; tuberculum sellae; vermilion border

Equipment
arch bars; Doppler probe; electrocautery; high-speed drill and diamond bit; interdental splint; microscope; osteotome; retention suture; Weitlaner or Gelpi retractors

Source
Adapted from Anson JA, Segal MN, Baldwin NG, Neal D. Resection of giant invasive pituitary tumors through a transfacial approach: technical case report. Neurosurgery Journal 1995;37:541-545.

 ## resection of undifferentiated embryonal sarcoma of the liver

Description
rare hepatic tumor occurring with highest incidence in children 6 to 10 years of age; undifferentiated embryonal sarcoma (UES) lesions have been diagnosed as malignant mesenchymoma, fibromyxosarcoma, embryonal hepatoma, or simple hepatic sarcoma; characterized by solid-to-cystic lesion usually in right hepatic lobe; cure rate improved with laparoscopy and laparotomy consisting of hepatic lobectomy and colon resection

Anatomy
liver; transverse colon

Equipment
standard surgery equipment

Source
Adapted from Johnson JA, White JG, Thompson AR. Undifferentiated (embryonal) sarcoma of the liver in adults. American Surgeon 1995;61:285-287.

 ## Resistex expiratory resistance exerciser

Description
expiratory resistance exerciser; creates positive expiratory pressure (PEP) in patients suffering from chronic obstructive pulmonary disease (COPD), cystic fibrosis (CF), and other lung diseases; sustained pressure may strengthen the breathing muscles to make breathing more efficient and comfortable, facilitate opening of the airways, and reduce air trapping in patients with secretory problems to improve physical endurance; symptoms may be relieved and medications may be dispensed through this device

Source
Mercury Medical product information. Clearwater, FL.

 ## RespiGam

Generic name
see respiratory syncytial virus IV immune globulin

 ## respiratory syncytial virus IV immune globulin

Brand name
RespiGam

Use
prevention of serious lower respiratory tract infection caused by respiratory syncytial virus (RSV) in children less than 24 months of age with abnormal tissue development of lungs or a history of prematurity (less than or equal to 35 weeks gestation)

Usual dosage
injectable: infused once a month during RSV season at 750 mg/kg, with the first dose being administered prior to RSV season, which usually occurs between November and April

Pharmaceutical company
Medimmune. Gaithersburg, MD.

Source
University of Pittsburgh Drug Information and Pharmacoepidemiology Center. Pittsburgh, PA.

Respitrace inductive plethysmograph

Description
respiratory transducer for monitoring respirations using circumferential Respibands (part of polysomnographic instrument system for sleep monitoring)

Source
Ambulatory Monitoring Inc. product information. Ardsley, NY.

Resposable Spacemaker surgical balloon dissector

Description
quickly and atraumatically dissects the pocket for placement of a breast implant

Source
General Surgical Innovations Inc. product information. Cupertino, CA.

Res-Q arrhythmia control device (ACD)

Description
cardiac device intended for long-term detection and termination of treatable ventricular tachycardia and ventricular fibrillation; for use in patients who are at high risk of sudden death due to ventricular arrhythmias

Source
Intermedics Inc. product information. Angleton, TX.

Restore CalciCare dressing

Description
most absorbent of the leading calcium alginates and Hydrofiber dressings; transforms into a protective gel when it comes in contact with wound exudate; conforms to wound bed; provides moist healing environment; maintains its integrity when saturated; easily removed from the wound in one piece

Source
Hollister Inc. product information. Libertyville, IL.

Restore Clean 'N Moist

Description
one-step application that cleanses, moisturizes, and protects skin; no-rinse formulation provides nonocclusive barrier ideal for incontinent patients

Source
Hollister Inc. product information. Libertyville, IL.

Retavase

Generic name
see reteplase

 reteplase

Brand name
Retavase

Use
for the treatment of acute myocardial infarction (AMI) in adults for the improvement of ventricular function following AMI, the reduction of the incidence of congestive heart failure and the reduction of mortality associated with AMI

Usual dosage
injectable: 10 unit bolus injection over two minutes followed by additional 10 unit bolus after 30 minutes; administer as soon as possible after the onset of AMI symptoms

Pharmaceutical company
Boehringer Mannheim Pharmaceuticals. Gaithersburg, MD.

Source
Stadtlanders Managed Pharmacy Services. Pittsburgh, PA.

 Retin-A Micro

Generic name
see tretinoin gel

 retinoblastoma protein detection

Synonyms
Rb detection; Rb immunohistochemistry

Use
detection of mutated retinoblastoma protein in tissue sections of suspected tumors

Method
immunohistochemical staining

Specimen
tissue biopsy

Normal range
staining pattern consistent with normal cell proliferation

Comments
retinoblastoma protein is the product of the Rb tumor-suppressor gene

Source
Oncogene 1993;8:279-288.

retinoic acid

Brand name
Vitinoin

Use
liquid polymer of retinoic acid for the treatment of acne

Usual dosage
topical: as TopiCare liquid polymer delivery system in gel and cream formulation; apply once daily

Pharmaceutical company
Penederm/Schering-Plough Corp. Kenilworth, NJ.

Source
Stadtlanders Managed Pharmacy Services. Pittsburgh, PA.

 Retinomax refractometry instrument

Description
ophthalmic diagnostic hand-held instrument to be used like a retinoscope; gives fast readings for objective refractometry

Source
Nikon Inc. Ophthalmic Instrument Division product information. Melville, NY.

 retrograde cholecystectomy from fundus downward

Description
a method has been designed of suturing the liver bed to the diaphragm in severe inflammatory cases of cholecystitis in order to safely perform laparoscopic cholecystectomy; it is composed of six steps: establishing access with creation of a pneumoperitoneum, exposing the porta hepatis by lifting the gallbladder fundus and liver edge, dissecting the cystic artery and duct, performing cystic duct cholangiography, releasing gallbladder from attachments, and removing the gallbladder from the abdomen

Anatomy
abdomen; anterior axillary line; Calot triangle; cystic artery and duct; common bile duct; fundus; gallbladder; infundibulum; intrahepatic area; liver bed; midsubclavicular line; porta hepatis; parietal peritoneum; right costal margin; right hepatic lobe; serosa; umbilicus; xiphoid process

Equipment
drain; electrocautery; flexible laparoscope; Gazayerli knot pusher; forward oblique-viewing telescope; flexible telescope; forceps; Ligaclip; needle holder; ski needle; trocars

Source
Adapted from Uyama I, Iida S, Ogiwara H, Takahara T, Kato Y, Furuta T, Kikuchi K. Laparoscopic retrograde cholecystectomy (from fundus downward) facilitated by lifting the liver bed up to the diaphragm for inflammatory gallbladder. Surgical Laparoscopy and Endoscopy 1995;5:431-436.

retroperitoneoscopic vein ligation

Description
procedure is minimally invasive, extraperitoneal approach to bilateral spermatic vein ligation; clearly identifies vascular structures and limits potential for damage to intraperitoneal organs, spermatic arteries, and lymphatics; may have fewer risks than transperitoneal laparoscopic techniques

Anatomy
scrotum; bladder; abdomen; genitalia; rectus abdominis muscles; linea alba; rectus fascia; peritoneum; retroperitoneum; Cooper ligaments; pubic symphysis; properitoneal tissues; spermatic vein; spermatic arteries; line of Douglas

Equipment
standard surgery equipment; Foley urethral catheter; blunt trocar; 10 mm endoscope with camera; Endoclip; absorbable sutures

Source
Adapted from Gurpinar T, Sariyuce O, Balbay MD, Ozkan S, Gurel M. Retroperitoneoscopic bilateral spermatic vein ligation. Journal of Urology 1995;153:127-128.

 retroviral transduction for gene therapy

Synonyms
gene transduction; cell transduction; retroviral-mediated transduction

Use
correction of genetic deficiency disease by insertion of the missing gene into cells of patients or donors

Method
genetically modified retrovirus introduces a missing gene into cultured cells prior to transfusion

Specimen
blood; bone marrow; peripheral blood cytapheresis product; umbilical cord blood

Normal range
acceptable level of gene expression

Comments
investigational use, currently limited to correction of genetic deficiency but likely to develop into correction of gene dysregulation

Source
University of Minnesota Department of Laboratory Medicine and Pathology. Minneapolis, MN.

484

 reusable laparoscopic electrode

Description
laparoscopic electrodes for cholecystectomy and other minimally invasive procedures; available electrodes include spatula tip (long or short), needle tip, spoon tip, hook tip (flat), and J hook tip

Source
Accurate Surgical & Scientific Instruments Corp. product information. Westbury, NY.

 Revase

Generic name
see desirudin

 Reveal single lens reflex (SLR) camera

Description
constant-focus intraoral camera with an arc lamp-based lighting system

Source
Welch Allyn product information. Skaneateles Falls, NY.

 Revex

Generic name
see nalmefene hydrochloride

 Rezulin

Generic name
see troglitazone

 Rhein cautery pen

Description
ophthalmic reusable device with different tip designs; 23 gauge with tapered tip, 18 gauge with 45 degree bevel, and 18 gauge with broad tip

Source
Rhein Medical Inc. product information. Tampa, FL.

 Rheumox

Generic Name
see azapropazone

Rhinocort

Generic name
see budesonide

Rhinoline endoscopic sinus surgery system

Description
rhinolaryngofiberscopes and hand instruments; scopes have a unique, flat field of view; hand instruments feature the Luer-Lok (Luer lock) cleaning system

Source
Olympus America Inc. product information. Lake Success, NY.

Rhinotec shaver

Description
ENT surgical instrument that cuts cleanly and accurately while preserving surrounding tissue; straight or bent blades; variety of tip styles; used with Apex universal drive system

Source
Linvatec Corp. product information. Largo, FL.

rho (D) immune globulin intravenous (human)

Brand Name
WinRho SD

Use
treatment of idiopathic thrombocytopenia purpura (ITP) and suppression of Rh isoimmunization in Rh-negative women

Usual Dosage
intravenous: for the treatment of ITP the dose is 250 IU/kg (50 µg/kg) and for Rh isoimmunization the dose is 1500 IU (300 µg) at 28 weeks gestation followed by a second dose of 600 IU (120 µg) within 72 hours of delivery

Pharmaceutical company
Univax Biologics Inc. Rockville, MD.

Source
University of Pittsburgh Drug Information and Pharmacoepidemiology Center. Pittsburgh, PA.

ribavirin

Brand Name
Virazole

Use
antiviral agent used in the treatment of chronic active hepatitis C (non-A and non-B)

Usual Dosage
oral: 1,000-1,200 mg/day for 6 months

Pharmaceutical company
Viratek Division of ICN Pharmaceuticals Inc. Costa Mesa, CA.

Source
University of Pittsburgh Drug Information and Pharmacoepidemiology Center. Pittsburgh, PA.

 rifaximin

Brand name
Normix

Use
treatment of gastrointestinal infections, antibiotic-associated colitis, and uncomplicated diverticular disease of colon

Usual dosage
oral: 400 mg twice a day for gastrointestinal infections or antibiotic-associated colitis, and for symptomatic relief in uncomplicated diverticular disease of colon; the dose 400 mg twice a day for 7 days every month was used during the clinical trials

Pharmaceutical company
Salix. Palo Alto, CA.

Source
Stadtlanders Managed Pharmacy Services. Pittsburgh, PA

 RIK fluid mattress

Description
non-powered, fluid-filled mattress to relieve pressure and prevent heel break-down

Source
RIK Medical product information. Boulder, CO.

 Rilutek

Generic Name
see riluzole

riluzole

Brand Name
Rilutek

Use
glutamate transmission modulator for use in the treatment of amyotrophic lateral sclerosis (ALS/Lou Gehrig disease)

Usual Dosage
oral: 100 mg daily was used in clinical trials

Pharmaceutical company
Rhone-Poulenc Rorer Pharmaceuticals Inc. Collegeville, PA.

Source
University of Pittsburgh Drug Information and Pharmacoepidemiology Center. Pittsburgh, PA.

 rimexolone

Brand name
Vexol

Use
treatment of postoperative inflammation following ocular surgery and treatment of anterior uveitis

Usual dosage
ophthalmic: 1% rimexolone suspension
postoperative inflammation: 1-2 drops in affected eye 4 times daily from 24 hours after surgery through 2 weeks
anterior uveitis: 1-2 drops in affected eye every hour while awake for first week followed by 1 drop every 2 hours while awake for 1 additional week

Pharmaceutical company
Alcon Laboratories Inc. Ft Worth, TX.

Source
University of Pittsburgh Drug Information and Pharmacoepidemiology Center. Pittsburgh, PA.

 ring clip

Description
ring clips with laterally curved blades for carotid cave aneurysm; left and right differentiation; modification of Sugita straight-angled fenestrated clips

Source
Adapted from Okudera H, Kobayashi S, Kyoshima K, Nitta J. Ring clip with laterally curved blades for carotid cave aneurysm. Neurosurgery 1996;39:614-616.

risedronate

Brand name
Actonel

Use
bisphosphonate used in the treatment of osteoporosis and Paget disease of the bone

Usual dosage
oral: 2.5-5 mg daily for osteoporosis and 30 mg daily for Paget disease in clinical trials

Pharmaceutical company
Procter and Gamble Pharmaceuticals. Cincinnati, OH.

Source
Stadtlanders Managed Pharmacy Services. Pittsburgh, PA.

 Ritch nylon suture laser lens

Description
laser lens that provides compression of the conjunctiva and blanches overlying blood vessels while allowing improved view of scleral flap sutures; used for suture lysis of subconjunctival nylon sutures after trabeculectomy, or to relax cataract wound sutures that cause astigmatism

Source
Ocular Instruments Inc. product information. Bellevue, WA.

 ritonavir

Brand name
Norvir

Use
protease inhibitor used in combination with nucleoside analogues or as monotherapy for the treatment of HIV infection when therapy is warranted

Usual dosage
oral: 600 mg twice a day, slow escalation of ritonavir regimen is recommended for side effect of nausea; ritonavir may be initiated with 300 mg b.i.d. for 1 day, 400 mg b.i.d. for 2 days, 500 mg b.i.d. for 1 day, and then 600 mg b.i.d. thereafter

Pharmaceutical company
Abbott Laboratories. Abbott Park, IL.

Source
University of Pittsburgh Drug Information and Pharmacoepidemiology Center. Pittsburgh, PA.

rizatriptan benzoate

Brand name
Maxalt

Use
oral serotonin-1D receptor agonist for treatment of migraine headaches

Usual dosage
oral: one 10 or 20 mg tablet to relieve migraine

Pharmaceutical company
Merck & Co. Inc. West Point, PA.

Source
Stadtlanders Managed Pharmacy Services. Pittsburgh, PA.

 ## roaming optical access multiscope (ROAM)

Description
right-angle scope that allows expansion of the optical cavity without changing retractor position or compromising exposure

Source
Snowden Pencer DSP product information. Fall River, MA.

 ## Robertazzi nasopharyngeal airway

Description
nasopharyngeal airway anesthesia device of soft, flexible Ultrasil material and silicone-coated latex for maximum patient comfort

Source
Rusch Inc. product information. Duluth, GA.

 ## rocuronium bromide

Brand name
Zemuron

Use
nondepolarizing neuromuscular blocking (paralytic) agent used as an adjunct to general anesthesia to facilitate both rapid sequence and routine intubation; skeletal muscle relaxant during surgery or mechanical ventilation

Usual dosage
intravenous: 50 mg vials at a concentration of 10 mg/ml; 0.6 to 1.2 mg/kg for rapid sequence intubation and 0.6 mg/kg for tracheal intubation; repeated doses of 0.1 to 0.2 mg/kg should be administered to maintain relaxation during surgery; continuous infusion dose of 0.01 to 0.012 mg/kg/min should be initiated only after evidence of spontaneous recovery from intubating dose; dose is adjusted according to response and various disease states

490

Pharmaceutical company
Organon Inc. West Orange, NJ.
Source
University of Pittsburgh Drug Information and Pharmacoepidemiology Center. Pittsburgh, PA.

 Roeder manipulative aptitude test device

Description
board which includes T-bar for evaluating aptitude; numerous perforations arranged in predetermined patterns; measures hand, arm, and finger dexterity and speed
Source
Fred Sammons Inc. product information. Western Springs, IL.

 Roll-A-Bout

Description
mobility device for patients with injuries below the knee; allows mobility, stability, and comfort with less effort than a set of crutches; special knee and ankle pads give support and comfort; designed to support up to 250 pounds; hand-brake to control speed and parking brake; patient places knee of the injured leg on the knee pad, rests ankle on the rear support, and propels with good leg; steer by taking a step with good leg while gently lifting the handle and turning in the desired direction
Source
Roll-A-Bout Corp. product information. Dover, DE.

 Rolyan AquaForm wrist and thumb spica splint

Description
zippered splint that aids in aligning splint correctly during fabrication and providing quick removal during use; circumferential splint immobilizes wrist-thumb, reduces pain associated with trapeziectomy, metacarpophalangeal (MCP) fractures and reconstruction and cumulative trauma injuries such as deQuervain syndrome and gamekeeper's thumb
Source
Smith & Nephew Rolyan product information. Largo, FL.

Rolyan arm elevator

Description
combines splint and elevating support into one positioner; anatomically correct foam positioning splint helps reduce edema, helps prevent shoulder-hand syndrome and metacarpophalangeal (MCP) extension contusions; positions hand in resting position, wrist in 30-degree extension, MCPs in 60-degree flexion, and interphalangeals (IPs) slightly flexed; can be modified

Source
Smith & Nephew Rolyan product information. Largo, FL.

Rolz device

Description
scar massage tool to reduce adhesions and limitations in movement from scar formation; consists of a 1-inch ball with a handle

Source
Elford Group Ltd. product information. Green Bay, WI.

Rooke perioperative boot

Description
adjustable calf-high boot; inner layer of sheepskin; outer layer of fabric; provides protection and warmth after arteriovascular surgery

Source
Osborn Medical product information. Utica, MN.

ropinirole

Brand name
Requip

Use
dopamine D2 receptor agonist for the relief of symptoms associated with Parkinson disease

Usual dosage
oral: 0.25 mg 3 times a day initially, and then titrated to 1.5 mg, 3 times a day was investigated in clinical trials

Pharmaceutical company
Smith Kline Beecham Pharmaceuticals. Philadelphia, PA.

Source
Stadtlanders Managed Pharmacy Services. Pittsburgh, PA.

ropivacaine

Brand name
Naropin

Use
long-acting amide local anesthetic for obstetric procedures; provides local or regional anesthesia and postoperative pain management

Usual dosage
injectable 0.5% and 1.0%: 0.5% (75 mg) to 1% (150 mg) of ropivacaine has been used in clinical trials

Pharmaceutical company
Astra USA Inc. Freeport, NY.

Source
University of Pittsburgh Drug Information and Pharmacoepidemiology Center. Pittsburgh, PA.

 roquinimex

Brand name
Linomide

Use
quinoline derivative, an immune response regulator; used for prevention of relapse in patients with chronic myeloid leukemia after bone marrow transplantation (stem cells autografting)

Usual dosage
oral: doses of 0.05 mg/kg has been used after autologous bone marrow transplantation in chronic myeloid leukemia in the phase I clinical trials

Pharmaceutical company
Pharmacia Inc. Columbus, OH.

Source
Stadtlanders Managed Pharmacy Service. Pittsburgh, PA.

 Rosen phaco splitter

Description
splits and separates lens nucleus

Source
Katena Products Inc. product information. Denville, NJ.

Rotaglide total knee system

Description
orthopaedic three-part meniscal prosthetic instrumentation that maximizes contact areas while minimizing torsional loosening forces transmitted to the tibial component; rotates while maintaining total area contact

Source
Corin Orthopaedic Products product information. Tampa, FL.

Rotashield

Generic name
see rotavirus vaccine

rotavirus vaccine

Brand name
Rotashield

Use
oral vaccine for protection against rotaviral diseases

Usual dosage
oral: dose to be given to infants at 2, 4, and 6 months of age

Pharmaceutical company
American Home Products. Madison, NJ.

Source
Stadtlanders Managed Pharmacy Services. Pittsburgh, PA.

Roth retrieval net

Description
endoscopically passed polypectomy snare with a net; for entrapment and removal of soft food impactions; can be used to capture round or oval-type foreign bodies of esophagus and stomach with ease

Source
U. S. Endoscopy Group Inc. product information. Mentor, OH.

Rowen spatula

Description
ophthalmic surgical instrument that combines a Bechert nucleus rotator and Rosen phaco splitter; allows surgeon to manipulate and split nucleus with same instrument

Source
Katena Products Inc. product information. Denville, NJ.

roxatidine acetate

Brand name
Roxin

Use
treatment of gastric and duodenal ulcers

Usual dosage
oral: doses of 75 mg once daily at bedtime or twice daily have been studied

Pharmaceutical company
Hoechst-Roussel Pharmaceuticals Inc. Somerville, NJ.

Source
University of Pittsburgh Drug Information and Pharmacoepidemiology Center. Pittsburgh, PA.

 Roxin

Generic name
see roxatidine acetate

 Royl-Derm wound hydrogel dressing

Description
wet-to-dry nonadherent dressing for partial and full-thickness wounds; promotes healing of first- and second-degree burns

Source
Acme United Corp. product information. Fairfield, CT.

 Rubin planer

Description
cartilage planer severs cartilage away from nasal cavity; bone planer removes segments of bone away from the nasal cavity

Source
Neo-Contemporary Co. Inc. product information. Randolph, MA.

 Ruhof Biocide

Description
instrument cleaning solution that kills all pathogens and viruses including HIV and tuberculosis; environmentally safe

Source
Ruhof product information. Valley Stream, NY.

RUMI device for laparoscopic procedures

Description
Rowden uterine manipulator injector (RUMI) improves access to pelvic structures; anteversion and retroversion of uterus easily achieved; fundus can be placed against pelvic sidewalls; chromotubation effective from any position

Source
Blairden product information. Lenexa, KS.

 ## Ruschelit polyvinyl chloride (PVC) endotracheal tube

Description
low-pressure cuffed endotracheal tube; flexible and non-kinking with stainless steel reinforcement built into the tube wall; soft atraumatic tip designed so that it cannot fold back; connector is permanently fixed into the tube; graduated sizes in increments of 0.5 mm from 5 to 11 mm with lengths of 27 cm, 33 cm, and 37 cm

Source
Rusch Inc. product information. Duluth, GA.

 ## sabeluzole

Brand name
Reminyl

Use
axonal transport enhancer to improve cognitive symptoms of Alzheimer disease and to treat memory impairment of elderly

Usual dosage
oral: starting with 5 mg to a maximum of 20 mg twice a day was investigated in elderly patients with probable Alzheimer disease

Pharmaceutical company
Janssen Pharmaceutical. Titusville, NJ.

Source
Stadtlanders Managed Pharmacy Service. Pittsburgh, PA.

 ## Sabra OMS 45

Description
45-degree angle handpiece used to access third molar impaction

Source
Sabra Dental Products product information. Hauppauge, NY.

Sabril

Generic name
see vigabatrin

 sacral segmental nerve stimulation for urge incontinence: implantable neural prosthesis

Description
most patients with detrusor instability and urge incontinence are treated conservatively initially with bladder retraining, exercises, and biofeedback supplemented with anticholinergic drugs; unilateral sacral segmental nerve stimulation offers a nondestructive alternative for conditions not responding to conservative measures; a permanent sacral (S3) foramen electrode has been implanted in patients showing a good response during temporary stimulation

Anatomy
afferent somatic nerve fibers; afferent anorectal branches of pelvic nerve; afferent sensory fibers of pudendal nerve; bladder; detrusor muscle; dorsal roots of sacral nerve; efferent motor fibers; foramen and foramina (plural); levator ani muscle; muscle afferent; S3 (sacral root); sacral nerve; spinal cord

Equipment
neuromodulation equipment; angiographic catheter sheath; electrodes; external neuro-stimulator; implantable neural prosthesis; pulse generator; spinal needle

Source
Adapted from Bosch JL, Groen J. Sacral (S3) segmental nerve stimulation as a treatment for urge incontinence in patients with detrusor instability: results of chronic electrical stimulation using an implantable neural prosthesis. The Journal of Urology 1995;154:504-507.

 sacrocolpopexy

Description
reconstructive procedure corrects vaginal vault prolapse; elevation of vagina and uterosacral ligament plication prevents subsequent formation of enterocele below vault suspension; vaginal vault suspension; reconstruction with Teflon mesh sutured to anterior longitudinal ligament and periosteum over first sacral vertebra; reperitonealization

Anatomy
vagina; vaginal vault; uterosacral ligament; presacral peritoneum; first sacral vertebra; detrusor muscle

Equipment
standard surgery equipment; Hegar dilator; Teflon mesh

Source
Adapted from Valaitis SR, Stanton SL. Sacrocolpopexy: a retrospective study of a clinician's experience. Obstetrical and Gynecological Survey 1995;50:107-108.

sacrospinous vaginal vault suspension with in-line suturing device

Description

disposable suturing instrument used for sacrospinous vault suspension facilitates suture placement and retrieval; pararectal space dissected and the suturing device is placed medial to the lateral one-third of the sacrospinous ligament-coccygeus muscle complex; needle retrieved with a needle holder; second suture placed medial to the first suture; if holding strength is considered inadequate, subsequent bites are taken; procedure completed using standard methods

Anatomy

ischial spine; pararectal space; sacrospinous ligament-coccygeus muscle complex; vaginal vault; vaginal mucosa

Equipment

standard gynecologic surgery equipment; Laurus needle driver (ND-260)

Source

Adapted from Lind LR, Choe J, Bhatia NN. An in-line suturing device to simplify sacrospinous vaginal vault suspension. Obstetric and Gynecology Journal 1997;89:129-132.

 Saeed Six-Shooter multi-band ligator

Description

hemorrhoid ligation device which allows placement of six bands with one intubation; provides optimal suction of varix or hemorrhoid

Source

Wilson-Cook Medical Inc. product information. Winston-Salem, NC.

 SafeTrak ESP system

Description

combined spinal/epidural regional anesthesia system using a Sprotte spinal and/or epidural needle allowing for self-sealing entry point, minimizing possibility of epidural catheter penetration; kink-resistant catheter and SafeTrak adapter allow firm insertion, with possible disconnection greatly reduced

Source

Kendall Healthcare Products Co. product information. Mansfield, MA.

 Safe-T-Wheel pinwheel

Description

neurological pinwheel; a hand-held rotating wheel with very sharp spikes

Source

Safety Medical Systems Inc. product information. Littleton, CO.

498

 SAFHS ultrasound device

Description
sonic accelerated fracture healing system (SAFHS) uses specific, low-intensi-ty, ultrasound pressure waves in order to induce low level mechanical forces into fracture site; for acceleration of healing of distal radius and tibial diaph-ysis

Source
Exogen Inc. product information. West Caldwell, NJ.

 Saf-T-Intima intravenous catheter safety system

Description
features a patented safety shield that encases the needle as it is withdrawn from the catheter; catheter system that provides needle stick protection from IV start to tubing connection

Source
Becton Dickinson Vascular Access product information. Sandy, UT.

 saliva HIV-1 antibody detection

Use
detect antibodies to human immunodeficiency virus (HIV-1)

Method
enzyme-linked immunosorbent assay (ELISA)

Specimen
saliva

Normal range
negative

Comments
oral fluid testing is not as accurate as conventional blood testing; all positive tests should be followed up with blood-based confirmation test; testing has false-positive rate of 2% and false-negative rate of 1% to 2%

Source
Lexi-Comp Inc. database. Hudson, OH.

 Salman FES stent

Description
stent that fits between middle turbinate and lateral nasal wall to help pre-vent complications from functional endoscopic sinus (FES) surgery; two "fin-gers" arising from base placed in maxillary sinus through middle meatal antrostomy, preventing dislodgement of stent without sutures

Source
Boston Medical Products product information. Waltham, MA.

salmeterol xinafoate

Brand name
Serevent

Use
long-acting beta-agonist in a metered-dose inhaler used for the prevention of bronchospasm in patients with asthma; prevention of exercise-induced asthma

Usual dosage
inhalant: prevention of asthma, use 2 puffs twice daily; exercise-induced asthma use 2 puffs inhaled 30-60 minutes before exercise; not to be given more than twice daily

Pharmaceutical company
Glaxo Inc. Research Triangle Park, NC.

Source
University of Pittsburgh Drug Information and Pharmacoepidemiology Center. Pittsburgh, PA.

 ## Salmonella sulA-test

Synonyms
SOS-inducing potency measurement; SOSIP assay

Use
detection of DNA-damaging compounds

Method
colorimetric evaluation of genotoxin-induced sulA reporter gene expression

Specimen
compound of interest

Normal range
SOSIP activity below threshold

Comments
can be expected to augment, not replace the standard SOS Chromotest and umu-test

Source
Adapted from Elmzibri M, De Meo MP, Laget M et al. The Salmonella sulA-test: a new in vitro system to detect genotoxins. Mutation Research 1996;369:195-208.

 ## samarium-EDTMP

Brand name
Quadramet

Use
radiopharmaceutical for the treatment of severe and chronic pain associated with cancer that has metastasized to the bone

Usual dosage
intravenous: 18.5-37 MBq/kg injected over one minute has been studied

Pharmaceutical company
DuPont Merck. Wilmington, DE.

Source
University of Pittsburgh Drug Information and Pharmacoepidemiology Center. Pittsburgh, PA.

 ## SAM facial implant

Description
Gore-Tex subcutaneous augmentation material (SAM) facial implant for auriculoplasty, rhinoplasty, mentoplasty, maxilloplasty, malarplasty, facial slings, orbital repair, and frontal/forehead defects; nonabsorbable material provides long-lasting correction; available in 1, 2, and 4 mm thicknesses

Source
WL Gore & Associates Inc. product information. Flagstaff, AZ.

 ## SAM (sleep apnea monitor) system

Description
instrument for overnight sleep apnea diagnostic testing, analyzing, and interpreting results; channels include body position, snoring sounds, respiratory effort, respiratory airflow, pulse rate, and oxygen saturation

Source
Intercare Technologies Inc. product information. Waukesha, WI.

 ## SAM (smart anesthesia multi-gas) module

Description
instrument for analyzing gas; offers on-line monitoring of respiratory and anesthetic gas concentrations; agent identification is instantaneous; "fast" oxygen attained with oxygen sensor

Source
Marquette Electronics Inc. product information. Milwaukee, WI.

 ## Sandalthotics postural support orthotic

Description
custom-crafted orthotic soles

Source
Foot Levelers Inc. product information. Roanoke, VA.

 ## sandoparin

Brand name
Mono-Embolex NM

Use
prophylaxis of deep vein thrombosis

Usual dosage
subcutaneous: 3,000 IU daily for 5 to 20 days with an average of 10 days

Pharmaceutical company
Sandoz Pharmaceutical Co. East Hanover, NJ.

Source
University of Pittsburgh Drug Information and Pharmacoepidemiology Center. Pittsburgh, PA.

 ## Santorini duct sphincteroplasty

Description
patients with acute recurrent pancreatitis and pancreas divisum who will benefit from surgery are identified by clinical means; criteria are evidence of complete pancreas divisum by pancreatography, absence of pancreatic calcifications, endoscopic cholangiopancreatographic findings of ductal dilation, absence of biliary calculi, and documented episodes of unexplained acute pancreatitis with serum amylase at least twice normal; pancreatitis in patients with pancreas divisum is restricted to the ventral pancreas by the abnormal anatomy

Anatomy
ampulla of Vater; accessory papilla; duct of Santorini; ventral pancreas

Equipment
standard surgical equipment

Source
Adapted from Bradley EL, Stephan RN. Accessory duct sphincteroplasty is preferred for long-term prevention of recurrent acute pancreatitis in patients with pancreas divisum. Journal of American College of Surgeons 1996;183:65-69.

 ## saquinavir

Brand name
Invirase

Use
protease inhibitor for use in HIV-infected patients

Usual dosage
oral: 600 mg every 8 hours

Pharmaceutical company
Roche Laboratories. Nutley, NJ.

Source
University of Pittsburgh Drug Information and Pharmacoepidemiology Center. Pittsburgh, PA.

 ## Sarnol-HC

Generic name
see hydrocortisone

Sarns soft-flow aortic cannula

Description
improved cannula for bypass procedures; does not expel blood at velocities many times greater than systolic flow; reduces velocity by 50% without impeding flow; reduces jetting action

Source
3M Healthcare Specialties product information. Ann Arbor, MI.

Satellight needle holder forceps

Description
microsurgery forceps; counterbalanced; curved angle to side; also forceps with tying platform

Source
Accurate Surgical & Scientific Instruments Corp. product information. Westbury, NY.

Saunders cervical HomeTrac

Description
friction-free track and specially designed air cylinder allow smooth application of traction and stretching to the upper back and neck in supine position; helps relax and reduce neck muscle activity; unit is calibrated in pounds and kilograms of traction to provide feedback to user and promote consistency in treatment

Source
The Saunders Group, Inc. product information. Chaska, MN.

Save-A-Tooth

Description
patented product that protects, nourishes, and revives knocked-out teeth for replantation by dentists; EM Save-A-Tooth emergency tooth preserving system protects an avulsed tooth from 2 primary causes of replanted tooth loss: tooth cell crushing and tooth cell dehydration

Source
3M Health Care product information. St. Paul, MN.

Saverburger irrigation/aspiration (I/A) tip

Description
ophthalmic surgical instrument with irrigation sleeve that extends maximally so that the irrigation stream exits as far distally as possible for aspiration of subincisional cortex; tip useful for aspirating viscoelastics

Source
American Surgical Instruments Corp. product information. Westmont, IL.

Schoenrock laser instrument set

Description

instrument set for laser-assisted blepharoplasties: Teaser is for extraction of fatty tissue from blepharoplasty incision; uses high friction knurled tip to grasp, tease out and roll up fat; laser ball retractor has two curved prongs with atraumatic ball tips for retraction of tissue; also includes Castroviejo forceps, Trelles post-less metal scleral shield, Yeager metal lid plate, and delicate curved mosquito hemostat

Source

Byron Medical product information. Tucson, AZ.

 ## Scholten sternal retractor

Description

updated version of Canadian rib spreader; low profile retractor with compact size and increased rigidity

Source

Scholten Surgical Instruments Inc. product information. Redwood City, CA.

 ## scleral tunnel incision for trabeculectomy

Description

modified technique for construction of trabeculectomy flap which involves the creation of scleral tunnel; advantages include: edges of flap are never grasped during dissection which prevents the flap from being perforated, dissection of the scleral pocket is easily advanced into clear cornea by angling the crescent-shaped knife upward slightly, and dissection of the pocket into clear cornea allows production of an anterior scleral ostium; this method has been successfully used

Anatomy

cornea; corneoscleral limbus; conjunctiva; globe; interpalpebral fissure; lamella; limbal vascular arcade; orbit; sclera; Tenon capsule

Equipment

standard ophthalmic surgery instruments; Pocket II 55-degree angled micro-blade; Vannas scissors

Source

Adapted from Schumer RA, Odrich SA. A scleral tunnel incision for trabeculectomy. American Journal of Ophthalmology 1995;120:528-530.

 ## ScleroLASER

Description

laser treatment for leg telangiectasia up to 1-mm size without needles

Source

Candela Corp. product information. Wayland, MA.

scrotal sonography

Synonyms
duplex sonography

Indications
acute disease of scrotum requires early detection and treatment; high incidence of testicular malignancy compared to benign neoplasm, which occurs primarily in young men; testicular torsion

Method
patient supine; use of acoustic gel; study encompasses examination of spermatic cord, epididymis, testes, scrotal wall; Valsalva maneuver done to examine for varicocele; patient examined standing and maneuver repeated

Normal findings
no scrotal or testicular abnormal findings

Comments
ultrasound has strong presence in diagnostic imaging of acute scrotal disease and is usually first study chosen for delineation of diagnosis

Source
Adapted from Gooding G. Scrotal sonography in acute disease. Emergency Radiology 1995;2:56-66.

 SeamGuard staple line material

Description
reinforcement material indicated for use as a prosthesis for pulmonary wedge resection using linear cutter surgical staplers

Source
W.L. Gore & Asso. Inc. product information. Flagstaff, AZ.

 SeaSorb alginate dressing

Description
dressing that immediately creates a soft gel in the wound bed to maintain an optimal moist wound environment; easily removed

Source
Coloplast Corp. product information. Humlebaek, Denmark.

 Seated Cable Row exerciser

Description
exercise device with line of tension for seven possible sitting positions; improves efficiency of musculature; supports spine and promotes spinal stability; component of reliance rehabilitation system

Source
Chattanooga Group Inc. product information. Hixson, TN.

Seated Hamstring Curl

Description
exercise chair of Alliance rehabilitation system with large handles and pull-pin adjustments; strengthens hamstring muscle to stabilize knee, controlling swing phase of gait and sagittal plane of pelvis
Source
Chattanooga Group Inc. product information. Hixson, TN.

 ## Security+ self-sealing Urisheath external catheter

Description
male external catheter; external tab allows sheath to unroll easily; unique push ring makes connection to the bag easy; features an anti-kink port to prevent back flow and pooling; made of nonlatex material
Source
Coloplast Corp. product information. Marietta, GA.

 ## Seibel Nucleus Chopper

Description
ophthalmic surgical instrument; mirror polished distal olive tip provides maximum safety to posterior capsule and anterior capsular rim while engaging the nuclear periphery
Source
Rhein Medical Inc. product information. Tampa, FL.

 ## Seiff frontalis suspension set

Description
ophthalmic set with stainless steel needles, solid rods, and silicone tubing; useful for frontalis suspension in patients with significant ptosis and poor levator function
Source
Visitec Co. product information. Sarasota, FL.

 ## Seitzinger tripolar cutting forceps

Description
endoscopic instrument; multiple function allows grasping, coagulating, and transecting with single instrument; designed for laparoscopic-assisted vaginal hysterectomy (LAVH), colectomy, myomectomy, adhesiolysis, oophorectomy, and Nissen fundoplication
Source
Cabot Medical Technology product information. West Homestead, PA.

Selachii

Generic name
see shark cartilage

Selecor

Generic Name
see celiprolol

semi-nested polymerase chain reaction (PCR) for immunoglobulin H (IgH) monoclonality

Synonyms
semi-nested PCR

Use
diagnosis of nonfollicular lymphoma

Method
polymerase chain reaction with partially-nested primer sets immunoglobulin heavy-chain gene rearrangements

Specimen
biopsy specimens

Normal range
no evidence of immunoglobulin heavy-chain gene rearrangement

Comments
investigational

Source
Archives Pathology Lab Med 1996;120:357-363.

semitendinosus augmentation of patellar tendon repair

Description
supplements surgical repair of acute ruptured midsubstance patellar tendon; eliminates need for stabilization hardware and subsequent removal; allows postoperative mobilization immediately and reduces need for second surgery; harvest semitendinosus tendon as free graft, trim, and suture at each end; pass tendon graft through holes drilled in tibial tubercle and distal patellar pole in loop or figure-of-8 fashion; tie sutures together and repair patellar tendon ends

Anatomy
quadriceps; patella; patellofemoral joint; patellar tendon; semitendinosus tendon; gracilis tendon; pes anserinus; tibial tubercle

Equipment
standard surgery equipment; Brand tendon stripper; intraoperative radiograph; nonabsorbable suture material

Source
Adapted from Larson RV, Simonian PT. Semitendinosus augmentation of acute patellar tendon repair with immediate mobilization. American Journal of Sports Medicine 1995;23:82-86.

 Semprex-D

Generic Name
see acrivastine/pseudoephedrine

 Sensiv endotracheal tube

Description
intermediate low-pressure cuff, close fitting for ease of intubation; compliant material forms a low pressure seal with no folds or leaks; graduated size in 0.5-mm increments ranging from 5 to 11 mm

Source
Rusch Inc. product information. Duluth, GA.

 Sentinel HIV-1 (human immunodeficiency virus-1) urine EIA (enzyme immunoassay)

Synonym
none

Use
testing safer, easier and more accessible compared with standard blood test; detects antibodies to HIV present in simple plastic cup specimens of urine using an enzyme-linked immunosorbent assay (ELISA) method to detect the presence of antibodies to HIV-1; previous HIV tests use either blood or oral fluid samples; any initially reactive sample will be retested twice; for confirmation of a positive urine test, the patient must be tested with a more accurate blood test (Editor note: also marketed under Calypte HIV-1 urine EIA manufactured by Calypte Biomedical Corp. Berkeley, CA)

Method
urinalysis

Specimen
urine

Normal range
none

Source
Adapted from Altman LK. The Houston Chronicle, August 7, 1996:12A and Internet www.fda.gov.

Sentinel-4 neurological monitor

Description
provides cerebral and neurological analysis and feedback of functioning neural pathways at risk, allowing time to intervene before these structures may be permanently damaged

Source
Axon Systems Inc. product information. Hauppauge, NY.

 ## Seprafilm membrane

Description
bioresorbable membrane reduces postoperative adhesions in laparotomy for abdominal and pelvic surgery; applied to adhesiogenic tissue before surgical closure; remains in place without suturing for up to seven days

Source
Genzyme Corp. product information. Cambridge, MA.

 ## Sequel compression system

Description
prophylactic device used for deep vein thrombosis and pulmonary embolus; delivers 45 mmHg preset pressure delivered sequentially and maintained throughout compression of the leg; 60-second venting allows veins to completely refill and maximizes blood movement regardless of patient positioning

Source
Kendall Healthcare Products Co. product information. Mansfield, MA.

 ## Sequoia ultrasound system

Description
ultrasound imaging device that uses higher frequency than previously and increased frame rate

Source
Acuson Corp. product information. Mountain View, CA.

 ## Seradyn Color Vue

Synonyms
microsome thyroid peroxidase antibody test; TPO antibody test

Use
enzyme immunoassay for screening and detection of autoantibodies against human thyroid peroxidase (TPO) (microsome) in serum and is used as an aid in the diagnosis of thyroid disorders

Method
assay serum levels

Specimen
blood

Normal range
normal thyroid-stimulating hormone (TSH) levels

Comments
none

Source
Seradyn Clinical Diagnostics database. Indianapolis, IN.

 ## Serena and Serena Mx

Description
hand-held apnea recorder/analyzer; provides portable apnea detection and sleep diagnostic monitoring from infant to adult

Source
Aequitron Medical Inc. product information. Minneapolis, MN.

 ## Serevent

Generic name
see salmeterol xinafoate

 ## Serlect

Generic name
see sertindole

 ## Sermion

Generic name
see nicergoline

 ## sermorelin acetate

Brand name
Geref

Use
growth hormone-releasing hormone for use in pediatric growth hormone deficiency

Usual dosage
injectable: 30 µg/kg/day administered subcutaneously

Pharmaceutical company
Serono Labs Inc. Norwell, MA.

Source
University of Pittsburgh Drug Information and Pharmacoepidemiology Center. Pittsburgh, PA.

Serola sacroiliac belt

Description
by stabilizing the sacroiliac joint the belt allows the wearer to better utilize muscles in daily tasks

Source
Serola Biomechanics product information. Honolulu, HI.

 Seroma-cath wound drainage system

Description
bulb suction reservoir, continuous drainage system for removal of fluid; effective for treating seromas following surgery; continuously removes fluid and eliminates need for frequent aspirations and open drains

Source
Greer Medical product information. Santa Barbara, CA.

 Seroquel

Generic name
see quetiapine

 Serostim

Generic name
see mammalian cell-derived recombinant human growth hormone

 serotonin receptor assay

Synonyms
5-hydroxytryptamine receptor assay, 5-HT receptor assay

Use
detection and quantification of tissue serotonin receptors in patients with neurobehavioral disorders

Method
immunoassay, immunohistochemical staining

Specimen
blood, tissue biopsy

Normal range
investigational

Comments
serotonin receptors have been implicated in several neurobehavioral disorders

Source
Brain Research. Molecular Brain Research. 1994;23:163-178.

sertindole

Brand name
Serlect

Use
selective serotonin and dopamine receptor antagonist used to treat schizophrenia

Usual dosage
oral: 20 mg daily

Pharmaceutical company
Abbott Laboratories. Abbott Park, IL.

Source
University of Pittsburgh Drug Information and Pharmacoepidemiology Center. Pittsburgh, PA.

 serum cytokine panel in immune thrombocytopenic purpura

Synonyms
AITP cytokine levels

Use
evaluation of pediatric patients with autoimmune thrombocytopenic purpura

Method
solid phase enzyme-linked immunoabsorbent assay for cytokines IL-2, IL-4, IL-6, IL-10, and interferon-γ

Specimen
serum

Normal range
investigational; individual reference ranges are being established for each cytokine

Comments
investigational; use largely limited to clinician-researchers specializing in immune thrombocytopenic purpura

Source
Adapted from Semple JW, Milev Y, Cosgrave D, Mody M, Hornstein A, Blanchette V, Freedman J. Differences in serum cytokine levels in acute and chronic autoimmune thrombocytopenic purpura: relationship to platelet phenotype and antiplatelet T-cell reactivity. Blood 1996;87:4245-4254.

 Serzone

Generic name
see nefazodone hydrochloride

S.E.T. catheter

Description
over-the-wire triple-lumen catheter system for treatment of thrombosed hemodialysis access grafts; fragments clots with high-pressure saline and flowing through outflow port into collection bag; sizes 4 to 10 French; clinical trials beginning

Source
Convergenza AG press release on Internet.

 sevirumab

Brand name
Protovir

Use
treatment of cytomegalovirus (CMV) retinitis

Usual dosage
oral: 60 mg every 2 weeks

Pharmaceutical company
Protein Design Labs. Mountain View, CA.

Source
Stadtlanders Managed Pharmacy Services. Pittsburgh, PA.

 sevoflurane

Brand name
Ultane

Use
inhalation anesthetic to provide induction of anesthesia

Usual dosage
inhalational: administered in concentrations of 1.8 to 5% in nitrous oxide/oxygen; concentrations of 0.75 to 3% are generally used for anesthesia maintenance

Pharmaceutical company
Abbott Laboratories. Abbott Park, IL.

Source
University of Pittsburgh Drug Information and Pharmacoepidemiology Center. Pittsburgh, PA.

shape memory clamps in surgical treatment of mandibular fractures

Description
in the search for new and easier methods of internal fixation, shape memory clamps are being used; they have the advantage of allowing closure of the fracture gap after the device has been implanted; due to the clamp's ability to regain its programmed shape at the temperature which corresponds to body temperature, the operation is reduced to aligning bone fragments in the correct position, boring holes in each segment, and placing in the clamps; transoral access is used in place of the traditional transcervical approach

Anatomy
collagen fibers; fibrous connective tissue; fibroblast; mandible; mandibular angle, body, canal; roots of teeth

Equipment
standard oral maxillofacial surgery equipment; TiNiCo (titanium, nickel, cobalt) shape memory clamps; rosette drill; standard stainless steel clamp

Source
Adapted from Drugacz J, Lekston Z, Morawiec H, Januszewski K. Use of TiNiCo shape memory clamps in the surgical treatment of mandibular fractures. Journal of Oral Maxillofacial Surgery 1995;53:665-671.

 ## shark cartilage

Brand name
Selachii

Use
has been investigated to use as anticancer agent

Usual dosage
oral: 100 gm/day was investigated in early clinical trials

Pharmaceutical company
Simone Protective Cancer Center. Lawrenceville, NJ.

Source
Stadtlanders Managed Pharmacy Services. Pittsburgh, PA.

 ## Sharplan Sight System

Description
ultrasound/video imaging system for laparoscopic surgery

Source
Sharplan Lasers Inc. product information Allendale, NJ.

Sharpoint spoon blade

Description

angled, double-beveled, circular tip, 360 degree cutting surface, for cataract surgery

Source

Surgical Specialties Corp. product information. Reading, PA.

 ## Shearing suction kit

Description

suction kit for removal of cortex at 12-o'clock position during phaco-emulsification; includes handpiece, 3-way stop-cock, and cortex removal cannula

Source

Eagle Laboratories product information. Rancho Cucamonga, CA.

 ## ShiatsuBACK back support

Description

contoured back support featuring 96 integral "massaging thumbs" providing manual shiatsu massage effect

Source

Kenshin Trading Corp. product information. Torrance, CA.

 ## Shiley Phonate speaking valve

Description

system allows phonation for tracheostomy patients who are able to breathe independently without assisted mechanical ventilation; valve connects to tracheostomy tube and directs air flow past the vocal cords to give patients the ability to speak; permits vocalization without finger occlusion; also Shiley Phonate speaking valve with oxygen port

Source

Mallinckrodt Medical Inc. product information. St. Louis, MO.

 ## Shockmaster heel cushions

Description

soft, springy heel cushions made of Enduron foam to protect from heel and foot pain; acts by absorbing step-shock or shockwave up to 3 times body weight that walking or jogging inflicts on the heels

Source

Health Center for Better Living Inc. product information. Naples, FL.

Shoemaker intraocular lens (IOL) forceps

Description
ophthalmic surgical instrument designed to repeatedly implant superior haptic into capsular bag; lens inserted into eye; instrument released allowing haptic to slide into capsule

Source
Storz Ophthalmics product information. St. Louis, MO.

shoulder subluxation inhibitor brace

Description
shoulder subluxation inhibitor (SSI) orthosis stabilizes shoulder after glenohumeral joint subluxation injury; allows range of motion; prevents motion that may cause re-injury

Source
Alipro product information. Avon, MA.

ShowerSafe waterproof cast and bandage cover

Description
durable, reusable and pliable plastic covering that keeps casts dry during showering

Source
Trademark Medical product information. Fenton, MO.

Show'rbag

Description
watertight cast and dressing cover; allows patient to shower comfortably without worrying about water seepage that could damage casts or dressings; has self-adhering fasteners that provide rapid and easy placement and removal; reusable for many months; sizes include adult leg, adult short leg, adult arm, child leg/arm, and adult short arm

Source
Margue Company Inc. product information. Tucker, GA.

Shuttle-Relay suture passer

Description
suture passer designed to allow braided suture to be used in arthroscopic tissue repair procedures of shoulder or knee; used in conjunction with either a suture punch, suture hooks, or hollow needle

Source
Linvatec Corp. product information. Largo, FL.

sibutramine

Brand name
Meridia

Use
monoamine reuptake inhibitor used for long-term weight reduction treatment

Usual dosage
oral: 5 to 30 mg once daily

Pharmaceutical company
Knoll Pharmaceuticals. Whippany, NJ.

Source
University of Pittsburgh Drug Information and Pharmacoepidemiology Center. Pittsburgh, PA.

 Siemens Endo-P endorectal transducer

Description
multiplane, multifrequency imaging for high resolution, mid-range depth and high resolution imaging, and imaging deeper or enlarged structures and for general survey; transrectal and transperineal needle-guided tissue sampling and histologic analysis of the ultrasound findings

Source
Siemens Medical Systems, Inc. product information. Issaquah, WA.

 Sigma II hyperbaric system

Description
hyperbaric chamber with built-in breathing system that allows for ability to independently adjust each patient's oxygen supply

Source
Perry Baromedical product information. Riviera Beach, FL.

 SignaDRESS hydrocolloid dressing

Description
wound dressing with visual change indicator line to inform caregivers when dressing needs changed

Source
ConvaTec/Bristol-Myers Squibb Co. product information. Princeton, NJ.

signal-averaged electrocardiograph

Description
signal-averaged electrocardiographs are used to detect occult derangements of ventricular activation, or late potentials present during sinus rhythm that appear to be a hallmark for sustained ventricular arrhythmias

Source
Adapted from Cain M, Anderson J, Arnsdorf M, Mason J, Scheinman M, Waldo A. Signal-averaged electrocardiography. Journal of the American College of Cardiology 1996;27(1):238-249.

 ## Signature Edition infusion system

Description
leading infusion therapy; designed for use with IVAC 72 series administration sets

Source
IVAC Medical Systems Inc. product information. San Diego, CA.

 ## Sigosix

Generic name
see interleukin-6

 ## sildenafil

Brand name
Viagra

Use
treatment of male erectile dysfunction

Usual dosage
oral: studies used 10, 25, or 50 mg once daily or as needed basis, a single oral dose one hour or less before sexual activity

Pharmaceutical company
Pfizer Inc. New York, NY.

Source
Stadtlanders Managed Pharmacy Services. Pittsburgh, PA.

 ## Silhouette laser

Description
endoscopic facial laser allows finer, more precise surgery while significantly reducing intracavity bleeding; quicker healing; less trauma

Source
Cynosure Inc. product information. Bedford, MA.

silicone epistaxis catheter

Description

latex-free, AE-1970 epistaxis catheter 4.5-mm O.D., 9.7-cm L and 21-French and AE-1975 epistaxis catheter 5-mm O.D., 12-cm L and 22-French; cuffs do not adhere to nasal mucosa or clot formation; catheter's airway permits nasal breathing and access for suctioning

Source

Armstrong Medical Industries Inc. product information. Lincolnshire, IL and San Diego, CA.

 silicone textured mammary implant

Description

silicone gel-filled breast implant available in three different profiles, natural, moderate and high; available in 18 sizes from 60 cc to 600 cc

Source

Polytech-Silimed Europe GmbH product information. Dieburg, Germany.

 Silk Skin sheet

Description

advanced silicone treatment sheet that will conform to any body surface; softens scars and improves texture, color, and reduces thickness; used for treatment and prevention of scars

Source

IAT Medical Products Inc. product information. Glens Falls, NY.

 Silon silicone thermoplastic splinting (STS) material

Description

Silon-STS material used to fabricate transparent face-masks and other types of splints for the treatment of dermal scars resulting from burns, surgical incisions, and other types of trauma; applies both pressure and topical silicone therapy in one step; the polyfluorotetraethylene (PTFE) makes the composite strong and tough, while the silicone makes it soft and pliable and provides the desired therapeutic effects

Source

BioMed Sciences Inc. product information. Eden Prarie, MN.

Silon-TSR (temporary skin replacement)

Description

wound dressing following laser resurfacing or dermabrasion that creates a selective adhesive action; clings to the wound surface but does not integrate into the wound as healing occurs

Source

Bio Med Sciences Inc. product information. Bethlehem, PA.

 ## Silosheath

Description

below-the-knee gel liner laminated with tri-block polymer; absorbs body weight and shear forces that cause skin breakdown and blisters; elasticity and gentle compression for good anatomical fit; conforms around bony prominences; also called Silopad

Source

Silipos Advanced Polymer Technology product information. Niagara Falls, NY.

 ## Siloskin dressing

Description

sterile self-adhesive waterproof dressing; releases mineral oil gel onto skin to prevent infection; may be applied over sutured or scarred areas

Source

Silipos Inc. product information. Niagara Falls, NY.

 ## Sims Per-fit percutaneous tracheostomy kit

Description

designed to permit safe and rapid percutaneous insertion of a tracheostomy tube; system features two unique features including a custom-designed Portex tracheostomy tube and a straight obturator/dilator system

Source

Smiths Industries Medical Systems product information. Keene, NH.

 ## Simulect

Generic name

see basiliximab

simultaneous cannulation and needle-knife papillotomy using a large-channel duodenoscope

Description
a method of papillotomy whereby needle-knife sphincterotomy can be performed directly over the diagnostic cannula without use of catheter exchange over guidewire

Anatomy
common bile duct; duodenum; ampulla

Equipment
Wilson-Cook needle-knife papillotome; diagnostic cannula; manometry catheter; Olympus TJF100 duodenoscope

Source
Adapted from Banerjee B. Simultaneous cannulation and needle-knife papillotomy using a large-channel duodenoscope. Gastrointestinal Endoscopy 1996;44(2):189-190.

 single tooth root form implant

Description
use of surgical template, pilot osteotomy and abutment guide to evaluate labiolingual angulation and position of initial pilot osteotomy; pilot hole drilled into bone; implant placed 3 mm below crestal bone; osteotomy completed when position, projectory, and available space are satisfactory, thus effecting aesthetic improvement

Anatomy
incisal surface; crestal bone

Equipment
standard oral surgery equipment; surgical template, latch-type root canal reamer bur; abutment guide; pilot drill; vacuum former

Source
Adapted from Shepherd NJ, Morgan VJ, Chapman RJ. Angulation assessment of anterior single tooth root form implants: technical note. Implant Dentistry 1995;4:52-54.

 Singulair

Generic name
see montelukast

 Sintoclar

Generic name
see citicoline sodium

sinus lift osteotome

Description
an osteotome used in conjunction with the implant site dilator to enlarge the osteotomy site to the desired implant diameter and length; also used to perform the internal sinus lift procedure

Source
ACE Surgical Supply Company Inc. product information. Brockton, MA.

 sinus lift procedures and International Team Implantologists (ITI) implants

Description
insufficient bone height in lateral maxilla is frequent contraindication for oral implants; lack of vertebral dimension primarily caused by large maxillary sinuses; augmentation of floor of maxillary sinus creates adequate bone height for placement of endosseous implants

Anatomy
maxilla; maxillary sinus; floor of maxillary sinus

Equipment
ITI screw implants

Source
Adapted from Bruggenkate CM. Sinus lift procedures and ITI implants: results of a clinical study with 36 patients and 74 ITI implants. Implant Dentistry 1996;5:54.

 sirolimus

Brand name
Rapamune

Use
prevention of graft rejection in organ transplantation and for induction of disease remission in some autoimmune diseases

Usual dosage
oral: daily doses ranging from 0.5-5 mg/m^2/day have been used in clinical trials for the prevention of kidney transplant rejection

Pharmaceutical company
Wyeth-Ayerst Laboratories. Philadelphia, PA.

Source
Stadtlanders Managed Pharmacy Services. Pittsburgh, PA.

SJM X-Cell cardiac bioprosthesis

Description
cardiac porcine bioprosthesis uses a proprietary process to extract preserved porcine connective tissue cells in an attempt to interrupt the calcification cascade that leads to dysfunction; not yet available in United States

Source
St. Jude Medical Inc. product information. St. Paul, MN.

Skelid

Generic name
see tiludronate

Skinlight erbium yttrium-aluminum-garnet (YAG) laser

Description
YAG laser used for ablation, vaporization, and coagulation of skin tissue

Source
Candela Corp. product information. Wayland, MA.

SkinTech medical tattooing device

Description
plastic and reconstructive surgical tattooing device; used for facial scars, nipple-areola reconstruction, eyebrow reconstruction, vitiligo, and other abnormalities

Source
Mekka Medical Supplies product information. Elspeet, Holland.

Slick stylette endotracheal tube guide

Description
sterile Slick set endotracheal tube guides for adult, pediatric, and neonatal applications; low-friction coating eliminates need for lubrication; malleable stylette is adjustable to desired length or shape; ET-100 Slick stylette, ET-750 Pedilette small adult /child stylette, and ET-500 Pedilette pediatric/neonatal stylette

Source
Armstrong Medical Industries Inc. product information. Lincolnshire, IL and San Diego, CA.

slide agglutination test for *Mycobacterium tuberculosis*

Synonyms
MTB latex slide agglutination

Use
rapid diagnosis of infection with *Mycobacterium tuberculosis*

Method
agglutination reaction with immobilized antigens extracted from *Mycobacterium w*, which shares antigenic determinants with *Mycobacterium tuberculosis*

Specimen
serum

Normal range
no agglutination

Comments
may permit mass screening for pulmonary and extrapulmonary tuberculosis

Source
Adapted from Bhaskar S, Jain NK, Mukherjee R. Slide agglutination test for the diagnosis of pulmonary and extrapulmonary tuberculosis. Tuberculosis and Lung Diseases 1996;77:160-163.

 SlimLine cast boots

Description
used for fiberglass casts and has a dual rocker sole for ambulation with weatherproof upper

Source
Darco International Inc. product information. Huntington, WV.

 Slippery Slider

Description
patient Slippery Slider assists with safe movement of extremely large patients with minimal staffing requirements; flexible and ultra-smooth to ensure patient comfort; radiolucent for use during x-ray procedures, and chemical resistant; 3 models

Source
Armstrong Medical Industries Inc. product information. Lincolnshire, IL and San Diego, CA.

 Slow Fluoride

Generic name
see sodium fluoride

SLS Chromos long pulse ruby laser system

Description
hair removal laser system for treatment of unwanted body hair

Source
MEHL/Biophile International press release on Internet.

 SmartDose infusion system

Description
gives the flexibility to deliver medication from acute care to home care

Source
IVAC Corp. product information. San Diego, CA.

 Smart Scope

Description
digitally controlled microscope

Source
Moller Microsurgical product information. Waldwick, NJ.

 SmartSite needleless system

Description
reduces the chance of needle sticks; latex-free compliance

Source
IVAC Medical Systems product information. San Diego, CA.

 Smart System irrigation/suction system

Description
suction/irrigation system for laparoscopy that offers variable pressure up to 950 mmHg, digital display, automatic bottle switch over

Source
Leisegang Medical Inc. product information. Boca Raton, FL.

 Smart Trigger Bear 1000 ventilator

Description
critical care ventilator monitors both flow and pressure within 1 ventilator circuit; at the onset of patient effort, unit triggers on the fastest signal

Source
Allied Health Care Products product information. Riverside, CA.

SmiLine abutment system

Description
dental implants offering angulated abutment 17-degree giving an aesthetic cervical margin; MirusCone abutment allows for construction of fixed bridge restorations in areas with limited vertical height; fixture positioning guides provide for optimal fixture positioning

Source
Nobelpharma product information. Westmont, IL.

 ## Smirmaul nucleus extractor

Description
ophthalmic surgical instrument secures nucleus for atraumatic removal during extracapsular cataract extraction

Source
Visitec Co. product information. Sarasota, FL.

 ## snare beside-a-wire biliary stent exchange

Description
stent exchange technique; instead of cannulating the stent lumen with a guidewire, the bile duct itself is cannulated with a guidewire alongside the stent under fluoroscopic control; applying a snare beside-a-wire technique maintains access across the stricture and facilitates successful stent exchange

Anatomy
bile duct; biliary system

Equipment
standard sphincterotome equipment; sphincterotome cautery wire; Tracer-Wire guidewire with hydrophilic tip; standard polypectomy snare; standard endoscope equipment; rat-tooth forceps; standard snare equipment

Source
Adapted from Tarnasky PR, Morris J, Hawes RH, Hoffman BJ, Cotton PB, Cunningham JT. Snare beside-a-wire biliary stent exchange: a method that maintains access across biliary strictures. Gastrointestinal Endoscopy 1996;44(2):185-187.

 ## Snowden-Pencer insufflator

Description
computerized high-flow instrument for laparoscopic gynecological surgery; immediate venting of excess patient pressure and continuous monitoring of pressure; reduces chill effect of high-flow insufflation and scope fogging

Source
Snowden-Pencer Inc. product information. Tucker, GA.

526

 ## sodium benzoate/sodium phenylacetate

Brand name
Ammonilect

Use
treatment of hyperammonemia

Usual dosage
intravenous: 0.25-0.30 gm/kg/day

Pharmaceutical company
Ucyclyd Pharmaceuticals Inc. Atlanta, GA.

Source
Stadtlanders Managed Pharmacy Services. Pittsburgh, PA.

 ## sodium bicarbonate/sodium carbonate

Brand name
Carbicarb

Use
to correct metabolic acidosis associated with heart attack

Usual dosage
intravenous: an average of 1.277 mmol/dose as needed to correct metabolic acidosis or the dose can be calculated by using the following equation: (dose [mEq of Na] = base deficit [mEq/L] x 0.2 x body weight [kg])

Pharmaceutical company
International Medication Systems Limited. South El Monte, CA.

Source
Stadtlanders Managed Pharmacy Services. Pittsburgh, PA.

 ## sodium fluoride

Brand name
Slow Fluoride

Use
slow release of fluoride to strengthen bones in osteoporosis

Usual dosage
oral: 25 mg (with calcium citrate 400 mg twice daily)

Pharmaceutical company
Mission Pharmaceutical Co. San Antonio, TX.

Source
University of Pittsburgh Drug Information and Pharmacoepidemiology Center. Pittsburgh, PA.

sodium hyaluronate

Brand name
BioLon

Use
high-molecular-weight hyaluronic acid preparation; used to maintain intraocular pressure in the immediate and late postoperative phase following intraocular surgery, protecting corneal endothelium during intraocular surgery

Usual dosage
topical: 1% solution, apply weekly to the eye(s) after surgery

Pharmaceutical company
BioTechnology General Corp. Iselin, NJ.

Source
Stadtlanders Managed Pharmacy Services. Pittsburgh, PA.

 sodium phenylbutyrate

Brand name
Buphenyl

Use
hyperammonemia agent; for management of chronic urea cycle disorders

Usual dosage
oral: 20 gm/day

Pharmaceutical company
Ucyclyd Pharmaceuticals Inc. Atlanta, GA.

Source
Stadtlanders Managed Pharmacy Services. Pittsburgh, PA.

 sodium sulfacetamide

Brand name
Klaron

Use
an alcohol-free topical lotion for the treatment of acne vulgaris in patients with sensitive skin

Usual dosage
topical: 10% lotion applied as a thin film to the affected area(s) twice a day

Pharmaceutical company
Dermik Laboratories Inc. Collegeville, PA.

Source
Stadtlanders Managed Pharmacy Services. Pittsburgh, PA.

sodium tetradecyl sulfate

Brand Name
Sotradecol

Use
sclerosing agent used in the treatment of bleeding esophageal varices, orphan indication

Usual Dosage
injectable: 1% to 3%, depending on the size of the lesion, has been used in clinical trials

Pharmaceutical company
Whitehall Labs Division of American Home Products Corp. Madison, NJ.

Source
University of Pittsburgh Drug Information and Pharmacoepidemiology Center. Pittsburgh, PA.

 Sof Matt pressure relieving mattress

Description
powered low-air-loss mattress; benefits include alternating cells providing effective pressure relief, adjustable control, helping to reduce heat and moisture buildup on the patient's skin

Source
Gaymar Industries Inc. product information. Orchard Park, NY.

 Sofsorb dressing

Description
nonadherent, highly absorbent wound dressing with a stay-dry liner to prevent maceration of the periwound skin; has exceptional wet and dry strength so it can be soaked with saline or topical agents

Source
DeRoyal Industries Inc. product information. Powell, TN.

 SoftLight laser

Description
target-specific laser hair removal system

Source
ThermoLase Corp. product information. San Diego, CA.

SofTouch device

Description
vacuum erection device; nonpermanent and noninvasive solution for impotence

Source
Mission Pharmacal Co. product information. San Antonio, TX.

 ## SOLEutions custom orthosis

Description
features seven orthotic styles including Rigid, Sport, Women's Fashion, Men's Fashion, Casual Dress, Accommodative, and Basic; other orthotics include SOLEutions Prefabs and SOLEutions Sport Shell

Source
STJ Orthotic Services Inc. product information. Ridgewood, NY.

 ## Solitens transcutaneous electrical nerve stimulation (TENS) unit

Description
hand-held adjustable battery-powered TENS unit; symptomatic relief of acute postsurgical and post-traumatic pain and chronic intractable pain

Source
MedTech Group Inc. product information. Plainfield, NJ.

 ## Soll suture and incision marker

Description
ophthalmic instrument used for cataract, secondary intraocular lens, and other anterior segment procedures requiring incisions into the anterior chamber

Source
Visitec Co. product information. Sarasota, FL.

 ## Somagard

Generic Name
see deslorelin

530

 somatomedin C (IGF-1)

Brand Name
Myotrophin

Use
biosynthetic insulin-like growth factor I (IGF-1) used in the therapy of amyotrophic lateral sclerosis (ALS/Lou Gehrig disease), orphan indication

Usual Dosage
injection: 0.05 mg/kg to 0.1 mg/kg daily

Pharmaceutical company
Cephalon Inc. West Chester, PA.

Source
University of Pittsburgh Drug Information and Pharmacoepidemiology Center. Pittsburgh, PA.

 somatropin

Brand name
Bio-Tropin

Use
recombinant human growth hormone product for the long-term treatment of children who have growth failure due to an inadequate secretion of normal endogenous growth hormone

Usual dosage
injectable supplied in vials of 4.8 mg lyophilized drug with a 10-mg vial of bacteriostatic 0.9% sodium chloride for injection: 0.1 mg/kg of body weight injected subcutaneously three times weekly

Pharmaceutical company
Abbott Lab. Abbott Park, IL.

Source
University of Pittsburgh Drug Information and Pharmacoepidemiology Center. Pittsburgh, PA.

 somatropin (rDNA origin) for injection

Brand name
Genotropin

Use
polypeptide hormone of recombinant DNA origin used in long-term treatment of children who have growth failure due to an inadequate secretion of endogenous growth hormone

Usual dosage
subcutaneous: 1.3 mg/ml or 5 mg/ml strength solutions supplied in an IntraMix two-chamber cartridge with 1.5 mg and 5.8 mg somatropin cartridges to be reconstituted with diluent in the attached chamber; dosage must be adjusted for each patient; generally a dose of 0.16 to 0.24 mg/kg body weight per week is recommended with the weekly dose being divided into 6 to 7 injections

Pharmaceutical company
Pharmacia Inc. Columbus, OH.

Source
University of Pittsburgh Drug Information and Pharmacoepidemiology Center. Pittsburgh, PA.

 Sonablate system

Description
transrectal probe (Sonablate-2000) that provides imaging for tissue targeting and high-intensity focused ultrasound (HIFU) for tissue ablation; HIFU results in thermally-induced coagulative necrosis only in intraprostatic tissue, without affecting intervening tissue; during the process, updated ultrasound images allow confirmation of targeting accuracy

Source
FOCUS Surgery product information. Fremont, CA.

 sonicated vascular catheter-tip culture

Synonyms
sonicated catheter-tip culture

Use
diagnosis of suspected catheter-related sepsis

Method
sonication of catheter tip in nutrient broth; followed by solid-agar culture of broth

Normal range
<1,000 CFU in catheter sonication broth

Comments
a more useful test than either conventional catheter culture methods or cytocentrifuge Gram stain

Source
Adapted from Kelly M, Wunderlich Wciorka LR, McConico S, Peterson LR. Sonicated vascular catheter tip cultures: quantitative association with catheter-related sepsis and the non-utility of an adjuvant cytocentrifuge Gram stain. American Journal of Clinical Pathology 1996;105:210-215.

 Sonicath imaging catheter

Description
catheter-based ultrasound transducer used with Diasonics interventional ultrasound system; produces a 360-degree cross-sectional view of vessel size, anatomy, and plaque morphology from inside the lumen; designed to provide access to coronary arteries, peripheral vascular system and urologic structures

Source
Diasonics Ultrasound product information. Milpitas, CA.

532

 sonohysterography

Synonyms
none

Indications
detection of intrauterine pathology

Method
sterile normal saline inserted into uterine cavity through French catheter; ultrasound probe inserted vaginally

Comments
minimally invasive; less expensive alternative to hysteroscopy

Source
Adapted from Jancin B. Sonohysterography quick and minimally invasive. Ob.Gyn. News 1996;31:13.

 Sonopsy biopsy system

Description
ultrasound-guided breast biopsy system with three-dimensional imaging that can be compared with x-ray mammogram

Source
NeoVision Corp. product information. Seattle, WA.

 Sono-Stat Plus sound device

Description
combination sonography and electromyography device for capturing temporomandibular joint (TMJ) sounds; computer memory permanently stores them for replay; documents muscle activity, both at rest and in function

Source
Myo-Tronics Inc. product information. Tukwila, WA.

 Sophy mini pressure valve

Description
small programmable implantable valve to monitor cerebrospinal fluid pressure

Source
Sophysa product information. Orsay, France.

 Soriatane

Generic Name
see acitretin

sorivudine

Brand Name
Bravavir

Use
antiviral used in the treatment of herpes simplex virus

Usual Dosage
oral: 40 mg once daily was used in clinical trials

Pharmaceutical company
Bristol-Myers Squibb Company. Princeton, NJ.

Source
University of Pittsburgh Drug Information and Pharmacoepidemiology Center. Pittsburgh, PA.

 ## Sotradecol

Generic Name
see sodium tetradecyl sulfate

 ## Soules intrauterine insemination catheter

Description
catheter, 25-cm long, that has been innovatively used for fluid instillation into uterus allowing diagnostic enhancement when performing sonography

Source
Cook OB/GYN product information. Indianapolis, IN.

 ## Spanidin

Generic name
see deoxyspergualin

 ## sparfloxacin

Brand name
Zagam

Use
fluoroquinolone antibiotic being studied for the treatment of community-acquired infections and respiratory tract infections

Usual dosage
oral: doses of 200 to 400 mg daily have been used in clinical trials

Pharmaceutical company
Rhone-Poulenc Rorer Pharmaceuticals Inc. Collegeville, PA.

Source
University of Pittsburgh Drug Information and Pharmacoepidemiology Center. Pittsburgh, PA.

Spectra-System abutments

Description
1-degree tapered hex for friction-fit, which eliminates the 4 to 9 degrees of rotational wobble reported with external hex dental implants
Source
Dentsply Implant product information. Encino, CA.

 Spectra-System implants

Description
dental implants with internal hex-thread connection; provides three times the interdigitation of external hex and internal octagon implants
Source
Dentsply Implant product information. Encino, CA.

 Spectrum ruby laser

Description
Spectrum Q-switched ruby laser for removing cutaneous lesions, tattoos, and pigmented lesions with few side-effects and cross-contamination
Source
Spectrum Medical Technologies Inc. product information. Natick, MA.

 SpeedReducer instrument

Description
high-speed instrumentation that offers the benefit of a mechanical stop perforator in using the Black Max high-speed drill system
Source
The Anspach Co. product information. Palm Beach Gardens, FL.

 Spetzler lumbar-peritoneal shunt

Description
extracranial one-piece lumbar-peritoneal shunt; eliminates further invasion of a compromised brain and ventricular system; used for communicating hydrocephalus and suspected normal pressure hydrocephalus
Source
Heyer-Schulte NeuroCare product information. Pleasant Prairie, WI.

 Spexil

Generic name
see trospectomycin sulfate

SpF-XL stimulator

Description
spinal fusion extra level (SpF-XL) stimulator is a totally implantable spinal device; treats up to five-level fusions with one adjunct; specifically designed leads help treat extra-level fusions; stimulates bone growth as soon as implanted

Source
Electro-Biology Inc. product information. Parsippany, NJ.

 SpinaLase neodymium:yytrium-aluminum-garnet (Nd:YAG) surgical laser system

Description
surgical laser instrument for percutaneous laser disc decompression (PLDD)

Source
Heraeus Surgical Inc. product information. Milpitas, CA.

 Spine-Power belt

Description
intertrochanteric support device that allows healing of sacral/ilium ligamentous structure; made from Spinalon material; worn 2 inches below the tip of the iliac crest; protects back from stress/strain while working or exercising; effective means of relieving back pain; may be used by women following childbirth for stabilizing and returning the stretched pelvis ligaments back to normal

Source
Leander Health Technologies Corp. product information. Port Orchard, WA.

 Spiral Mark V portable ultrasonic drug inhaler

Description
compact, portable nebulizer; temperature controlled to protect the integrity of medication; Airflow-Assist simplifies treatments to small children; bacteria-free air; heated mist; large capacity vial with electronics which monitors the patient's demand and the unit's fluid level

Source
Medisonic U.S.A. Inc. product information. Clarence, NY.

spiral *Salmonella* assay

Synonyms
spiral Ames assay

Use
evaluation of potentially mutagenic agents

Method
bacterial growth measurement following metabolic activation in presence of varying doses of test compound

Specimen
drug of interest

Normal range
no evidence of mutagenicity

Comments
a simplified, automated approach to bacterial mutagenicity testing, with greater sensitivity than the standard pour-plate method

Source
Adapted from Diehl M, Fort F. Spiral *Salmonella* assay: validation against the standard pour-plate assay. Environmental Molecular Mutagenesis 1996;27:227-236.

 spirapril hydrochloride

Brand name
Renormax

Use
angiotensin-converting enzyme inhibitor used in the treatment of hypertension

Usual dosage
oral: 3, 6, 12, and 24 mg tablets; starting dose 12 mg daily in 1 or 2 divided doses; increases made at 2- to 4-week intervals according to response; most patients will eventually require 24 mg for adequate blood pressure control

Pharmaceutical company
Sandoz Pharmaceuticals Corp. East Hanover, NJ.

Source
University of Pittsburgh Drug Information and Pharmacoepidemiology Center. Pittsburgh, PA.

 Spirolite 201 spirometer

Description
instrument affording wide choice of lung function measurements; best efforts are determined and compared to predicted normal values for rendering a possible diagnosis; features automatic best test selection

Source
Medical Systems Corp. product information. Greenvale, NY.

Spirosense system

Description
in-office alternative to stand-alone spirometry systems with PC (personal computer) compatible software; hand-held flow sensor

Source
Burdick Inc. product information. Milton, WI.

 splenic microanatomical localization of lymphoma and leukemia

Synonyms
none

Indications
small lymphocytic lymphoma (SLL) and chronic lymphocytic leukemia (CLL) were considered together because of their cytology and indistinguishable pattern in the lymph node and spleen

Method
novel silver nitrate immunoperoxidase (SNIP) double-staining technique; Gordon and Sweet reticulin stain followed by immunoperoxidase staining for B-lineage marker using avidin-biotin

Normal findings
features identified by SNIP found only in SLL/CLL, but not in reactive lymphoid hyperplasia (RLH) or traumatized spleens, were trabecular infiltration and prominent sinus involvement

Comments
the spleen is highly compartmentalized, and many techniques have been used to study different aspects of splenic microanatomy

Source
Adapted from Edelman M, Evans L, Zee S, Gnass R, Ratech H. Splenic microanatomical localization of small lymphocytic lymphoma/chronic lymphocytic leukemia using a novel combined silver nitrate and immunoperoxidase technique. American Journal of Surgical Pathology 1997;21:445-451.

 Spline dental implant system

Description
dental implants available in cylinders and screws; precise fit reduces micro-movement of implant

Source
Calcitek product information. Carlsbad, CA.

 Sporanox

Generic name
see itraconazole

SporTX pulsed direct current stimulator

Description
palm-sized battery powered stimulator for first and second degree athletic injuries; promotes relief through increased circulation
Source
Staodyn Inc. product information. Longmont, CO.

 ## Sprotte spinal and epidural needles

Description
regional anesthesia device; pencil-point tip is designed to separate dural fibers instead of cutting, reducing the risk of post dural puncture headache; 90-mm length; 17 and 18 gauges
Source
Rusch Inc. product information. Duluth, GA.

 ## Stableloc II external fixator system

Description
lightweight, radiolucent fixator with threaded guide pins for correction of Colles fractures and distal radial osteotomies
Source
Acumed product information web site.

 ## StaphVAX

Generic Name
see *Staphylococcus aureus* vaccine

 ## *Staphylococcus aureus* typing by nested PCR ribosomal DNA amplification

Synonyms
nested PCR *Staphylococcus aureus* typing
Use
identification and typing of *Staphylococcus aureus* subspecies
Method
nested polymerase chain reaction with universal primers, followed by *Staphylococcus aureus*-specific primers
Specimen
bacterial culture specimen
Normal range
negative

Comments
useful in clinical epidemiologic studies of *Staphylococcus aureus* infection

Source
Adapted from Saruta K, Matsunaga T, Kono M, et al. Rapid identification and typing of *Staphylococcus aureus* by nested PCR amplified ribosomal DNA spacer region. FEMS Microbiology Letters 1997;146:271-278.

 Staphylococcus aureus vaccine

Brand Name
StaphVAX

Use
bivalent polysaccharide-protein conjugate vaccine for prevention of *Staphylococcus aureus* infections in patients with end-stage renal disease

Usual Dosage
intramuscular: clinical trials showed efficacy at 25 µg immunizing dose, but higher doses of 37 to 100 µg are being tested for possible extended response

Pharmaceutical company
Univax Biologics Inc. Rockville, MD.

Source
University of Pittsburgh Drug Information and Pharmacoepidemiology Center. Pittsburgh, PA.

 star enterocystoplasty

Description
a modification of sagittal cystoplasty that reconfigures the neuropathic bladder; star modification incorporates lateral cystotomies with anteroposterior cystotomy to defunctionalize any potential noncompliant hyperreflexic tendencies inherent to the neuropathic bladder before augmentation and increases the linear length of the edge available for anastomosis of bowel to bladder

Anatomy
bladder area; bladder; ileum; ileocecal segment; rectus and transversalis fascia; ureter; dome; bladder neck; trigone; detrusor; ureterovesical junction; stoma

Equipment
standard surgical, polyglycolic acid suture

Source
Adapted from Keating MA, Ludlow JK, Rich MA. Enterocystoplasty: the star modification. Journal of Urology 1996;155:1723-1725.

 STAR*LOCK multi-purpose submergible threaded implant

Description
dental implant that is radiofrequency plasma glow-discharged and gamma sterilized; anti-lock rotation on a 15-degree or 25-degree angled and straight abutment for removable restoration

Source
Park Dental Research Corp. product information. New York, NY.

540

 ## Stat-Temp II & WR (wide range)

Description
continuous display of patient's current body temperature; provides a measure of protection in alerting anesthesia to a potential problem when sudden temperature changes occur; circular shape accommodates blood flow areas on the forehead, temple, behind the ear, over the heart and along the limbs; from 95°F to 107°F or 35°C to 42°C

Source
Trademark Medical product information. Fenton, MO.

 ## stavudine

Brand name
Zerit

Use
antiretroviral agent used to treat HIV-infected adult patients who are intolerant or resistant to other approved antiretroviral agents such as zidovudine, didanosine, or zalcitabine

Usual dosage
oral: starting dose 30 mg twice daily for adults under 60 kg; 40 mg twice daily for adults over 60 kg; dosage adjustment required in patients with renal failure

Pharmaceutical company
Bristol-Meyers Squibb Co. Princeton, NJ.

Source
University of Pittsburgh Drug Information and Pharmacoepidemiology Center. Pittsburgh, PA.

 ## StealthStation image-guided system

Description
frameless stereotactic surgery LED image-guided tracking system that can be secured to the cranium by two small screws; freehand localization and real-time navigation technology

Source
Sofamor Danek Group Inc, Memphis, TN and adapted from Vrionis FD, Foley KT, Robertson JH, Shea JJ III. Use of cranial surface anatomic fiducials for interactive image-guided navigation in the temporal bone: a cadaveric study. Neurosurgery 1997;40:755-764.

Steiner electromechanical morcellator

Description
facilitates removal of relatively large sections of tissue; consists of a motor-driven cutting cannula that can be inserted directly into the peritoneal cavity or introduced through a standard trocar; tissue is morcellated and removed by applying uniform traction and varying the speed and direction of the cannula's rotation

Source
Karl Storz Endoscopy-America Inc. product information. Culver City, CA.

 ## Stellbrink fixation device

Description
fixation device consists of two threaded bars, eight wire blocks, and four K-wires; for external finger fixation, distraction of digits, joint arthrodesis, and osteotomy

Source
Link America Inc. product information. Denville, NJ.

 ## Step device

Description
device that has a radially expandable sleeve that fits over a Veress needle; the device uses a blunt dilator/cannula to expand the tract made by the needle, splitting each layer of tissue along the path of least resistance

Source
InnerDyne product information. Sunnyvale, CA.

 ## stereotactic microsurgical craniotomy

Description
microsurgical technique modification of transcortical approach for resection of colloid cyst in third ventricle; less operative time than standard craniotomy

Anatomy
third ventricle; lateral ventricle; foramen of Monro; coronal suture; dura; gyrus; gyral crest; sulcus; septum pellucidum

Equipment
Leksell model G stereotactic head frame; Mayfield adapter; Leksell arc; stereotactic retractor; stereotactic blunt probe; Apfelbaum retractor; obturator; operating microscope; cylindrical retractor; ventricular catheter

Source
Adapted from Cabbell KL, Ross DA. Stereotactic microsurgical craniotomy for the treatment of third ventricular colloid cysts. Neurosurgery 1996;38:301-307.

Steri-Dent dry heat sterilizer

Description
instrument sterilizing machine that does not dull sharp instruments or cause rust or corrosion

Source
Steri-Dent Corp. product information. Holbrook, NY.

Steri-Oss Hexlock implant

Description
external hexagonal extension threaded dental implant

Source
Steri-Oss product information. Yorba Linda, CA.

Steri-Oss implant system

Description
titanium screw type endo-osseous dental implants; clinically versatile system

Source
Bausch & Lomb Inc. product information. Rochester, NY.

STERIS endoscope leakage tester

Description
instrument used to confirm the watertight integrity of flexible endoscopes before immersion into reprocessing fluids

Source
STERIS Corp. product information. Mentor, OH.

Stetho-Dop stethoscope

Description
stethoscope adding Doppler technology by utilizing multiple heads for standard evaluation of sound as well as blood flow sensors

Source
Imex Medical Systems product information. Golden, CO.

Stiegmann-Goff Clearvue ligator

Description
endoscopic surgical cylinder ligator; application of an "o" ring obliterates esophageal varices by process of necrosis; minimizes potential for esophageal stricture or deep ulcers

Source
CR Bard Inc. product information. Tewksbury, MA.

 ## St. Jude medical heart valve Hemodynamic Plus (HP) series

Description
mechanical heart valve for patients requiring aortic prosthesis; particularly well suited for small aortic annulus; valve design places the sewing cuff above the annulus while keeping the pyrolytic carbon orifice within the annulus

Source
St. Jude Medical Inc. product information. St. Paul, MN.

 ## Stonetome stone removal device

Description
sphincterotomy and stone removal in a single pass; recanalization not necessary

Source
Boston Scientific Corp. product information. Boston, MA.

 ## Storz multifunction valve trocar/cannula system

Description
allows rapid, easy insertion of instrument with significant gas loss during endoscopy; cannula valve opens manually by finger pressure or automatically using a blunt instrument

Source
Karl Storz Endoscopy product information. Culver City, CA

 ## Storz rhinomanometer

Description
diagnostic meter used to measure the airflow through a nonoccluded nostril

Source
Storz Instrument Co. product information. St. Louis, MO.

Strasbourg-Fairfax in vitro fertilization needle

Description
uniquely designed needle for transvaginal, sonographically guided oocyte retrieval through follicle aspiration; alternative to laparoscopy

Source
Accurate Surgical & Scientific Instruments Corp. product information. Westbury, NY.

Strata hip system

Description
surgical hip prosthesis that in one fluid motion allows insertion, alignment, and pressurization

Source
Howmedica Inc. product information. Rutherford, NJ.

Stratus impact reducing pylon

Description
used with a prosthesis; a step up in comfort even stepping down; absorbs the jolt of every step, reducing trauma to the residual limb; amputees can walk, stand, shop, and work longer

Source
Ohio Willow Wood Co. product information. Mt. Sterling, OH.

Stress Echo bed

Description
specially designed bed for stress echocardiography studies; drop section (acoustical window) which increases image quality by bringing the apex closer to the chest wall; transects the true apex with proper positioning of patient

Source
American Echo Inc. product information. Kansas City, MO.

Stretch Net dressing

Description
tubular elastic dressing; used for patients with fragile skin, who are allergic to tape, and who require frequent dressing changes

Source
DeRoyal Industries Inc. product information. Powell, TN.

Stride cardiac pacemaker

Description
implantable, dual-chamber multiprogrammable cardiac pulse generator; designed to provide rate-adaptive pacing sequentially to the atrium and ventricle; specifically indicated for treatment of conduction disorders

Source
Intermedics Inc. product information. Angleton, TX.

Stromectol

Generic name
see ivermectin
▶ *Mectizan trade name is used outside of the U.S.*

Stronghands hand exerciser

Description
hand exerciser with variable resistance for each finger

Source
HDS Inc. product information. Bolingbrook, IL.

subpectoral implantation of cardioverter defibrillator

Description
Medtronic Jewel pacer-cardioverter-defibrillator (PCD) is a small-size implantable cardioverter-defibrillator (ICD); a technique for the subpectoral implantation has been successful; small infraclavicular incision made; defibrillator leads placed using a modified Seldinger technique into subclavian vein under fluoroscopic guidance; pulse generator positioned beneath pectoralis muscle; final electrophysiologic testing performed to verify device function

Anatomy
anterior thorax; areolar complex; infraclavicular area; inframammary crease; latissimus dorsi muscle; left hemithorax; pectoralis fascia and muscle; subclavian vein; serratus anterior muscle

Equipment
standard cardiovascular surgery equipment; Medtronic Jewel PCD

Source
Adapted from Eastman DP, Selle JG, Reames MK. Technique for subpectoral implantation of cardioverter defibrillators. Journal of American College of Surgeons 1995;181:475-476.

subscapularis tendon transfer

Description

massive tears of the rotator cuff that were not suited to direct tendon-to-bone or tendon-to-tendon repair were reconstructed; repair consisted of transfer of subscapularis tendon in conjunction with subacromial decompression; anterior acromioplasty and resection of coracoacromial ligament was also done; dissection of the subscapularis muscle is made easier by the fact that it receives its innervation from the superior and inferior subscapular nerves; the muscle can be divided for a short distance without substantial risk of loss of function

Anatomy

acromioclavicular joint; subacromial space; bicipital groove; coracoacromial, coracoclavicular, and coracohumeral ligaments; glenohumeral joint; infraspinatus fossa; lesser tuberosity of humerus; raphe; rotator cuff; suprascapular neurovascular pedicle; teres minor

Equipment

standard orthopaedic surgery equipment

Source

Adapted from Karas SE, Giachello TL. Subscapularis transfer for reconstruction of massive tears of the rotator cuff. The Journal of Bone and Joint Surgery 1996;78-A:239-244.

 sub-Tenon anesthesia cannula

Description

ophthalmic anesthesia curved instrument to ensure delivery of anesthetic solution to the posterior sub-Tenon space; technique provides anesthesia for cataract, corneal, vitreoretinal, trabeculectomy and strabismus procedures

Source

Visitec product information. Sarasota, FL.

 subxiphoid laparoscopic approach for resection of mediastinal parathyroid adenoma

Description

symptomatic primary hyperthyroidism is treated by surgical resection; a high percentage will have a solitary parathyroid tumor; a new technique is reported for resection of ectopic parathyroid adenomas after radiologic localization, a minimally invasive subxiphoid laparoscopic approach; Tc-99m sestamibi is used for improved localization of parathyroid adenomas

Anatomy

anterior cervical area; carotid sheath; embryologic descent of parathyroid glands; fourth branchial pouch; innominate vein; internal mammary vein; inferior mediastinal space; lymph nodes; mediastinum; pericardial fat pad; parathyroid tissue; pleura; retroesophageal space; sternum; subxiphoid area; third branchial pouch; thymic tissue; thyroid gland; superior submanubrial area; suprasternal notch

Equipment
Allis clamp; blunt dissector; cannula; angled endoscope; fiberoptic instruments; end-view laparoscope; grasper; irrigating solution; sternal retractor; suction-irrigation instrument; 18 French straight mediastinal tube

Source
Adapted from Wei JP, Gadacz TR, Weisner LF, Burke GJ. The subxiphoid laparoscopic approach for resection of mediastinal parathyroid adenoma after successful localization with Tc-99m sestamibi radionuclide scan. Surgical Laparoscopy and Endoscopy 1995;5:402-406.

suction sclerotherapy

Description
a hybrid of band ligation and sclerotherapy; does not require an overtube and may minimize local complications of sclerotherapy; ethanolamine is used as the injection material

Anatomy
gastroesophageal junction; esophagus

Equipment
Olympus GIF-100 endoscope; Bard Interventional friction fit adaptor; sclerotherapy needle

Source
Adapted from Blackard WG, Marks RD, Baron TH. Suction sclerotherapy for the treatment of esophageal varices. Gastrointestinal Endoscopy 1996;44(6):725-728.

Sugita multipurpose head frame

Description
device designed specifically for microneurosurgery; angle of head of patient easily adjusted during surgery without disturbing brain retractor system

Source
Mizuho America Inc. product information. Beverly, MA.

Sular

Generic name
see nisoldipine

sulfatide antibody

Synonyms
none

Use
sulfatide is the major acidic glycosphingolipid in myelin; antibodies to sulfatide are primarily associated with sensory neuropathies but may also be detected in patients with Guillain-Barré syndrome, chronic inflammatory demyelinating polyradiculoneuropathy, and in some patients with sensorimotor peripheral neuropathy

Method
enzyme-linked immunosorbent assay (ELISA)

Specimen
blood

Normal range
IgG: less than 1:100; IgM: 1:800

Comment
IgG antibodies to sulfatide are typically polyclonal, whereas IgM antibodies may be present as either polyclonal or monoclonal protein. Up to 50% of patients with sulfatide antibodies will also have myelin-associated glycoprotein (MAG) antibodies

Source
Lexi-Comp Inc. database. Hudson, OH.

 ## Sullivan III nasal continuous positive air pressure (CPAP) device

Description
specifically designed to improve patient compliance; lightweight and portable with disposable foam mask insert that traps patient's heat and moisture and returns it with the next inspired breath for occasional humidification or when travelling to reduce nasal dryness, sore throat, and sinus problems associated with CPAP therapy

Source
ResCare Inc. product information. San Diego, CA.

 ## Sullivan nasal variable positive airway pressure (VPAP) unit

Description
variable positive airway pressure (VPAP) unit senses when patient breathes in and out and adjusts pressure accordingly; unit automatically starts when patient puts mask on and stops when patient takes it off; bi-level device in unit provides a delay timer allowing patient to fall asleep before receiving full pressure; also Sullivan VPAP II

Source
Rescare Inc. product information. San Diego, CA.

 ## Sully shoulder stabilizer brace

Description
immobilizes and stabilizes anterior instabilities, multi-directional instabilities, inferior instabilities, posterior instabilities, rotator cuff deceleration, shoulder separations, and pectoralis muscle strains

Source
Saunders Group product information. Chaska, MN.

sumatriptan

Brand name
Imitrex

Use
intranasal formulation for the treatment of migraine headaches

Usual dosage
intranasal: doses of 5, 10, or 20 mg intranasally at the onset of migraine attacts were studied in the clinical trials

Pharmaceutical company
Glaxo Wellcome Inc. Research Triangle Park, NC.

Source
Stadtlanders Managed Pharmacy Services. Pittsburgh, PA.

 Super ArrowFlex sheath

Description
polyurethane-wrapped stainless steel wire coil extends the entire length of the sheath allowing it to flex in any direction without kinking or collapsing; for angioplasty catheters and vascular stents; post-percutaneous transluminal coronary angioplasty (PTCA) patients can sit up at a 60-degree angle with sheath in place

Source
Arrow International product information. Reading, PA.

 Super* ClearPro suction socket

Description
dual-durometer liner as well as silicone suction socket; aluminum distal umbrella for locking devices and suspension systems; transparent elastic proximal region provides comfort and easy monitoring of socket pressure and tension; sizes 14 cm-44 cm

Source
ALPS South Corp. product information. St. Petersburg, FL.

 superficial liposculpture

Description
body contouring procedure where more superficial layers of fat beneath the intact dermis are removed in order to achieve skin retraction; also known as subdermal liposculpture; primarily used in facial and neck areas

Anatomy
preauricular region; nasolabial fold; labial commissure; submental region; forehead

Equipment

Texas cannula or other blunt-end cannula with a single aperture at the tip bisected by a curved septum or bridge; scalpel

Source

Adapted from Goodstein WA. Superficial liposculpture of the face and neck. Plastic and Reconstructive Surgery 1996;98:988-996.

superior oblique muscle and trochlear luxation

Description

superior oblique luxation and trochlear luxation have been used as new procedures for acquired Brown syndrome, and superior oblique muscle overaction; these two procedures have been developed to weaken the superior oblique muscle by inactivating the trochlea; the superior oblique tendon fibers are relaxed ("desagittalization") without changing the tendon insertion in relation to the equator; this is an advantage over the superior oblique muscle recession

Anatomy

anteronasal area; bony orbit; cartilaginous trochlear saddle; equator; inferior oblique muscle; levator, lateral rectus, medial rectus, and orbicularis muscles; periosteum; superior orbital margin; subperiosteal space; superior oblique tendon; superior oblique muscle; trochlea; trochlear fossa

Equipment

standard ophthalmic surgery equipment; cyclophorometer of Franceschetti (Maddox rod graded in degrees and equipped with a spirit level); muscle hook; periosteal elevator; silicone; viscoelastic product

Source

Adapted from Mombaerts I, Koornneef L, Everhard-Halm Y, Hughes DS, Wenniger-Prick, LJJ. Superior oblique luxation and trochlear luxation as new concepts in superior oblique muscle weakening surgery. American Journal of Ophthalmology 1995;120:83-91.

Super "M" vacuum extractor cup

Description

soft polyethylene flexible cup; fits over infant's scalp for vacuum extraction delivery

Source

Mityvac Obstetrical product information. Rancho Cucamonga, CA.

Super punctum plug

Description

tapered-shaft punctum plug; easy insertion and plug retention; holds securely in the punctum; soft and flesh-like and can be easily monitored and removed

Source

Eagle Vision product information. Memphis, TN.

SuperSkin thin film dressing

Description
liquid skin sealant that cures upon application to unbroken skin; strengthens natural skin integrity; dries in seconds; can last 24-36 hours

Source
MedLogic Global Corp. product information. Colorado Springs, CO.

 SupraFoley suprapubic introducer

Description
suprapubic introducer with bevelled sheath; any Foley catheter of correct gauge can be inserted down the peel-off sheath

Source
Rusch Inc. product information. Duluth, GA.

 sural island flap for foot and ankle reconstruction

Description
one-stage operative procedure with creation of a distally based flap to cover medium to large soft tissue defects in the distal leg or foot; the distally based flap has an excellent vascular supply, reducing the possibility of nonviability

Anatomy
foot; lateral malleolus; medial malleolus; Achilles tendon; sural nerve

Equipment
standard orthopaedic instruments

Source
Adapted from Jeng S, Wei F. Distally based sural island flap for foot and ankle reconstruction. Plastic and Reconstructive Surgery 1997;99:744-750.

 Sure-Closure skin stretching system

Description
unique combination of needles and controls distribute tension and relax skin; used for primary closure of skin deficit wounds that previously required grafts or flaps

Source
MedChem Products Inc. product information. Woburn, MA.

 SurePress high compression bandage

Description
reusable, lightweight, durable bandages with visual application guides to ensure appropriate compression

Source
ConvaTec product information. Princeton, NJ.

SureScan system

Description

scanning system for cosmetic skin resurfacing that reduces erythema and scarring

Source

Luxar Corporation product information. Seattle, WA.

 SureStep glucose meter

Description

easy to use glucose meter (glucometer) designed for diabetics who also suffer from physical limitations such as vision and dexterity problems, inexperienced testers, and children; indicates adequate blood on the strip before they test

Source

LifeScan Inc. product information. Milpitas, CA.

 Sur-Fit Natura pouch

Description

drainable and closed-end ostomy pouch with exclusive flange design with an audible clicking system that ensures the user of a secure, accurate closure; the body-side wafer features a low-profile design incorporating rounded and contoured edges and unique flange attachment for greater comfort and security; double-sided comfort panels designed to provide softer, quieter wear

Source

Bristol-Myers Squibb Co. product information. Princeton, NJ.

 Surgica K6 laser

Description

HGM EDO laser technology; 100-watt continuous-wave Nd:YAG laser; contact tip or free beam with exposure pulse modes of auto repeat, single pulse, and continuous; exposure times from 0.1 to 60 seconds as well as continuous

Source

HGM product information. Salt Lake City, UT.

 Surgicraft Copeland fetal scalp electrode

Description

fetal scalp electrode designed to instantly and continuously monitor fetal distress

Source

Accurate Surgical Instruments Corp. product information. Westbury, NY.

Surgicutt incision device

Description
automated skin-incision device for collecting small blood samples; used in neonatal units, blood banks, and laboratories

Source
Thermo Electron product information. Waltham, MA.

 ## SurgiFish viscera retainer

Description
patented viscera retainer that protects the bowel from injury and promotes easy closure of the peritoneal cavity; one size; imprinted with contour lines for easy cutting

Source
Greer Medical product information. Santa Barbara, CA.

 ## Surgilast tubular elastic dressing

Description
retainer holds primary dressings in place; it is a stretch net of nylon and rubber that is knitted in a continuous seamless tube

Source
Glenwood Inc. product information. Tenafly, NJ.

 ## SurgiPeace analgesia pump

Description
ambulatory pump provides continuous infusion of local analgesia into surgical wound site; may be used for nonsurgical chronic pain conditions

Source
Sgarlato Labs product information. San Jose, CA.

 ## Surgitube tubular gauze

Description
made from 100% cotton that is knitted in a continuous, seamless tube; holds bandages in place and is capable of accommodating small toes to an entire leg

Source
Glenwood Inc. product information. Tenafly, NJ.

Surgiwand suction/irrigation device

Description

disposable surgical instrument used for suction or irrigation; available with or without cautery

Source

United States Surgical Corp. product information. Norwalk, CT.

Surveyor CPAP Monitor system

Description

CPAP monitoring system provides a 365-day histogram of patient compliance. Used with Horizon nasal CPAP unit, also from DeVilbiss

Source

DeVilbiss Sunrise Medical product information. Somerset, PA.

Sustain dental implant system

Description

cylinder implants with hex-top interface offers prosthetic components for difficult restorative situations; grooves increase the stimulus to bone in crestal region; antirotational dimples prevent stress-shielded bone loss or poor osseous ingrowth from limited vascularization

Source

Sustain Dental Implants Inc. product information. Chaska, MN.

Swede-Vent taper-lock (TL)

Description

dental device for self-tapping external hex implant; gives press-fit that eliminates micromovement, the main cause of screw loosening

Source

Dentsply Implant product information. Encino, CA.

Swiss Therapy eye mask

Description

moist, cold compress eye mask that is pliable and conforming, non-adherent; cools by skin contact and evaporation; excellent for blepharoplasty and rhinoplasty

Source

Invotec International Inc. product information. Jacksonville, FL.

Swivel-Strap ankle brace

Description
innovative ankle strap that "swivels;" wraps anatomically to support the
ankle and permit counter-rotation; hook always covered by strap to prevent
snags

Source
Aircast Inc. product information. Summit, NJ.

Sygen

Generic name
see GM-1 ganglioside

Symcor

Generic name
see tiamenidine

Syme Dycor prosthetic foot

Description
a single-axis prosthesis that provides ankle articulation with forefoot inver-
sion/eversion with an average 9-ounce component weight and is available in
1-1/2 to 2 inches of ground clearance

Source
Knit-Rite Inc. product information. Kansas City, MO.

Synaptic 2000 pain management system

Description
noninvasive synaptic electronic activation (SEA) system that activates the
descending inhibitory pathways and modulates secretion of neurotransmitters,
i.e., endorphins, serotonins, ACTH, epinephrine, norepinephrine, and somato-
statins; produces immediate, profound, and lasting anesthesia/analgesia

Source
Hessco product information. Minnetonka, MN.

Synercid

Generic Name
see quinupristin/dalfopristin

Synovir

Generic name
see thalidomide

 tacrolimus

Brand name
Prograf

Use
macrolide immunosuppressive compound used for prophylaxis of organ rejection in patients receiving an allogenic liver transplant

Usual dosage:
intravenous: 0.15 mg/kg daily for 3 days
oral: 0.15 mg/kg twice daily

Pharmaceutical company
Fujisawa Pharmaceutical Co. Deerfield, IL.

Source
University of Pittsburgh Drug Information and Pharmacoepidemiology Center. Pittsburgh, PA.

 TACTICON peripheral neuropathy screening device

Description
portable hand-held device to screen for subclinical peripheral neuropathy of fingers and toes

Source
Tacticon Medical Enterprises Inc. product information. Westtown, PA.

 talonavicular arthrodesis

Description
talonavicular arthrodesis was utilized as the primary stabilizing procedure for acquired painful foot, a syndrome that has come to be known as posterior tibial tendon insufficiency; other surgeries performed at the time of arthrodesis included transfer of the flexor digitorum longus into the medial cuneiform and associated arthrodesis of the first tarsometatarsal joint

Anatomy
calcaneocuboid joint; flexor digitorum longus; forefoot; hindfoot; medial cuneiform; navicular tuberosity; naviculocuneiform joint; posterior tibial tendon; subtalar joint; tarsometatarsal joint; talar body; transverse tarsal joint; talonavicular joint

Equipment
standard orthopaedic surgery equipment; cannulated screws; self-retaining retractor

Source
Adapted from Harper MC, Tisdel CL. Talonavicular arthrodesis for the painful adult acquired flatfoot. Foot and Ankle International Journal 1996;17:658-661.

 Tamarack flexure joint

Description
a self-alignment flexure joint with high-strength inner core which increases tensile strength

Source
Tamarack Rehabilitation Technologies, Inc. product information. St. Paul, MN.

 tamsulosin

Brand name
Flomax

Use
alpha adrenergic receptor antagonist used in benign prostatic hypertrophy

Usual dosage
oral: 0.4 mg taken 30 minutes after the same meal once daily, may increase dose to 0.8 mg daily after 2 to 4 weeks

Pharmaceutical company
Boehringer Ingelheim Pharmaceuticals. Ridgefield, CT.

Source
Stadtlanders Managed Pharmacy Services. Pittsburgh, PA.

 Tano device

Description
double mirror peripheral vitrectomy lens allows for right-side-up visualization; field-of-view up to 158 degrees in the aphakic eye making it easier to detect extremely small retinal holes; fits in the Landers vitrectomy ring

Source
Ocular Instruments Inc. product information. Bellevue, WA.

 Tapscope esophageal stethoscope

Description
esophageal pacing stethoscope offers heart rate control for intraoperative bradycardia; transesophageal atrial pacing (TAP); faster and more controllable than drug therapy

Source
Arzco Medical Systems Inc. product information. Tampa, FL.

Targocid

Generic name
see teicoplanin

 Tarka

Generic name
see trandolapril/verapamil HCl ER

 tarsoconjunctival composite graft

Description
autogenous tarsal grafts have been used for management of ectropion; ancillary procedures included combined laterocanthal suspension (tarsal tongue technique), upper lid gold weight loading, and medial canthopexy; undersurface of the free tarsal graft marked with surgical marker and wrapped in saline-soaked gauze for later use; eyelid returned to normal position; no surgical repair necessary at donor site; subcilial incision made in recipient lower lid and carried into a crow's foot wrinkle; graft is oriented so that the conjunctival surface faces the globe

Anatomy
autologous graft tissues: auricular, conchal, fossa triangularis, and septal cartilage; superior-based myocutaneous flap; hard palate; mucosa recipient area: laterocanthal angle; orbicularis muscle; levator aponeurosis; Muller (Mueller) muscle; orbital rim and septum; preseptal plane; periosteum; superior fornix; subcilial area; tarsal plate; tarsus

Equipment
Adson forceps; delicate cutting cautery or bipolar cautery; Desmarres retractor; double-armed chromic suture; Frost suture; saline-soaked gauze; surgical marker; Stevens tenotomy scissors

Source
Adapted from Shaw GY, Khan J. The management of ectropion using the tarsoconjunctival composite graft. Archives of Otolaryngology Head/Neck Surgery 1996;122:51-55.

 Tasmar

Generic name
see tolcapone

 Taxotere

Generic name
see docetaxel

tazarotene

Brand name
Zorac

Use
topical retinoid gel for the treatment of acne and psoriasis

Usual dosage
topical: 0.05% and 0.1% gel applied once a day (acne) or twice a day (psoriasis)

Pharmaceutical company
Allergan Inc. Irvine, CA.

Source
Stadtlanders Managed Pharmacy Services. Pittsburgh, PA.

 TBird ventilator

Description
turbine-powered intensive care unit (ICU) ventilator system decreases need
to change ventilators when transporting patient becomes necessary

Source
Bird Products Corp. product information. Palm Springs, CA.

 3TC

Generic name
see lamivudine

 T-cell depletion by elutriation

Synonyms
counterflow elutriation; countercurrent elutriation

Use
depletion of T-lymphocytes from allogeneic bone marrow to reduce risk or
severity of graft-vs.-host disease in transplant recipient

Method
T-lymphocytes are separated from other cells in allogeneic bone marrow
using a combined centrifuge fluid-flow system

Specimen
allogeneic bone marrow

Normal range
investigational use

Comments
indicated for some patients receiving imperfectly matched bone marrow
transplants

Source
University of Minnesota Department of Laboratory Medicine and Pathology. Minneapolis, MN.

560

 Teaser

Description

surgical instrument for laser blepharoplasty; features knurled tip that grasps, teases out, and rolls up exposed fatty tissue

Source

Byron Medical product information. Tucson, AZ.

 technetium 99m (Tc-99m) hexamethylpropylamine oxine-labeled (HMPAO) white blood cell (WBC) scintigraphy

Synonyms

Ceretec-labeled leukocyte scintigraphy

Indications

noninvasive diagnosis of osteomyelitis in patients with pre-existing pedal abnormalities

Method

radiolabeled WBC was prepared from venous blood; after reinjection of Tc-99m HMPAO-labeled WBCs images of the feet were acquired on a large field-of-view gamma camera using a low-energy, high-resolution collimator and a 15% energy window; anterior, both lateral and plantar images of the feet were acquired 3-4 hours after radiopharmaceutic injection for 60,000 counts each

Normal findings

no focal bony uptake of labeled cells greater than soft tissue background

Comments

positive Tc-99m HMPAO-labeled leukocyte scan required focal bony uptake of labeled cells greater than soft tissue background at the site of the suspected osteomyelitis

Source

Adapted from Blume PA, Dey HM, Daley LJ, Arrighi JA, Soufer R, Gorecki GA. Diagnosis of pedal osteomyelitis with Tc-99m HMPAO labeled leukocytes. The Journal of Foot and Ankle Surgery 1997;36:120-126.

 technetium 99m labeled antigranulocyte Fab' fragment

Brand name

LeukoScan

Use

diagnostic agent used to image infection in long bones, patients with diabetic foot ulcers, and acute atypical appendicitis in patients with right lower quadrant disease

Usual dosage

injectable: clinical trials used three dose ranges: 0.1-0.5 mg, 0.5-0.9 mg, and 0.9-1.0 mg with results obtained 1-6 hours after injection

Pharmaceutical company
Immunomedics. Morris Plains, NJ.
Source
Stadtlanders Managed Pharmacy Services. Pittsburgh, PA.

 technetium pertechnetate-anti-carcinoembryonic antigen monoclonal antibody BW 431/26; Scintimun (Behring-Werke, Marburg, Germany) used to image colorectal cancer

Synonyms
none

Indications
persistent rise in serum carcinoembryonic antigen (CEA) levels of unknown origin and/or questionable findings by other imaging studies

Method
tomography scans performed up to 24 hours after intravenous antibody injection

Normal findings
not applicable

Comments
highly reliable diagnostic procedure in detecting colorectal cancer recurrence and is especially useful for diagnosis of patients with rising CEA blood levels of unknown origin

Source
Adapted from Zwas ST, Goshen EG, Rath P, Brenner H, Klein E, Ben-Ari G. Detection efficiency of colorectal carcinoma recurrence using technetium pertechnetate-anti-carcinoembryonic antigen monoclonal antibody BW 431/26. Cancer 1995;76:215-222.

 Techni-Care surgical scrub

Description
provides 99.99% bacterial reduction in 30 seconds without dermal irritation; eliminates Gram-negative and Gram-positive bacteria with active ingredient 3% chloroxylenol (PCMX)

Source
Care-Tech Laboratories product information. St. Louis, MO.

 Technicon Immuno 1 free thyroxine assay

Synonyms
Technicon Immuno 1 fT4

Use
thyroid function evaluation

Method
sequential magnetic separation competitive assay performed on an automated random access analyzer

Specimen
serum

Normal range
9.5-16.4 ng/L

Comments
an automated, rapid, highly sensitive and specific means of evaluating thyroid function

Source
Adapted from Bock JL, Morris D, Cheng J, Ehresman D. Evaluation of the Technicon Immuno 1 free thyroxine assay. American Journal of Clinical Pathology 1996;105:583-588.

 Teczem

Generic name
see diltiazem maleate/enalapril maleate

 Tefcat intrauterine insemination catheter

Description
surgical instrument used for introduction of washed spermatozoa into uterine cavity; flexible hub and adjustable positioner

Source
Cook OB/GYN product information. Spencer, IN.

 TefGen-FD guided tissue regeneration membrane

Description
nonporous full density (FD) membrane; used in a variety of guided tissue regeneration applications; effective as biocompatible barrier membrane when used in dental bony defect regeneration

Source
American Custom Medical Inc. product information. Lubbock, TX.

 teicoplanin

Brand name
Targocid

Use
glycopeptide antibiotic used in the therapy of serious Gram-positive infections

Usual dosage
injection: loading dose; 400 to 600 mg intravenous; maintenance dose: 200 to 600 mg intramuscular or intravenous once daily

Pharmaceutical company
Marion Merrell Dow. Kansas City, MO.

Source
University of Pittsburgh Drug Information and Pharmacoepidemiology Center. Pittsburgh, PA.

Tenderlett device

Description
finger incision devices provide safe, automated, pain-free blood sampling from the finger; customized to age and vasculature of the patient; adult size incises to a hollow 1.75-mm depth; Tenderlett Junior for pediatric patients incises to 1.25-mm depth; Tenderlett Toddler for older infants and toddlers incises to 0.85-mm depth; shallow, standardized incisions result in little discomfort in younger patients

Source
International Technidyne Corp. product information. Edison, NJ.

 tenidap

Brand name
Enable

Use
nonsteroidal anti-inflammatory agent demonstrating efficacy in patients with rheumatoid arthritis and osteoarthritis

Usual dosage
oral: doses of 120 mg daily have been studied

Pharmaceutical company
Pfizer Inc. New York, NY.

Source
University of Pittsburgh Drug Information and Pharmacoepidemiology Center. Pittsburgh, PA.

 tenoxicam

Brand name
Tilcotil

Use
nonsteroidal anti-inflammatory agent effective in the treatment of rheumatoid arthritis, osteoarthritis, ankylosing spondylitis, and nonarticular rheumatic conditions

Usual dosage
oral: 20 mg once daily; rectal: 20 mg once daily

Pharmaceutical company
Roche Laboratories. Nutley, NJ.

Source
University of Pittsburgh Drug Information and Pharmacoepidemiology Center. Pittsburgh, PA.

tension-control suture technique in open rhinoplasty

Description
suture technique for correction of nasal tip cartilage concavities using inter-locking mattress sutures in a chain-link fashion; each stitch creates a minia-ture convexity and the combined linkages form the complete convex arch

Anatomy
alar cartilage; middle crus; lateral crus; alar dome; nostrils; septum

Equipment
standard rhinoplasty equipment; cotton-tipped applicator

Source
Adapted from Neu BR. Suture correction of nasal tip cartilage concavities. Plastic and Reconstructive Surgery 1996;98:971-979.

 ## Tension Isometer

Description
assists in detection of graft bone placement sites; facilitates adjustment of graft tension to control surgically reconstructed ligament length and normal knee motion

Source
MEDmetric Corp. product information. San Diego, CA.

 ## Teq-Trode electrode

Description
oval-shaped electrodes used with transcutaneous electrical nerve stimulator (TENS) devices and portable muscle stimulators

Source
AdvanTeq product information. Westlake Village, CA.

 ## terbinafine hydrochloride

Brand name
Lamisil

Use
an antifungal agent used for treatment of nail infections (onychomycosis)

Usual dosage
oral: 250 mg every day for 6 weeks for treatment of the toenail and 250 mg every day for 12 weeks for treatment of the fingernail

Pharmaceutical company
Sandoz Pharmaceutical Corp. East Hanover, NJ.

Source
University of Pittsburgh Drug Information and Pharmacoepidemiology Center. Pittsburgh, PA.

terlipressin

Brand Name
Glypressin

Use
long-acting analogue of lysine-vasopressin used in the treatment of bleeding esophageal varices and nosebleeds

Usual Dosage
intravenously: 2 mg every 4 hours for 24 hours was used in clinical trials

Pharmaceutical company
Ferring Laboratories Inc. Suffern, NY.

Source
University of Pittsburgh Drug Information and Pharmacoepidemiology Center. Pittsburgh, PA.

 terodiline hydrochloride

Brand Name
Micturin

Use
non-selective anticholinergic used in the treatment of urinary incontinence, nocturia, and urinary frequency

Usual Dosage
oral: 12.5 mg to 25 mg twice a day

Pharmaceutical company
Forest Pharmaceutical Inc. St. Louis, MO.

Source
University of Pittsburgh Drug Information and Pharmacoepidemiology Center. Pittsburgh, PA.

 Terumo syringe

Description
latex-free, plastic disposable syringes with gaskets made of special thermo-plastic synthetic elastomer

Source
Terumo Medical Corp. product information. Somerset, NJ.

 Teslascan

Generic name
see mangafodipir trisodium

testicular sperm extraction (TESE)

Description
testicular parenchyma retrieval

Anatomy
testis; tunica albuginea; seminiferous tubules

Equipment
loupes or operating microscope; curved iris scissors; angiocatheter

Source
Adapted from Sheynkin Y, Schlegel PN. Sperm retrieval for assisted reproductive techniques. Contemporary OB/GYN 1997;42:113-129.

 testosterone

Brand name
AndroTest-SL

Use
another testosterone formulation; androgenic hormone replacement therapy for treatment of hypogonadism

Usual dosage
sublingual: 2.5 or 5 mg three times a day was used in clinical trials

Pharmaceutical company
Bio-Technology General. Iselin, NJ.

Source
Stadtlanders Managed Pharmacy Services. Pittsburgh, PA.

 testosterone transdermal patch

Brand name
Androderm

Use
testosterone replacement therapy for men; used for conditions associated with deficiency or absence of endogenous testosterone

Usual dosage
transdermal extended-release film applied to abdomen, back, thighs, or upper arms: delivers 2.5 mg/24 hrs; normal usage is 2 patches or 5 mg/day

Pharmaceutical company
SmithKline Beecham. Philadelphia, PA.

Source
University of Pittsburgh Drug Information and Pharmacoepidemiology Center. Pittsburgh, PA.

Test-Size orchidometer

Description
graduated series of 12 different size and shape models of testes; allows pediatrician, endocrinologist, or andrologist to make necessary comparison and evaluation; eliminates use of calipers

Source
Accurate Surgical and Scientific Instruments Corp. product information. Westbury, NY.

Teveten

Generic name
see eprosartan

Tew cranial/spinal retractor

Description
patient-based retractor system designed for use during posterior fossa and spinal cord surgery

Source
OMI Surgical Products product information. Cincinnati, OH.

ThAIRapy vest

Description
airway clearance system that improves mucus clearance by using high-frequency chest wall oscillation to enhance mucus mobilization; high-frequency compression pulses are applied to the chest wall via air-pulse generator and inflatable vest

Source
American Biosystems product information. Saint Paul, MN.

thalidomide

Brand name
Synovir

Use
immune modulator for the treatment of cachexia associated with HIV/AIDS infection

Usual dosage
oral: 100 mg 4 times a day was used in clinical trials

Pharmaceutical company
Celgene Corp. Warren, NJ.

Source
Stadtlanders Managed Pharmacy Services. Pittsburgh, PA.

thallium breast imaging

Synonyms
thallium-201 breast scintigraphy

Indications
evaluate palpable breast lesions; effective means of differentiating benign from malignant lesions

Method
inject thallium-201 intravenously in the arm on the opposite side of the known breast lesion; perform imaging 2 minutes and 1 hour postinjection

Normal findings
not applicable

Comments
patient must cooperate and be capable of sitting for 45 minutes in order for study to be adequate

Source
Lexi-Comp Inc. database. Hudson, OH.

 The Original Backnobber massage tool

Description
hand-held deep muscle massager

Source
The Pressure Positive Co. product information. Gilbertsville, PA.

 The Original Index Knobber II massage tool

Description
hand-held deep muscle massager to apply pressure to trigger points

Source
The Pressure Positive Co. product information. Gilbertsville, PA.

 The Original Jacknobber massage tool

Description
hand-held deep muscle massager

Source
The Pressure Positive Co. product information. Gilbertsville, PA.

TheraBeads moist heat pack

Description
form-fitting pack delivers moist therapeutic heat; warmed in microwave; reusable; avoids danger of leaking gels or exposure to wiring or chemicals as with other heat packs; includes a skin temperature monitor strip

Source
Bruder Healthcare Co. product information. Marietta, GA.

 ## Thera-Boot bandage

Description
provides graduated compression therapy for burns, venous leg ulcers, and lymphedema; nonelastic; adjustable; reusable for same-patient treatments

Source
CircAid Medical Products product information. San Diego, CA.

 ## Thera Cane

Description
therapeutic massager that applies pressure to treat muscle dysfunction; looks like a shepherd's staff with extra projections

Source
Thera Cane Co. product information. Denver, CO.

 ## Therafectin

Generic name
see amiprilose

 ## Theraform Selectives

Description
prefabricated foot orthotics; consists of ten advanced laminate shells; these shells possess distinctive functional properties ranging from protective and accommodative to functional and controlling

Source
Benefoot Inc. product information. Edgewood, NY.

Thera-Med cold pack

Description
device for treatment by RICE (rest, ice, compression, and elevation) method for a wide variety of injuries or sore muscles; Velcro straps compress the pack around the affected area to help reduce swelling; Crylon Gel remains flexible; fitted models for sprains, pulled muscles, stiffness, and swelling; universal pad for ankles, knees, wrists, and elbows; also includes a back pad, shoulder pad, headache band, sinus mask, wrist band, and collar pad

Source
Thera-Med product information. Waco., TX.

 ## Thera-Medic shoe

Description
custom shoe; features a base flare, extra-rigid counter, solid ankle cushioned heel, metatarsal pads, and heel wedge

Source
Tru-Mold Shoes Inc. product information. Buffalo, NY.

 ## Theramini 1 electrotherapy stimulator

Description
electrotherapy with a 2-channel, single waveform stimulator that comes in 6 different modes including quadpolar classic interferential, bipolar premodulated interferential, monophasic high-volt, microcurrent, biphasic low volt, and Russian; liquid crystal display (LCD) screen provides treatment information; set up is simplified by use of a control dial; system can change waveforms by having them downloaded via Theratouch stimulator; also Theramini 2 with QuickSets comes with programs for most common treatments; both fit into custom carrying case for easy portability

Source
Rich-Mar Corp. product information. Inola, OK.

 ## TheraPatch

Generic name
see methyl salicylate patch

TheraPEP pre-respiratory therapy treatment

Description
positive expiratory pre-therapy system; employs positive expiratory pressure to improve clearance of secretions and facilitate opening of airways; reduces need for postural drainage; features an integral pressure indicator for immediate, visual feedback; used with either a mask or a mouthpiece

Source
Diemolding Healthcare Division product information. Canastota, NY.

 ## Thera*Press

Description
trigger point release tool made of plastic with a contoured hand grip for pressure point therapy

Source
Integrated Health Concepts Inc. product information. Gainesville, FL.

 ## Therasound transducer

Description
therapy hammer transducer; rugged, lightweight, portable, full power unit for electrotherapy

Source
Rich-Mar Corp. product information. Inola, OK.

 ## ThermoFlex unit

Description
water-induced thermotherapy (WIT) prostate treatment for benign prostatic hypertrophy (BPH); nonsurgical treatment with 18F Foley balloon catheter from bladder neck to verumontanum; increases urinary flow, decreases postvoid residual urine, and improves urinary symptoms; can be administered simultaneously with ionizing radiation therapy for treatment of carcinoma of the prostate; (in the U.S. for investigational use only at this time)

Source
Argomed product information. Herzla, Israel.

Thermo-Flo irrigation system 3

Description
irrigation device includes pump, probe, and tube set that can be used for irrigation during laparoscopic and general surgical procedures; regulates irrigation solution temperature which prevents hypothermia

Source
Sanese Medical product information. Columbus, OH.

thermography testing with breast carcinoma

Synonyms
none

Indications
to determine relation of thermal abnormality with ductal carcinoma of the breast

Method
liquid crystal (contact) thermography; vascularity assessed with Doppler ultrasound; microvessel density by immunohistochemical staining with factor VIII-related antigen; tumor proliferation rate measured using Ki-67 monoclonal antibody

Normal findings
abnormal thermogram is associated with large tumors, high grade, and lymph node positivity, but not proliferation rate or microvessel density

Comments
thermography is not an independent prognostic indicator

Source
Adapted from Sterns EE, Zee B, SenGupta S, Saunders FW. Thermography: its relation to pathological characteristics, vascularity, proliferation rate, and survival of patients with invasive ductal carcinoma of the breast. Journal of American Cancer Society 1996;77:1324-1328.

Thermoskin heat retainer

Description
wrap-around heat therapy for pain relief and prevention that allows skin to ventilate and contains wicking fibers that keep moisture off skin

Source
United Pacific Inc. product information. Columbia, SC.

The Rope stretch and traction device

Description
attaches to any door to provide gentle traction for the shoulders and thoracolumbar spine

Source
PrePak Products product information. Carlsbad, CA.

Thero-Skin gel padding

Description
gel padding that can be applied to splinting materials before placing in hot water to form; conforms to all body contours and eliminates friction; moisturizes skin

Source
Fred Sammons Inc. product information. Western Springs, IL.

Thomas Long-Term (LT) endotracheal tube holder

Description
holder designed to be secure, yet extremely comfortable for long-term patient care

Source
STI Medical Products product information. Costa Mesa, CA.

Thomas subretinal instrument set II

Description
set of subretinal instruments including an angled cannula, pick, horizontal scissors, and horizontal forceps

Source
Synergetics Inc. product information. Chesterfield, MO.

thrombopoietin (TPO) level

Synonyms
TPO assay

Use
evaluation of persistent thrombocytopenia

Method
TPO receptor capture enzyme immunoassay

Specimen
serum or plasma

Normal range
undetectable, or <200 pg/mL

Comments
differentiates thrombocytopenias due to peripheral destruction from those due to production disorders

Source
Adapted from Emmons RVB, Reid DM, Cohen RL, Meng G, Young NS, Dunbar CE, Shulman NR. Human thrombopoietin levels are high when thrombocytopenia is due to megakaryocyte deficiency and low when due to increased platelet destruction. Blood 1996;87:4068-4071.

thymidine kinase gene transduction

Synonyms
suicide gene transfer

Use
allows destruction of donor marrow cells after transplant, to limit severity of graft-versus-host disease

Method
retroviral-mediated gene transfer

Specimen
donor marrow leukocytes

Normal range
not applicable

Comments
may provide a means of controlling otherwise lethal graft-versus-host disease

Source
Department of Laboratory Medicine and Pathology, University of Minnesota, Minneapolis, MN.

 Thymoglobulin

Generic name
see antithymocyte immunoglobulin

 thymopentin

Brand name
Timunox

Use
synthetic pentapeptide used in the treatment of HIV infection in asymptomatic patients

Usual dosage
subcutaneous: 50 mg three times weekly

Pharmaceutical company
Johnson & Johnson. New Brunswick, NJ.

Source
University of Pittsburgh Drug Information and Pharmacoepidemiology Center. Pittsburgh, PA.

thymosin alpha 1

Brand name
Zadaxin

Use
stimulates T-cell proliferation and function, when used in combination with alpha interferon in the treatment of chronic, active hepatitis C

Usual dosage
injectable: 900 µg/m^2 twice weekly was studied in clinical trials

Pharmaceutical company
SciClone Pharmaceuticals Inc. San Mateo, CA.

Source
Stadtlanders Managed Pharmacy Services. Pittsburgh, PA.

 Thyrogen

Generic name
see recombinant thyroid stimulating hormone

 tiagabine

Brand name
Gabitril

Use
specific gamma aminobutyric acid (GABA) reuptake inhibitor used as adjunctive therapy for epilepsy and partial seizures

Usual dosage
oral: mean doses of 32 mg and 24 mg daily were used in clinical trials

Pharmaceutical company
Abbott Laboratories. Abbott Park, IL.

Source
University of Pittsburgh Drug Information and Pharmacoepidemiology Center. Pittsburgh, PA.

 tiamenidine

Brand name
Symcor

Use
centrally acting antihypertensive agent

Usual dosage
oral: 1 to 3 mg daily

Pharmaceutical company
Hoechst-Roussel. Somerville, NJ.

Source
University of Pittsburgh Drug Information and Pharmacoepidemiology Center. Pittsburgh, PA.

 Tiazac

Generic name
see diltiazem hydrochloride (HCl)

 tibolone

Brand name
Livial

Use
synthetic steroidal agent with estrogenic, progestogenic, and androgenic activity for the treatment of menopausal symptoms and in the prevention of bone loss in postmenopausal patients

Usual dosage
oral: 2.5 mg daily

Pharmaceutical company
Organon. West Orange, NJ.

Source
University of Pittsburgh Drug Information and Pharmacoepidemiology Center. Pittsburgh, PA.

 Tielle hydropolymer dressing

Description
synthetic polymer gel absorbent dressing; adhesive waterproof backing; permeable to water vapor; creates a moist wound environment; absorbs wound exudate without leaking; wicks exudate away from wound; controls odor; easily removed

Source
Johnson & Johnson Medical Inc. product information. Arlington, TX.

 tight-to-shaft (TTS) Aire-Cuf tracheostomy tube

Description
TTS cuff design provides benefits of a cuff with profile of a cuffless tube; Aire-Cuf can be deflated or re-inflated for patients requiring cuff inflation for managed, controlled leaks; provides protection from potential aspiration during feeding or for short periods of total pressure tracheal seal

Source
Bovina Medical Technologies product information. Gary, IN.

Tilcotil

Generic name
see tenoxicam

 # Tilt-In-Space wheelchair conversion

Description
better wheelchair patient control in forward flexion and increase in chair time versus bed time; infinite number of recline positions, adjustable leg supports

Source
Suiter Medical product information. McCook, NE.

 # tiludronate

Brand name
Skelid

Use
hormone replacement therapy used in the treatment of Paget disease

Usual dosage
oral: 400 mg daily

Pharmaceutical company
Sanofi. New York, NY.

Source
University of Pittsburgh Drug Information and Pharmacoepidemiology Center. Pittsburgh, PA.

 # TiMesh titanium bone plating system

Description
rigid fixation bone plating systems for craniomaxillofacial and neurosurgery; 1 mm micro system, 1.5 mm midface and cranial system, 1.5 mm system for small bone grafts, 2.2 mm craniofacial system; 1, 2.2, and 2.5 mm combination system; all systems include implants and high torque thread cutting screws

Source
TiMesh Inc. product information. Las Vegas, NV.

 # Timunox

Generic name
see thymopentin

Tina-quant [a] digoxin assay

Synonyms
turbidimetric digoxin assay

Use
therapeutic drug monitoring for digoxin

Method
turbidimetric inhibition immunoassay

Specimen
blood

Normal range
investigational

Comments
does not require sample pretreatment or dedicated analyzers, and is more resistant to digoxin-like immunoreactive factor (DLIF) interference than current methods

Source
Adapted from Scholer A, Boecker J, Engelmayer U, et al. Comparability of a new turbidimetric digoxin test with other immunochemical tests and with HPLC—a multicenter evaluation. Clinical Chemistry 1997;43:92-99.

 ## tinzaparin

Brand name
Logiparin

Use
low molecular weight heparin being studied for use in blood coagulation disorders including deep vein thrombosis (DVT)

Usual dosage
subcutaneous: low molecular weight heparin dosing has ranged from 2400 to 3200 anti-factor Xa units, once to twice daily for prophylaxis of DVT

Pharmaceutical company
Novo Nordisk Pharmaceuticals Inc. Princeton, NJ.

Source
University of Pittsburgh Drug Information and Pharmacoepidemiology Center. Pittsburgh, PA.

 ## tirilazad mesylate

Brand name
Freedox

Use
investigation for treatment of traumatic head injury, spinal cord injury, subarachnoid hemorrhage, or stroke

Usual dosage
intravenous: 0.6 to 15 mg/kg daily used during clinical trials

Pharmaceutical company
Upjohn Co. Kalamazoo, MI.
Source
University of Pittsburgh Drug Information and Pharmacoepidemiology Center. Pittsburgh, PA.

tirofiban

Brand name
Aggrastat

Use
reduce adverse cardiac events in treatment of unstable angina and angioplasty

Usual dosage
intravenous: doses of 5, 10, and 15 µg/kg were used in clinical trials

Pharmaceutical company
Merck & Company Inc. West Point, PA.
Source
Stadtlanders Managed Pharmacy Services. Pittsburgh, PA.

tissue band ligation followed by snare resection (band and snare)

Description
technique for tissue acquisition in the esophagus; this procedure predictably
delivers submucosal tissue which has both diagnostic and therapeutic implications

Anatomy
esophagus

Equipment
ligator adaptor; standard endoscope equipment; standard electrocoagulator
equipment; polypectomy snare; overtube

Source
Adapted from Fleischer DE, Wang GQ, Dawsey S, Tio TL, Newsome J, Kidwell J. Tissue band ligation followed
by snare resection (band and snare): a new technique for tissue acquisition in the esophagus. Gastrointestinal
Endoscopy 1996;44(1):68-72.

tissue-based monoamine oxidase assay

Synonyms
MAO spectrophotometric assay

Use
measurement of MAO inhibition induced by antidepressant and antiparkin-
sonian drugs

Method
spectrophotometric absorbance at wavelength 498 nm

Specimen
biological tissue homogenate

Normal range
monoamine oxidase activity consistent with untreated control tissue

Comments
permits monitoring of patients treated with monoamine-oxidase-inhibiting drugs, as well as screening potential drugs for monoamine oxidase inhibition

Source
Adapted from Holt A, Sharman DF, Baker GB, Palcic MM. A continuous spectrophotometric assay for monoamine oxidase and related enzymes in tissue homogenates. Analytical Biochemistry 1997;244:384-392.

 tissue expansion vaginoplasty

Description
construction of neovagina in patients with congenital vaginal agenesis; normal saline tissue expanders placed bilaterally under labia majora; expanders removed after several weeks; neovagina created by dissection between bladder and rectum; newly created tissue sutured as bipedicle flap to create vaginal wall

Anatomy
labia majora; vulva; urethra; bladder; rectum

Equipment
standard surgery equipment; vaginal stent

Source
Adapted from Chudacoff RM, Alexander J, Alvero R, Segars JH. Tissue expansion vaginoplasty for treatment of congenital vaginal agenesis. Obstetrics & Gynecology 1996;87:865-868.

 tissue plasminogen activator detection

Synonyms
plasminogen activator detection; tissue plasminogen activator antigen; TPA

Use
evaluate hypercoagulable state, Crohn disease, ulcerative colitis, and myocardial infarction

Method
chromogenic substrate

Specimen
blood

Normal range
1-12 ng/ml

Comments
abnormally high levels of hemoglobin, bilirubin, or lipid levels present concurrently in the plasma sample may affect results

Source
Lexi-Comp Inc. database. Hudson, OH.

titanium aneurysm clip

Description
titanium aneurysm clip; superior imaging characteristics and create less imaging artifacts than conventional clips made of cobalt-based alloys

Source
Adapted from Lawton MT, Ho JC, Bichard WD, Coons SW, Zabramski JM, Spetzler RF. Titanium aneurysm clips: part I—mechanical, radiological, and biocompatibility testing. Neurosurgery 1996;38:1158-1164.

 titanium plasma sprayed (TPS) dental implants

Description
commercially pure titanium sprayed over a dental implant fabricated from titanium alloy for superior strength; allows for 32% more bone volume between the threads than in standard V thread designs

Source
Steri-Oss Bausch & Lomb Co. product information. Yorba Linda, CA.

 tizanidine hydrochloride

Brand name
Zanaflex

Use
centrally acting muscle relaxant for spasticity associated with multiple sclerosis and cerebrovascular or spinal cord disorders; also shown to be useful in chronic tension headache

Usual dosage
oral: 6 to 36 mg daily in three divided doses has been used in treating spasticity of multiple sclerosis, low back pain, and other disorders; doses of up to 18 mg daily have been used for tension headache

Pharmaceutical company
Athena Neurosciences, Inc. South San Francisco, CA.

Source
University of Pittsburgh Drug Information and Pharmacoepidemiology Center. Pittsburgh, PA.

 TOBI

Generic name
see tobramycin for inhalation

tobramycin for inhalation

Brand name
TOBI

Use
treatment of chronic lung infections caused by Gram-negative bacteria
(*Pseudomonas aeruginosa*) in patients with cystic fibrosis

Usual dosage
inhale: 300 mg twice a day for 4 weeks

Pharmaceutical company
Pathogenesis. Seattle, WA.

Source
Stadtlanders Managed Pharmacy Services. Pittsburgh, PA.

 tolcapone

Brand name
Tasmar

Use
a catechol-O-methyl transferase inhibitor used to augment the actions of levodopa in the treatment of Parkinson disease

Usual dosage
oral: 200, 400, and 800 mg 3 times a day have been studied in clinical trials

Pharmaceutical company
Hoffman La Roche. Nutley, NJ.

Source
Stadtlanders Managed Pharmacy Services. Pittsburgh, PA.

 tolrestat

Brand name
Alredase

Use
aldose reductase inhibitor used in the treatment of diabetic complica-
tions/prevention of complications induced by elevated sugar levels in nerve,
kidney, and lens

Usual dosage
oral: 200 mg daily has been frequently used in clinical trials

Pharmaceutical company
Wyeth Ayerst Laboratories. Philadelphia, PA.

Source
University of Pittsburgh Drug Information and Pharmacoepidemiology Center. Pittsburgh, PA.

tolterodine

Brand name
Detrusitol

Use
muscarinic receptor antagonist for treatment of urinary incontinence

Usual dosage
oral: 1 or 2 mg twice daily in clinical trials

Pharmaceutical company
Pharmacia and Upjohn Co. Kalamazoo, MI.

Source
Stadtlanders Managed Pharmacy Services. Pittsburgh, PA.

 Topamax

Generic Name
see topiramate

 topiramate

Brand Name
Topamax

Use
anticonvulsant for the treatment of epilepsy

Usual Dosage
oral: up to 800 mg daily was used in clinical trials

Pharmaceutical company
Johnson & Johnson. Arlington, TX.

Source
University of Pittsburgh Drug Information and Pharmacoepidemiology Center. Pittsburgh, PA.

 topodermatography

Synonyms
computerized image analysis screening

Indications
identify and evaluate changes of cutaneous lesions in melanoma screening or follow-up of patients with cancer

Method
digitized measurements of skin surface image parameters performed using high speed processor, high-resolution video camera, and image processing software

Normal findings
not applicable

Comments
topodermatographic image analysis helps to optimize screening and follow-up procedures for patients with melanoma and populations at risk for melanoma

Source
Adapted from Voigt H, Claben R. Topodermatographic image analysis for melanoma screening and the quantitative assessment of tumor dimension parameters of the skin. Cancer 1995;75:981-987.

 topographic scanning/indocyanine green (TopSS/ICG) angiography combination instrument

Description
ICG ophthalmic angiography that works with TopSS; confocal scanning laser tomograph uses fluorescence detection system eliminating need for multiple illumination sources; continuous live fundus image

Source
Laser Diagnostic Technologies Inc. product information. San Diego, CA.

 topotecan

Brand name
Hycamtin

Use
chemotherapeutic agent being studied in the treatment of colorectal, ovarian, breast, and small-cell lung cancer

Usual dosage
intravenous: phase I studies have used 1.25 to 1.5 mg/m^2 infused daily for 5 days as a single cycle of chemotherapy

Pharmaceutical company
SmithKline Beecham. Philadelphia, PA.

Source
University of Pittsburgh Drug Information and Pharmacoepidemiology Center. Pittsburgh, PA.

 toremifene citrate

Brand name
Fareston

Use
anti-androgen agent for use in advanced metastatic breast cancer in post-menopausal women

Usual dosage
oral: 10 mg/day to 400 mg/day are being used in clinical trials with the greatest response being found with a 60-mg dose and the median time to progression around 6.3 to 7.3 months

Pharmaceutical company
Schering-Plough. Kenilworth, NJ.

Source
University of Pittsburgh Drug Information and Pharmacoepidemiology Center. Pittsburgh, PA.

 ## total laparoscopic hysterectomy with transvaginal tube

Description
placement of wide-bore plastic tube to expose cervicovaginal junction and stretch vaginal fornices; allows hysterectomy to be performed totally by laparoscopy; tube used to guide incision and protect adjacent structures

Anatomy
cervix; vagina; cervicovaginal junction; vaginal fornices; uterus; ovaries; bladder; uterosacral ligaments

Equipment
standard laparoscopic surgery equipment; transparent polypropylene tube; endoscopic scissors; surgical stapler-cutting device; coagulation diathermy; Spacman cannula; Vulsellum clamp

Source
Adapted from McCartney AJ, Johnson N. Using a vaginal tube to separate the uterus from the vagina during laparoscopic hysterectomy. Obstetrics & Gynecology 1995;85:293-296.

 ## Total Synchrony System

Description
electronic impedance patient-triggered system for very low birth weight infants; Sechrist IV-200-SAVI system is exhalation-on-demand, in the event of active exhalation such as coughing, the positive pressure breath is immediately terminated; feature displays include mean airway pressure, high and low pressure alarm limits, trigger rate, impedance signal bar graph, trigger and control breath indicators, and sensitivity control; if patient efforts fail to initiate the inspiratory phase, the system immediately operates at the back-up respiratory rate

Source
Sechrist Industries. Inc. product information. Anaheim, CA.

 ## Townsend endocervical biopsy curette

Description
endocervical biopsy curette that allows tissue sampling without dilation of the cervix

Source
Miltex Instrument Co. product information. Lake Success, NY.

TrachCare multi-access catheter (MAC)

Description
MAC directs delivery of surfactant on the liquid-to-liquid interface and maintains ventilation; provides postive end expiratory pressure (PEEP) and oxygen therapy throughout the delivery procedure; allows access to the distal airway without loss of ventilation for fluid sampling, pressure monitoring, and drug delivery; has a 5-French 7.5-mm port plug with 2- to 4-mm Y-adapter

Source
Ballard Medical Products product information. Draper, UT.

 TRACOEflex tracheostomy tube

Description
features include full rotation neck plate that swivels 60 degrees horizontally and 30 degrees vertically to allow freedom of movement

Source
Boston Medical Products product information. Westborough, MA.

 TRAKE-fit system

Description
tracheostomy tube holders provide maximum patient comfort with a 1-inch cotton-lined neck-band; easily installed with hook-and-loop tabs

Source
Ackrad Laboratories Inc. product information. Cranford, NJ.

 tramadol

Brand name
Ultram

Use
opioid-type analgesic used to treat acute and chronic pain

Usual dosage
oral: 50 to 100 mg every 4 to 6 hours as needed

Pharmaceutical company
McNeil Pharmaceutical. Raritan, NJ.

Source
University of Pittsburgh Drug Information and Pharmacoepidemiology Center. Pittsburgh, PA.

trandolapril

Brand name
Mavik

Use
angiotensin-converting enzyme inhibitor used in the treatment of hypertension; under investigation for its effects on mortality following acute myocardial infarction; positive effects on reducing urinary albumin loss in diabetic, hypertensive patients

Usual dosage
oral: usual starting dose is 2 mg daily; 0.5 mg daily in patients with hepatic or renal insufficiency

Pharmaceutical company
Knoll Pharmaceuticals. Whippany, NJ.

Source
University of Pittsburgh Drug Information and Pharmacoepidemiology Center. Pittsburgh, PA.

 # trandolapril/verapamil HCl ER

Brand name
Tarka

Use
combination of angiotensin converting enzyme (ACE) inhibitor and calcium channel blocker for the treatment of moderate-to-severe hypertension

Usual dosage
oral: available as 2/180, 1/240, 2/240, 4/240 mg trandolapril/verapamil tablets; administered as once a day dose; daily dose is slowly titrated in individual patient with hypertension

Pharmaceutical company
Knoll Pharmaceutical Co. Mount Olive, NJ.

Source
Stadtlanders Managed Pharmacy Services. Pittsburgh, PA.

 # Tranquility Quest continuous positive air pressure (CPAP)

Description
compact CPAP features advanced blower design and optional compliance meter that records actual use; coupled with Soft Series Mask; fits in an overnight bag or on a nightstand

Source
Healthdyne Technologies product information. Marietta, GA.

transanal resection by rectal advancement and rectoanal anastomosis

Description

most anastomotic colorectal or ileoanal strictures are manageable by dilatation with a digit, bougie, or proctoscope; in some cases stenosis recurs and resection becomes mandatory; transanal pouch advancement with neoileoanal anastomosis has been proposed for anastomotic strictures; technique described is a simple method for transanal resection in a patient with a low rectal stricture resulting from suppository abuse

Anatomy

anal canal; dentate line; internal anal sphincter; presacral space; perirectal tissue; supralevator space; rectum

Equipment

standard surgical equipment; anal retractor; cautery; Hegar dilator

Source

Adapted from Panis Y, Ettorre G, Valleur P. Transanal resection of a low rectal stenosis by rectal advancement and rectoanal anastomosis. British Journal of Surgery 1997;84:92-93.

 transcranial resection of paranasal sinuses

Description

transcranial approach can achieve removal of tumors of sinuses, nasal cavity, orbit, and anterior cranial fossa; may be considered whenever sinus tumors extend beyond the reach of conventional approaches; transcranial approach performed first to prevent intradural contamination by bacteria or tumor cells; criteria generally used for transfacial approach were invasion of floor or maxillary sinus, base of nasal septum, soft tissues of face, and orbital involvement requiring orbital exenteration

Anatomy

cribriform plate; epidural space; epipericranial area; ethmoid maxillary and sphenoid sinuses; frontonasal dura; hard palate; olfactory rootlets; nasion; planum sphenoidale

Equipment

standard neurosurgical equipment; lumbar subarachnoid drainage tube

Source

Adapted from McCutcheon IA, Blacklock JB, Weber RS et al. Anterior transcranial (craniofacial) resection of tumors of the paranasal sinuses: surgical technique and result. Neurosurgery Journal 1996;38:471-480.

Transeal dressing

Description
transparent wound dressing, acts like a second skin controlling the environment in which the wound will heal; has a high moisture vapor transmission rate and was specifically designed to address the problems associated with moisture accumulation under films; impermeable to water and bacteria

Source
DeRoyal Industries Inc. product information. Powell, TN.

transesophageal echocardiography

Synonyms
TEE

Indications
confirm diagnosis of endocarditis; identify cardiac sources of embolization; evaluate chronically implanted prosthetic valves

Method
advance endoscope-mounted transducer into esophagus; crystals at end of the transesophageal echocardiography (TEE) transducer activate to produce ultrasound beam; views of the heart captured

Normal findings
mitral and aortic valves free of vegetations; exclusion of atrial thrombi; absence of mitral valve regurgitation and sinus venosus defects; normal functioning aortic valve cusps

Comments
TEE is useful intraoperatively; provides continuous observation of cardiac function during cardiovascular surgery

Source
Adapted from Webber JD, Schiller NB. Clinical application of transesophageal echocardiography. Internal Medicine 1995;16:58-65.

transfacial transclival approach

Description
surgical approach to midline posterior circulation aneurysm

Anatomy
nasal complex; clivus; ethmoids; sphenoids; vertebral and basilar arteries

Equipment
Mayfield or radiolucent headrest; Doppler flow probe; high-speed air drill; MRI; scimitar blade; Crockard transoral clip applier; Sano clip applier

Source
Adapted from Ogilvy CS, Barker FG, Joseph MP, Cheney ML, Swearingen B, Crowell RM. Transfacial transclival approach for midline posterior circulation aneurysms. Neurosurgery 1996;39:736-742.

transient evoked otoacoustic emission (TEOAE) test

Synonyms
none

Indications
diagnosis of deafness in infants

Method
otoacoustic-specific evoked potential measurement

Normal findings
detectable neuroelectric response to otoacoustic stimulation

Comments
used as a screening test, to be followed by auditory brainstem response test if needed

Source
Adapted from Watkin PM. Neonatal otoacoustic emission screening and the identification of deafness. Archives of Diseases of Children and Fetal and Neonatal Education 1996;74:F16-F25.

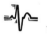

transjugular intrahepatic portosystemic shunt

Synonyms
TIPS; TIPSS

Indications
transjugular intrahepatic portosystemic shunt (TIPS, TIPSS) provides treatment for severe portal hypertension including treatment of severe variceal bleeding unresponsive to standard therapies

Method
a permanent communication between the portal and hepatic veins is achieved through the placement of a metallic stent inserted percutaneously via the jugular vein

Normal findings
intrahepatic metallic stent bridging portal and hepatic veins; diminished portal venous pressures and decompression of portal venous collaterals responsible for variceal bleeding

Comments
provides alternative to traditional high-risk surgical technique

Source
University of Maryland Department of Diagnostic Radiology. Baltimore, MD.

transpapillary pancreatoscopy

Synonyms
none

Indications
exploration of the entire main pancreatic duct

Method
Optiscope C-type CFS-B20SL miniscope

Normal findings
none

Comments
permitting peroral transpapillary endoscopic exploration of the entire main pancreatic duct

Source
Adapted from Özkan H, Saisho H, Yamaguchi T, et al. Clinical usefulness of a new miniscope in the diagnosis of pancreatic disease. Gastrointestinal Endoscopy 1995;17(1):480-485.

 ## transrectal ultrasound-guided transperineal cryoablation

Description
ultrasound-guided percutaneous cryoablation is being effectively used in the treatment of prostatic carcinoma; can be performed rapidly with minimal blood loss; modern ultrasound affords the advantage of precise cryoprobe placement, and accurate regulation of the freezing zone, resulting in maximal prostate destruction with minimal ablation of surrounding tissues; it is a relatively new procedure and requires further evaluation

Anatomy
anterior abdominal wall; bladder; pelvic lymph node; perineum; peripheral posterior prostate; prostate; prostatic urethra; rectum; scrotum; suprapubic area; urethra; urethrorectal area

Equipment
standard surgery equipment; Accuprobe System cryosurgery instrument; cryoprobes; cannulas; Councill tip Foley catheter; dilators; J-tip guide; 18-gauge needles with perineal biopsy guide; percutaneous suprapubic catheter; stylets; 7.5-MHz transducer; transrectal ultrasound; urethral warming device

Source
Adapted from Wieder J, Schmidt JD, Casola G, vanSonnenberg E, Stainken BF, Parsons CL. Transrectal ultrasound-guided transperineal cryoablation in the treatment of prostate carcinoma: preliminary results. The Journal of Urology 1995;154:435-440.

 ## transscleral neodymium:yytrium-aluminum-garnet (Nd:YAG) laser cyclophotocoagulation for glaucoma

Description
noncontact Nd:YAG laser cyclophotocoagulation is effective in lowering intraocular pressure in eyes with refractory glaucoma after keratoplasty; retrobulbar anesthesia given; laser set in multiple mode, 20 milliseconds duration, maximum offset, and single pulse per burst; approximately 30 evenly spaced burns applied 1.0 to 1.5 mm from the corneoscleral limbus for 360 degrees

Anatomy
anterior chamber lens; corneoscleral limbus; cornea; epithelium; optic nerve; posterior chamber lens; retrobulbar area; subconjunctival area; vitreous

592

Equipment

Nd:YAG laser (Lasag Microruptor II)

Source

Adapted from Threlkeld AB, Shields MB. Noncontact transscleral cyclophotocoagulation for glaucoma after penetrating keratoplasty. American Journal of Ophthalmology 1995;120:569-575.

 transsyndesmotic bolt in tibiofibular diastasis

Description

diastasis, in relation to the ankle, is described as a splaying of the fibula away from the tibia beyond the normal yield allowed by the fibrous structure binding the distal ends together; various forms of fixation have been utilized; the authors found the use of transsyndesmotic bolt to be more successful than a transmalleolar screw

Anatomy

distal tibiofibular articulation; fibula; lateral malleolus; ligaments: anterior inferior and posterior inferior tibiofibular; transverse tibiofibular, and interosseous; lateral dorsal cutaneous and sural nerves; tendon of peroneus longus; tibiofibular syndesmosis; tibia; talus; talar dome; tibial plafond; transmalleolar area

Equipment

bone clamp; fiberglass cast; neutralization plate; nut and washer; screws; staples; transmalleolar screw; transsyndesmotic bolt

Source

Adapted from Grady JF, Moore CJ. The use of a transsyndesmotic bolt in the treatment of tibiofibular diastasis: two case studies. Journal of Foot and Ankle Surgery 1995;34:571-576.

 transurethral collagen injection

Description

minimally invasive treatment for type III urinary incontinence; injection of collagen periurethrally via cystourethroscopy

Anatomy

external sphincter; urethra; "drain-pipe" urethra; urethral mucosa; bladder neck; detrusor muscle

Equipment

purified bovine dermal collagen cross-linked with glutaraldehyde; spinal needle; Wolf panendoscope; Bard implant syringe; Contigen (purified collagen implant)

Source

Adapted from Perone N. A simple, yet effective, treatment for intrinsic sphincteric deficiency. Contemporary OB/GYN 1996;41:73-77.

transvaginal fine-needle biopsy

Synonyms
none

Indications
gynecological mass

Method
ultrasound-guided fine-needle biopsy performed through a vaginal approach

Normal findings
not applicable

Comments
can be done more accurately and as safely as a transabdominal puncture of a mass

Source
Adapted from Boschert S. Transvaginal fine-needle biopsies appear safe, accurate. Ob.Gyn. News 1996;31:13.

 transversus and rectus abdominis musculoperitoneal (TRAMP) flap

Description
vulvovaginal reconstruction technique following radical exenterative pelvic surgery; flap of rectus muscle and transversus abdominis muscle created; blood supply from inferior epigastric artery preserved; flap sutured into tube; flap rotated downward to vagina

Anatomy
vagina; vaginal mucosa; rectus abdominis muscle; transversus abdominis muscle; posterior rectus fascia; transversalis fascia; parietal peritoneum; inferior epigastric artery; anterior rectus sheath; linea semilunaris; arcuate line

Equipment
standard surgery equipment

Source
Adapted from Hockel M. The transversus and rectus abdominis musculoperitoneal (TRAMP) composite flap for vulvovaginal reconstruction. Plastic and Reconstructive Surgery 1996;97:455-459.

 TRAUMEX

Description
fully integrated radiographic system which performs all standard radiographic views of both ambulatory and traumatized patients

Source
Fischer Imaging product information. Denver, CO.

594

 Trelex natural mesh

Description
high strength monofilament polypropylene mesh for hernia repair
Source
Meadox Medicals Inc. product information. Oakland, NJ.

 Trelles metal scleral shield

Description
used for protection of sclera, cornea, and conjunctiva during facial laser procedures; ideal for blepharoplasty and skin resurfacing procedures
Source
Byron Medical product information. (*Editor note:* advertising uses byron but company name correctly is Byron) Tucson, AZ.

 Treponema pallidum recombinant antigen-based enzyme immunoassay (EIA)

Synonyms
TPA-EIA
Use
detection of treponemal immunoglobulin G antibodies in blood bank syphilis screening
Method
EIA with two major *Treponema pallidum* recombinant antigens
Specimen
serum
Normal range
negative
Comments
sensitivity and specificity equal to, or greater than, *Treponema pallidum* hemagglutination assay (TPHA) and nontreponemal Venereal Disease Reference Laboratory test (VDRL)
Source
Adapted from Zrein M, Maure I, Boursier F, Soufflet L. Recombinant antigen-based enzyme immunoassay for screening of *Treponema pallidum* antibodies in blood bank routine. Journal of Clinical Microbiology 1995;33:525-527.

tretinoin

Brand name
Vesanoid

Use
second-line treatment of refractory acute promyelocytic leukemia

Usual dosage
oral: recommended dosage is 45 mg/m^2/day administered as a single daily dose or divided into twice daily doses until complete remission is documented; therapy should be discontinued 30 days after the achievement of complete remission or after 90 days of treatment whichever comes first

Pharmaceutical company
Roche Laboratories. Nutley, NJ.

Source
University of Pittsburgh Drug Information and Pharmacoepidemiology Center. Pittsburgh, PA.

 # tretinoin cream

Brand Name
Renova

Use
retinoid that is used to reduce fine wrinkling, surface roughness, and mottled hyperpigmentation caused by photo damage

Usual Dosage
topical cream 0.05%: once daily application

Pharmaceutical company
Ortho Pharmaceutical Corp. Raritan, NJ.

Source
University of Pittsburgh Drug Information and Pharmacoepidemiology Center. Pittsburgh, PA.

 # tretinoin gel

Brand name
Retin-A Micro

Use
formulation for treatment of acne vulgaris that is less irritating to the skin

Usual dosage
topical: applied once daily in the evening; available as microsphere 0.1% topical preparation

Pharmaceutical company
Ortho Pharmaceutical Corp. Raritan, NJ.

Source
Stadtlanders Managed Pharmacy Services. Pittsburgh, PA.

Trichomonas vaginalis one-tube, nested-PCR assay

Synonyms
Trichomonas vaginalis PCR

Use
diagnosis of vaginal trichomoniasis

Method
nested PCR targeting a series of 650 base-pair specific DNA repeats

Specimen
vaginal discharge fluid

Normal range
290 base-pair PCR reaction product not detected

Comments
simple, rapid, accurate, and sensitive method for the diagnosis of vaginal trichomoniasis

Source
Adapted from Lin PR, Shaio MF, Liu JY. One-tube, nested-PCR assay for the detection of *Trichomonas vaginalis* in vaginal discharges. Annals of Tropical Medicine and Parasitology 1997;91:61-65.

TriggerWheel Wand

Description
wand used directly on skin or through light clothing to locate latent trigger points to inactivate them; allows user to maintain constant contact with muscle being treated

Source
RPI product information. Atlanta, GA.

Trileptal

Generic name
see oxcarbazepine

Triple Care antifungal

Description
light, water-based antifungal cream cures athlete's foot, jock itch, ringworm and provides relief of itching, scaling, redness, burning, and irritation

Source
Smith & Nephew Rolyan Inc. product information. Largo, FL.

triple test

Synonyms
triple screen

Use
detect problems in pregnancy

Method
beta human chorionic gonadotropin (B-HCG) and estriol by radioimmunoassay (RIA); alpha-fetoprotein (AFP) by enzyme immunoassay (EIA)

Specimen
blood

Normal range
each component's range is dependent on number of weeks gestation

Comments
none

Source
Lexi-Comp Inc. database. Hudson, OH.

 triptorelin

Brand name
Decapeptyl

Use
luteinizing hormone-releasing hormone (LHRH) agonist that demonstrated efficacy in the treatment of ovarian carcinoma, prostatic carcinoma, endometriosis, uterine leiomyomata, fibrocystic breast disease, and precocious puberty

Usual dosage
intramuscular: usual doses are 3.2 or 3.75 mg once monthly; for central precocious puberty, 50 to 100 mcg/kg every 25 to 30 days

Pharmaceutical company
Organon Inc. West Orange, NJ.

Source
University of Pittsburgh Drug Information and Pharmacoepidemiology Center. Pittsburgh, PA.

trisegmentectomy of liver

Description
hepatic surgical techniques include many types; usually indicates right or left trisegmentectomy without exclusive preservation of the anterior segment; a new alternative form of trisegmentectomy of the liver includes removal of the left lobe, posterior segment, and caudate lobe; this was performed in patients with atrophy of the left lobe and posterior segment due to hepatolithiasis; the procedure is indicated only in a small number of patients

Anatomy
Arantius ligament; Cantlie line; caudate lobe of liver; hepatoduodenal ligament; hilar plate; hepatic hilum; hepatic duct; inferior vena cava; parenchyma; portal venous branch; portal vein; Spigelius lobe; vena cava ligaments

Equipment
standard surgical equipment

Source
Adapted from Miyagawa S, Kawasaki S, Satoh A, Hayashi K, Harada H, Kitamura H, et al. A new alternative for trisegmentectomy of the liver. Journal of American College of Surgeons 1995;181:270-271.

 trisomy 12 detection in chronic lymphocytic leukemia

Synonyms
trisomy 12 testing in CLL

Use
evaluation of patients with CLL prior to morphologic transformation

Method
fluorescence in situ hybridization with DNA probe specific for chromosome 12 centromere

Specimen
blood, bone marrow

Normal range
diploid pattern only; no evidence of trisomy

Comments
may be used to predict which patients will experience poorer prognosis morphologic tranformation

Source
American Journal of Clinical Pathology 1995;104:199-203.

TriStander

Description
Tumble Forms TriStander 45 adjusts prone, supine, and vertical standing; adjustable modules cushion and secure the user at trunk, knees, hip, head, and foot; pneumatic tilt mechanism adjusts from 15 to 90 degrees; foot rests can be tilted 5 degrees forward or backward; includes activity tray, shoes with bar, hip support, and support pads for trunk support
Source
J.A. Preston Corp. product information. Jackson, MI.

 # Tritec

Generic name
see ranitidine bismuth citrate

 # troglitazone

Brand name
Rezulin
Use
first in new generation of diabetes medications known as glitazones; approved for treatment of type II diabetes in patients who are on over 30 units of insulin per day and having uncontrolled glucose levels
Usual dosage
200 and 400 mg tablets
Pharmaceutical company
Parke-Davis Division of Warner-Lambert. Morris Plains, NJ.
Source
Warner-Lambert press release on Internet.

 # Troilius capsulotomy knife

Description
surgical instrument for performing open capsulotomy for capsular contracture occurring after subpectoral breast augmentation; instrument has also been used for dissection in primary breast augmentation
Source
Padgett Instruments product information. Kansas City, MO.

Trovan

Generic name
see trovafloxacin

 True Sheathless catheter

Description
balloon catheter designed to be used without a sheath; less obstruction to blood flow, better peripheral circulation, staged guidewire

Source
Datascope Corp. product information. Fairfield, NJ.

 Tru-Pulse carbon dioxide (CO_2) laser

Description
laser with the potential to produce a pulse varying from 30 μsec to 1 μsec and pulse energy of over 5J/cm²; has shorter pulse duration than the UltraPulse and SilkTouch lasers, which affords faster healing time

Source
Tissue Technologies product information. Albuquerque, NM.

 Trusopt

Generic name
see dorzolamide

 TruZone peak flow meter

Description
peak flow meter (PFM) with logarithmic scale to simplify reading of peak expiratory flow rate (PEFR) with ColorZone tapes that are transparent for actual zones, not end points, preventing inadvertent changes in the PEFR readings, and providing reliable and accurate readings

Source
Monaghan Medical Corp. product information. Plattsburgh, NY.

602

 ## TSI ligature device

Description
hand-held double-needle device for loop ligature placement; permits one-hand operation; needles placed simultaneously into skin; one needle is hollow and suture is passed through it; device handle is squeezed until other needle is locked into place to capture the suture; disposable unit; used for closure of trocar wounds, ligating bleeding vessels

Source
Tahoe Surgical Instruments product information. San Juan, PR.

 ## TubeCheck esophageal intubation detector

Description
used for confirming proper endotracheal tube placement in the emergency-intubated patient; device depends on anatomical features which are constant; when used prior to ventilation gives an immediate answer for appropriate intubation and does not pose the risk of carbon dioxide detection devices

Source
Ambu Inc. product information. Linthicum, MD.

 ## TubeGauz bandage

Description
elastic net bandage conforms to body contours; covers fingers, toes, hands, feet, elbows, and knees

Source
Acme United Corp. product information. Fairfield, CT.

 ## TubiFast bandage

Description
tubular retention bandage holds wound dressings firmly in place; encourages ventilation and freedom of movement

Source
Acme United Corp. product information. Fairfield, CT.

 ## TubiGrip bandage

Description
elastic tubular bandage used for tissue support; indicated for strains/sprains, soft tissue injuries, joint effusions, edema, pressure dressings, post burn scarring, arm fixation, and/or rib cage injuries

Source
Acme United Corp. product information. Fairfield, CT.

tubing introducer forceps

Description
used in glaucoma drainage implant surgery in cases of refractory glaucoma; when closed, the jaw of the forceps forms a channel that holds the tube without crushing it

Source
Accurate Surgical & Scientific Instruments Corp. product information. San Diego, CA.

 Tuf Nex neck exerciser

Description
portable prosthetic device for neck exercise including flexion, extension, abduction, and rotation

Source
Lifeline International product information. Madison, WI.

 Tulip syringe system

Description
large volume aspiration syringe with precision injection capabilities

Source
The Tulip Co. product information. San Diego, CA.

 tumor necrosis as a prognostic factor in glioblastoma multiforme classification

Synonyms
none

Indications
presence of glioblastoma multiforme

Method
multivariate proportional hazards survival analysis was used to assess importance of tumor necrosis after adjustment for other prognostic factors

Normal findings
not applicable

Comments
absence of necrosis was associated with younger age and with less extensive surgical resection; absence of necrosis predicted longer survival in univariate analysis and after adjustments for age

Source
Adapted from Barker II FG, Davis RL, Chang SM et al. Necrosis as a prognostic factor in glioblastoma multiforme. Cancer 1996;77(6):1161-1166.

tumor necrosis factor level

Synonyms
TNF

Use
elevated tumor necrosis factor (TNF) levels have been described in cancer, septic shock, graft rejection, parasitic infections, systemic lupus erythematosus, posthemofiltration products, and during in vivo cytokine therapy; elevations have also been found in human immunodeficiency virus (HIV) infections, malaria, meningococcal meningitis, and kalaazar; TNF acts as a multipotent mediator of the body's defense mechanisms to viral, bacterial, and parasitic infections

Method
immunoradiometric assay (IRMA)

Specimen
blood

Normal range
0-10 pg/ml; investigational use

Comments
performance characteristics have not been established

Source
Lexi-Comp Inc. database. Hudson, OH.

 tumor suppressor gene-inactivating mutation assay

Synonyms
germ-line specimen mutational screening

Use
genetic diagnosis for individuals at high risk for diseases associated with germ-line mutations in cancer susceptibility genes, such as early-onset breast cancer and familial adenomatous polyposis

Method
PCR-amplified gene sequence of interest inserted into a yeast fusion protein, and transformed yeast cells tested for growth characteristics

Specimen
any biological tissue

Normal range
no evidence of mutation

Comments
more rapid and reliable than other screening methods will be valuable in screening high-risk families

Source
Adapted from Ishioka C, Suzuki T, FitzGerald M, et al. Detection of heterozygous truncating mutations in the BRCA1 and APC genes by using a rapid screening assay in yeast. Proceedings of the National Academy of Sciences USA 1997;94:2449-2453.

Turapy device

Description
radiofrequency device for thermal tissue ablation for benign prostatic hypertrophy; heating element and two thermoprobes are mounted on a Foley-like
catheter for simultaneous treatment, administration, and monitoring; treatment administered at a maximum temperature of 70 to 75° C for 1 hour
under local anesthesia

Source
Direx Medical Systems product information. Edinburgh, Scotland.

TurnAide therapeutic system

Description
TurnAide 1000 cover helps protect against adverse effects of external
mechanical forces, including pressure, friction and shearing; resistant to
moisture, abrasion, punctures, and tearing; antimicrobial coating to increase
water resistance and decreased bacteria buildup; promotes positive out-
comes, including reduced risks for pulmonary complications, reduced risk of
urinary tract infection, and decreased risk of developing decubitus ulcers or
pressure ulcers; maintains proper position and body alignment

Source
Dermacare Products Inc. product information. Louisville, KY.

Turner syndrome mosaic analysis

Synonyms
PCR/HUMARA-based Turner syndrome mosaic analysis

Use
detection of cryptic mosaicism in patients with phenotypic variations of
Turner syndrome

Method
Y-chromosome-derived fragments detected by polymerase chain reaction
using three Y-specific primer pairs, and X chromosome mosaicism detected
by modified HUMARA (human androgen receptor assay)

Specimen
blood

Normal range
no evidence of X or Y chromosome mosaicism

Comments
permits detection of low-frequency X- or Y-chromosome fragments in
patients with the genetic disorder Turner syndrome

Source
Adapted from Yorifuji T, Muroi J, Kawai M, Sasaki H, Momoi T, Furusho K. PCR-based detection of mosaicism
in Turner syndrome patients. Human Genetics 1997;99:62-65.

Tuwave unit

Description
pulsed galvanic waveform stimulator to increase blood circulation to site plus transcutaneous electrical nerve stimulator (TENS) for pain control; reduces swelling and pain following knee, ankle, elbow, and hand surgery, bunionectomies, liposuction, pain control from sprains or strains, or muscle spasms

Source
Staodyn Inc. product information. Longmont, CO.

 twin-peak sign

Synonyms
lambda sign

Indications
undetermined chorionicity in multiple pregnancy

Method
ultrasound evaluation for the presence or absence of a triangular projection of placental tissue extending between the layers of the intertwin membrane in multiple pregnancy

Normal findings
not applicable

Comments
none

Source
Adapted from Wood SL, St. Onge R, Connors G, Elliott PD. Evaluation of the twin peak or lambda sign in determining chorionicity in multiple pregnancy. Obstetrics & Gynecology 1996;88:6-9.

 type II collagen

Brand name
Colloral

Use
treatment of adult and juvenile rheumatoid arthritis

Usual dosage
oral liquid: 2 drops in juice, 15 minutes before breakfast

Pharmaceutical company
Autoimmune Inc. Lexington, MA.

Source
Stadtlanders Managed Pharmacy Services. Pittsburgh, PA.

Typhim Vi

Generic name
see typhoid vaccine

 typhoid vaccine

Brand name
Typhim Vi

Use
prevention of typhoid fever

Usual dosage
intramuscular: a single 0.5 ml injection 2 weeks prior to expected exposure

Pharmaceutical company
Connaught Laboratories Inc. Swiftwater, PA.

Source
University of Pittsburgh Drug Information and Pharmacoepidemiology Center. Pittsburgh, PA.

 Typhoon cutter blade

Description
endoscopic sinus surgery blade that works with the microdebrider hand-piece; targeted irrigation prevents clogging; no irrigation occurs during cutting

Source
TreBay Medical Corp. product information. Clearwater, FL.

 Tyshak catheter

Description
microthin peripheral balloon dilatation catheter; low deflation profile; rapid inflation/deflation time; wide selection of sizes

Source
Braun Cardiovascular Division product information. Bethlehem, PA.

 Ultair

Generic name
see pranlukast

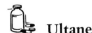 Ultane

Generic name
see sevoflurane

Ultima mammography system

Description
Ultima CR (computed radiography) encompasses all benefits of digital imaging; wide dynamic range allows detection of lesions in dense breasts and permits visualization of wide density differences from chest wall to skin line

Source
Fuji Medical Systems USA Inc. product information. Stamford, CT.

 Ultiva

Generic name
see remifentanil

 Ultraflex esophageal stent

Description
Microvasive esophageal stent maintains patency, resists tumor compression; less traumatic design simplifies implantation and fluoroscopic placement for obstructive esophageal malignancy; 18 mm diameter with 7.5, 10, and 15 cm stent lengths

Source
Microvasive Boston Scientific Corp. product information. Watertown, MA.

 Ultraflex self-adhering male external catheter

Description
flexible, latex-free external catheter to reduce irritation and odor; built-in adhesive is part of the catheter wall and allows easy application providing a strong bond for increased patient confidence and longer wear time; transparent material permits frequent skin inspection; kink-proof funnel ensures uninterrupted urine flow; available in 5 sizes; also Ultraflex pop-on catheter; ideal for long-term external catheter uses

Source
Rochester Medical Corp. product information. Stewartville, MN.

 Ultrafyn cautery tip

Description
thermal cautery tip used in vasectomy

Source
Advanced Meditech International product information. Flushing, NY.

Ultraject contrast media syringe

Description
prefilled syringe for use with radiography and computed tomography exams; avoid delays; prelabeled, eliminating misadministration; save unused Ultraject syringe for future use rather than discard

Source
Mallinckrodt Medical Inc. product information. St. Louis, MO.

 ## Ultra Low resistance voice prosthesis

Description
used in the rehabilitation of patients post total laryngectomy; features a very thin retention collar and a rounded tip for ease of insertion and an auxiliary airflow port; available in 16 and 20 French sizes

Source
Bivona Medical Technologies product information. Gary, IN.

 ## Ultram

Generic name
see tramadol

 ## Ultra-Neb nebulizer

Description
ultrasonic stand-alone aerosol generator designed to meet aerosol therapy needs, including bronchoprovocation testing, drug delivery, and high-volume humidification

Source
DeVilbiss Health Care Inc. product information. Somerset, PA.

 ## UltraPower drill system

Description
surgical drill system with a vast array of cutters

Source
Zimmer product information. Largo, FL.

Ultrata forceps

Description
capsulorrhexis forceps with flat or round handles with ultra-thin 11.5-mm blades to eliminate incision grasping and prevent iris pickup; forceps jaws are angled at 45 degrees to provide a secure grasp of the anterior capsular flap; tongue and groove slot in the iris stop for stable tip closure
Source
Rhein Medical product information. Tampa, FL.

 ## Ultravist

Generic Name
see iopromide

 ## Ultra Voice speech aid

Description
speech aid for laryngeal-impaired individuals, status post laryngectomy, status post ventilator support, or with laryngeal paralysis; worn like a denture or retainer; transmitter is held in the hand and sends the speech signal through the mouth, not through the neck tissues
Source
Ultra Voice product information. Paoli, PA.

 ## Umbrella punctum plug

Description
ultra-thin, slanted collarette with flexible bulb that collapses for easy insertion and then expands to resist expulsion
Source
FCI product information. Marshfield Hills, PA.

 ## Unicat knife

Description
diamond knives for clear corneal procedures; features a single footplate with 7 preset depth settings at 0.25, 0.30, 0.50, 1.50, and 6 mm; ideal for the initial groove followed by entry into the anterior chamber; also 1 mm for initial groove and/or side port incision
Source
American Surgical Instruments Corporation product information. Westmont, IL.

UniFile Imaging and Archiving system

Description
windows-based computerized digital photography and archiving; automatically names, dates, and stores each patient's pictures together in an individual patient file

Source
United Imaging Inc. product information. Winston-Salem, NC.

 ## unilateral laminotomy for bilateral ligamentectomy

Description
degenerative central lumbar stenosis has traditionally been considered to be due to bony narrowing of the spinal canal; lumbar spinal stenosis may have several causes; preoperative radiographic evaluation can point to a markedly thickened ligamentum flavum as the cause of the stenosis; a method has been devised where the ligamentum flavum can be excised with minimal destruction of normal spinal anatomy; the facet joints or intraspinous ligaments are not destroyed when this is done unilaterally through a wide laminotomy

Anatomy
bony canal; cartilage; caudal lamina; cauda equina; disk space; epidural fat; facets; interpedicular lamina; interspinous ligaments; lamina; ligamentum flavum; paraspinal muscles; rostral pedicle, rim and vertebra; spinal canal; spinous process; supraspinous ligaments

Equipment
standard neurosurgery equipment; air drill; straight curette; straight pituitary forceps; angled kerasin rongeur

Source
Adapted from Poletti CE. Central lumbar stenosis caused by ligamentum flavum: unilateral laminotomy for bilateral ligamentectomy: preliminary report of two cases. Neurosurgery Journal 1995;37:343-347.

 ## Unipass endocardial pacing lead

Description
single-pass lead designed for use with implantable pulse generator; used exclusively with Intermedics pulse generators as part of permanent transvenous pacing system

Source
Intermedics Inc. product information. Angleton, TX.

Uniplane rocker

Description

balance device for subconscious control of muscles responsible for postural maintenance and gait; also wooden wobble device and exercise sandals; emphasizes systematic response of the locomotor system influencing musculoskeletal pain

Source

OPTP product information. Minneapolis, MN.

 UniPlast Imaging and Archiving system

Description

windows-based computerized video imaging

Source

United Imaging Inc. product information. Winston-Salem, NC.

 Uniretic

Generic name

see moexipril/hydrochlorothiazide

 Unity-C cardiac pacemaker

Description

implantable, multiprogrammable rate-adaptive cardiac pulse generator that uses a single-pass lead to sense the atrium, and sense and pace the ventricle; primarily intended to provide VDD (atrial synchronous, ventricular inhibited) pacing

Source

Intermedics Inc. product information. Angleton, TX.

 Unity System biopsy handling

Description

portable all-in-one system for ease in organization of accessories and handling biopsies in GI suite

Source

Chek-Med Systems Inc. product information. Camp Hill, PA.

 Univasc

Generic name

see moexipril hydrochloride

Unna-Flex Plus venous ulcer kit

Description
includes 4-inch wide Unna Boot with self-adherent bandage for compression and nonslip support

Source
ConvaTect product information. Princeton, NJ.

 Up and About system

Description
stance and reciprocating gait orthosis designed to give individuals with paraplegia, spina bifida, and other similar disorders, the ability to stand and to move about unassisted; ability to conceal system under patient's clothing

Source
Cascade Orthopaedic Supply Co. product information. Dallas, TX.

 Urban Walkers

Description
diabetic/arthritic shoe designed to give biochemical support, reduce shear force, and provide maximum comfort; moldable multi-density insert included

Source
Acor Orthopaedic Inc. product information. Cleveland, OH.

 ureteral nipple construction

Description
creation of a leak-proof valve in ureteral diversions to prevent reflux; technically demanding due to handling requirements of delicate ureteral tissues

Anatomy
pelvic area; ureters; bladder, adventitia, stoma, ileum, ileocecal segment, rectus and transversalis fascia, ureter, dome, bladder neck, trigone, detrusor, ureterovesical junction

Equipment
standard surgical equipment

Source
Adapted from Atta MA. The everting suture: a new technical aid for ureteral nipple construction. Journal of Urology 1996:155;1372-1373.

urinary glycosaminoglycan (GAG) measurement assay

Synonyms
urinary GAG assay

Use
patient monitoring following diagnosis of hyperthyroidism

Method
enzyme-linked immunosorbent assay (ELISA)

Specimen
urine

Normal range
investigational

Comments
may become useful in follow-up of ophthalmopathy due to thyroid dysfunction

Source
Adapted from Reinhardt MJ, Moser E. An update on diagnostic methods in the investigation of diseases of the thyroid. European Journal of Nuclear Medicine 1996;23:587-594.

 ## urinary gonadotropin peptide detection

Synonyms
UGP; urinary gonadotropin fragment detection (UGF); beta core

Use
monitor clinical status and aid in early detection of serous as well as mucinous, endometroid, and other nonserous ovarian cancer

Method
enzyme immunoassay (EIA)

Specimen
urine

Normal range
less than 4.5 fmol/mg creatinine

Comments
urinary gonadotropin peptide (UGP) has molecular weight of 10.4 kilodaltons and is cleared rapidly from the circulation, therefore, it is measured only in the urine and is not detectable in serum

Source
Lexi-Comp Inc. database. Hudson, OH.

urinary neutrophil elastase (NE) assay

Synonyms
none

Use
diagnosis of urethritis, *Neisseria gonorrhoeae* or *Chlamydia trachomatis* infection

Method
immunoassay

Specimen
urine

Normal range
no detectable neutrophil elastase

Comments
investigational

Source
Adapted from Fraser PA, Teasdale J, Gan KS, Eglin R, Scott SC, Lacey CJ. Neutrophil enzymes in urine for the detection of urethral infection in men. Genitourinary Medicine 1995;71:176-179.

 ## urinary NTx assay

Synonyms
Osteomark

Use
detection of changes in human bone resorption rates

Method
spectrophotometrically-measured immunoassay for N-telopeptides of collagen type I

Specimen
urine

Normal range
5-65 nM NTx/mM creatinine

Comments
primarily for use in women receiving hormone replacement therapy

Source
Journal of Clinical Endocrinology 1994;79:1693-1700.

 ## URIprobe

Description
combination of tests for chlamydial and gonorrheal infections packaged together

Source
Abbott Laboratories product information. Abbott Park, IL.

Uriscreen

Synonyms
none

Use
detection of clinically significant bacteriuria

Method
enzyme-linked immunosorbent assay (ELISA)

Specimen
urine

Normal range
negative

Comments
may represent a sensitive, although less specific alternative to culture screening of all pregnant patients; results in 1 minute; also ideal for geriatrics

Source
Adapted from Hagay Z, Levy R, Miskin A, Milman D, Sharabi H, Insler V. Uriscreen, a rapid enzymatic urine screening test: useful predictor of significant bacteriuria in pregnancy. Obstetrics & Gynecology. 1996;87:410-413.

 Uri-Two

Synonyms
none

Use
used to detect urinary tract infection from a urine sample

Method
split petri dish in which one side contains cystine-lactose-electrolyte-deficient agar to detect Gram-negative and some Gram-positive organisms; the other side has MacConkey II agar to detect Gram-negative bacteria

Specimen
urine

Normal range
presence or absence of growth

Comments
none

Source
Culture Kits product information. Norwich, NY.

 UroCystom unit

Description
computer-based machine for urodynamic tests; determines post void residual

Source
Browne Medical Systems Inc. product information. White Bear Lake, MN.

uroflowmetry curve interpretation

Synonyms
none

Indications
routine investigation in patients with symptoms of lower urinary tract and patients with no symptoms

Method
panel of urologists questioned about relevance of visual inspection and flow parameters for interpretation; parameters included voiding time, flow time, time to maximum flow rate, average flow rate, and voided volume

Normal findings
large differences existed between panel opinions

Comments
results necessitate reconsideration of the diagnostic use of uroflowmetry in daily urologic practice

Source
Adapted from Van De Book C, Stoevelaar HJ, McDonnell J et al. Interpretation of uroflowmetry curves by urologists. Journal of Urology 1997;157:164-168.

 ## urofollitropin

Brand name
Fertinex

Use
stimulation of follicular recruitment and development, and the induction of ovulation in women with polycystic ovary syndrome; also indicated to treat infertility in women who have failed to respond or conceive following adequate clomiphene citrate therapy

Usual dosage
subcutaneous: dosage range from 75 to 300 IU per day

Pharmaceutical company
Serono Laboratories Inc. Randolph, MA.

Source
Stadtlanders Managed Pharmacy Services. Pittsburgh, PA.

 ## UroGold laser

Description
right-angle laser treatment for prostate enlargement; this provides shorter, cheaper procedure for treating benign prostatic hyperplasia

Source
Trimedyne Inc. product information. Irvine, CA.

618

 ## Uroloop electrode

Description
urologic surgical vaporizing instrument; surface combines innovative rolling elements with individual grooved areas for simultaneous cutting and vaporization
Source
Endocare Inc. product information. Irvine, CA.

 ## Urso

Generic name
see ursodeoxycholic acid

 ## ursodeoxycholic acid

Brand name
Urso
Use
solubilizing agent for the treatment of primary biliary cirrhosis
Usual dosage
oral: 13-15 mg/kg/day
Pharmaceutical company
Axcan. Plattsburgh, NY.
Source
Stadtlanders Managed Pharmacy Services. Pittsburgh, PA.

 ## vacuolating cytotoxin gene of *Helicobacter pylori* significance

Synonyms
vacA

Indications
study done to determine the association of vacA genotype with gastric inflammation, in vitro cytotoxin activity, and peptic ulceration
Method
endoscopy and gastric biopsy; biopsies processed for culture and histology; *H. pylori* vacA typed by polymerase chain reaction and colony hybridization; cytotoxin activity assessed by HeLa cell vacuolation assay
Normal findings
tests with different strains of vacA showed duodenal ulcer disease occurring in 89% of 18 patients

Comments
H. pylori strains of vacA signal sequence type s1a are associated with enhanced gastric inflammation and duodenal ulceration; vacA s2 strains are associated with less inflammation and lower ulcer prevalence

Source
Adapted from Atherton JC, Peek RM, Tham KT, Cover TL, Blaser MJ. Clinical and pathological importance of heterogeneity in vacA, the vacuolating cytotoxin gene of *Helicobacter pylori*. Gastroenterology Journal 1997;112:92-99.

 vacuum assisted closure (V.A.C.) dressing

Description
applies negative pressure to specialized dressing positioned in wound cavity or over flap or graft; excess wound fluid collected in disposable canister; applies universal force to draw edges of wound to center, thus assisting wound closure; helps reduce edema, increase blood supply and decrease bacterial colonization; effective with pressure ulcers, chronic wounds, and grafts

Source
Kinetic Concepts Inc. product information. San Antonio, TX.

 vaginal cuff closure

Description
sagittal closure of vaginal cuff during abdominal hysterectomy; reduces enterocele formation and blood loss without compromising vaginal depth; primary modification is use of side-to-side hemostatic sutures instead of traditional front-to-back closure

Anatomy
abdominal cavity; vaginal cuff; uterosacral fold; round ligaments; broad ligament; adnexal structures; bladder peritoneum; bladder; uterine vessels; cervix; posterior fornix

Equipment
standard surgery equipment; Allis clamp; polyglactin suture

Source
Adapted from Watson T. Vaginal cuff closure with abdominal hysterectomy: a new approach. Obstetrical and Gynecological Survey 1995;50:354-356.

620

 ## vaginal wall tube for cystocele repair and treatment of stress urinary incontinence

Description

vaginal wall tube for cystocele repair and treatment of stress urinary incontinence; vaginal wall tube created with base in bladder neck and fixation to periurethral tissues or suspension to suprapubic area

Anatomy

vagina; bladder

Equipment

standard surgical equipment

Source

Adapted from Benizri E, Volpe P, Pushkar D. A new vaginal procedure for cystocele repair and treatment of stress urinary incontinence. The Journal of Urology 1996;156:1623-1625.

 ## valacyclovir

Brand name

Valtrex

Use

acyclovir prodrug for the treatment of herpes simplex and herpes zoster

Usual dosage

oral: 1000 mg 2-3 times daily

Pharmaceutical company

Burroughs Wellcome Co. Research Triangle Park, NC.

Source

University of Pittsburgh Drug Information and Pharmacoepidemiology Center. Pittsburgh, PA.

 ## valproate sodium

Brand name

Depacon

Use

injectable formulation of antiepileptic drug used to temporarily treat certain types of epilepsy when oral administration is not possible

Usual dosage

intravenous: 500 mg four times a day

Pharmaceutical company

Abbott Laboratories. Abbott Park, IL.

Source

Stadtlanders Managed Pharmacy Services. Pittsburgh, PA.

valsartan

Brand name
Diovan

Use
angiotensin-converting enzymes II (ACE II) receptor subtype-1 inhibitors for the treatment of hypertension

Usual dosage
oral: one daily dosing of valsartan in doses of 40 to 80 mg per day investigated in phase I clinical trial

Pharmaceutical company
Novartis (Ciba-Geigy and Sandoz). Summit, NJ.

Source
Stadtlanders Managed Pharmacy Services. Pittsburgh, PA.

 Valtrex

Generic name
see valacyclovir

 VAPORloop

Description
electrosurgical tool used for resection of tissue with added benefit of hemostasis

Source
ENDOcare Inc. product information. Irvine, CA.

 VaporTrode

Description
vaporization electrode for use in standard transurethral resection of prostate; provides rapid vaporization of soft tissue of the urinary tract and prostate; shorter catheterization time and no laser-type irritative symptoms

Source
Circon ACMI product information. Stamford, CT.

Vapor Vac II

Description

second generation smoke plume evacuator used when performing laser surgery, electrosurgery, radiosurgery, and electrocautery procedures; removes noxious odor of smoke plume and the particulate matter, providing staff fresh air and protection against microbes and carbonized tissue, micro-organisms, and viral-DNA

Source

Ellman International Inc. product information. Hewlett, NY.

Vaqta

Generic name

see hepatitis A vaccine

varicella vaccine

Brand name

Varivax

Use

prevention of varicella-zoster virus or chickenpox

Usual dosage

subcutaneous: one 0.5 ml injection which is equivalent to 1000 to 1625 plaque-forming units of live attenuated virus

Pharmaceutical company

Merck Human Health Division. West Point, PA.

Source

University of Pittsburgh Drug Information and Pharmacoepidemiology Center. Pittsburgh, PA.

Varigrip spine fixation system

Description

provides multidirectional support; attaches to lamina without pedicle screws; manufactured by Advance and distributed by Paragon

Source

Food and Drug Administration Internet site.

Varivax

Generic name
see varicella vaccine

 Vasceze Vascular Access Flush Device (VAFD)

Description
enables the delivered pressure to be less than syringes and other flush devices; a safe alternative for peripheral, CVC (central venous catheter), PICC (peripherally inserted central catheter), and midline catheter flush sequences

Source
Vital Signs Inc. product information. Totowa, NJ.

 vascular bundle implantation into bone

Description
implantation of vascular bundle containing the ramus carpeus dorsalis of the interosseal anterior artery into the lunate bone for aseptic necrosis; vascular bundle ligated, severed, and inserted into the lunate bone; the two ligated ends of the vascular bundle tied to straight needles, pushed through drill holes, and continued forward obliquely to the palm of the hand; the two ends were ligated to the skin with a button padded to immobilize the vascular bundle

Anatomy
arterial radialis; dorsal articular capsule; extensor digitorum communis muscles; lunate bone; metacarpophalangeal joint; nervus medianus; nervus ulnaris; perivascular connective tissues; processus styloideus; ramus carpeus dorsalis of the interosseal anterior artery and vein; ulna

Equipment
button; Kirschner wire; pneumatic tourniquet; straight needle; drill; plaster cast

Source
Adapted from Jing-hua Guo. Vascular bundle implantation into bone for aseptic necrosis of the lunate. Annals of Plastic Surgery 1996;36:133-138.

vascularized split calvarial cranioplasty

Description
diagnose intrasphenoidal temporal encephalocele with radionuclide cisternography and beta$_2$-transferrin assay; frontotemporal incision creates calvarial graft with vascularized pedicle attached to temporalis muscle; perform craniotomy and zygomatic osteotomy; amputate pedicle of the encephalocele; split calvarial graft, trim to fit sphenoid sinus defect, and hold with microplate and screws; intradural patch and fibrin glue used to close dural defect

Anatomy
sphenoid sinus; sphenoid wall; calvarium; temporalis muscle; zygoma; zygomatic arch and root; frontozygomatic suture; orbital rim; temporal lobe; temporalis fascia; cranial base; dura; foramen rotundum; foramen ovale

Equipment
standard neurosurgery equipment; four-hole Lorenz titanium microplate; fibrin glue

Source
Adapted from Clyde BL, Stechison MT. Repair of temporosphenoidal encephalocele with a vascularized split calvarial cranioplasty: technical case report. Neurosurgery 1995;36:202-206.

 ## Vasomax

Generic name
see phentolamine

 ## VasoView balloon dissection system

Description
for vascular and cardiovascular procedures; incorporates BiCOAG product line of bipolar cutting forceps and scissors for endoscopic harvesting of saphenous vein; manufactured by Guidant/Everest Medical Minneapolis, MN

Source
Internet news sources.

 ## VaxSyn

Generic Name
see AIDS vaccine

Vector low back analysis system

Description
documents pain accurately and objectively; measures low back range of motion in 3D with patient input switch

Source
Baltimore Therapeutic Equipment Co. product information. Hanover, MD.

VectorVision surgical tracking system

Description
wireless surgical tracking system that establishes a three-dimensional link between computed tomography, magnetic resonance, patient anatomy, and all instrumentation

Source
BrainLAB USA Inc. product information. Moorestown, NJ.

velnacrine maleate

Brand name
Mentane

Use
centrally acting cholinesterase inhibitor used to enhance cognition and memory in patients with Alzheimer disease

Usual dosage
oral: 30 to 225 mg daily in divided doses

Pharmaceutical company
Hoechst-Roussel Pharmaceuticals Inc. Somerville, NJ.

Source
University of Pittsburgh Drug Information and Pharmacoepidemiology Center. Pittsburgh, PA.

Veni-Gard stabilization dressing

Description
dressing with transparent window which provides visibility of IV insertion site; provides maximum catheter stabilization; minimizes pullouts and restarts; several styles available AP (all purpose), ML (multi-lumen catheter), SP (special port), TM (transparent membrane), TM JR. (transparent membrane junior size), TPN (total parenteral nutrition), and IV (intravenous) describe the types of stabilization

Source
CONMED Andover Medical Inc. product information. Haverhill, MA.

venlafaxine

Brand name
Effexor

Use
serotonin, norepinephrine, and dopamine reuptake inhibitor used in the treatment of depression

Usual dosage
oral: 25, 37.5, 50, 75, and 100 mg tablets; initial dose of 75 mg daily in 2-3 divided doses; may be increased to 150 or 225 mg daily depending upon tolerance and need; maximum daily dose is 375 mg

Pharmaceutical company
Wyeth-Ayerst Laboratories. Philadelphia, PA.

Source
University of Pittsburgh Drug Information and Pharmacoepidemiology Center. Pittsburgh, PA.

 venous arterial blood management protection system (VAMP)

Description
closed blood sampling system; eliminates the threat of needle sticks and minimizes blood spatter while increasing blood conservation; a direct draw unit with preattached cannula allowing quick and easy filling of laboratory tubes

Source
Baxter Healthcare Corp. product information. Santa Ana, CA.

 Ventrix tunnelable ventricular intracranial pressure (ICP) monitoring system

Description
the sensor at the tip accurately measures ICP; tunnelability enables utilization of favored technique for catheter placement; large lumen facilitates CSF (cerebrospinal fluid) drainage

Source
NeuroCare Group product information. San Diego, CA.

 vermiform appendix as internal urinary device in oncology

Description
urinary obstruction is frequent in gynecologic malignancy; resection of a damaged ureter sometimes is required; to avoid complications of common techniques, the use of vermiform appendix as an internal device is proposed for repair of a resected ureter; the distal tip of the appendix is amputated; the appendix mesentery vascularization is protected, and rotated toward either end of the resected ureter; the ends of the ureter and appendix are anastomosed; pigtail stent is placed in lumen of repaired ureter; one end is in the renal pelvic area, and the other in the bladder

Anatomy

appendix; appendix mesentery; bladder; cecum; juxtavesical portion of ureter; lumen; mesentery; psoas muscle; rectovaginal area; renal pelvic area; ureter; vermiform appendix; vesicovaginal area

Equipment

standard surgery equipment; pigtail stent

Source

Adapted from Scarabelli C, Giorda G, Zarrelli A, Campagnutta E. Use of the vermiform appendix as an internal urinary device in gynecologic oncology. American College of Surgeons 1995;181:171-173.

 ## Verruca-Freeze freezing system

Description

a freezing system without the hassles of liquid nitrogen; simple bloodless procedure that takes less than a minute; treats 21 types of benign skin lesions including hard-to-treat plantar warts

Source

Cryosurgery Inc. product information. Nashville, TN.

 ## VertaAlign spinal support system

Description

two-piece constuction of rigid plastic shell; delivers external spinal support in as little as 10 minutes; compatible with diagnostic imaging modalities

Source

Bremer Group Co. product information. Jacksonville, FL.

 ## Vertetrac ambulatory traction system

Description

unique ambulatory traction system for treatment of lower back pain; requires no connection to a power source and no drugs

Source

Meditrac product information. Palm Desert, CA.

 ## Vesanoid

Generic name

see tretinoin

vesicovaginal Holter

Synonyms
none

Indications
a specially designed vaginal transducer, used as part of continuously ambu-latory monitoring to detect occult bladder instability; reveals occult detrusor contraction and thus facilitates diagnosis

Method
uses a microtip vaginal transducer and a modified continuous ambulatory monitor

Normal findings
not given

Comments
early detection to determine the degree of vaginal prolapse, cystorectocele, and bladder incontinence; still in testing stage

Source
Adapted from Jill M, Rabin MD, Copal H, Badlani MD, Albert Einstein College of Medicine of Yeshiva University, Bronx, NY. Detecting bladder instability with the vesicovaginal Holter. Contemporary OB/GYN, April 1996.

 vesnarinone

Brand name
Arkin-Z

Use
inotropic agent used in the treatment of symptomatic congestive heart fail-ure (CHF)

Usual dosage
oral: 60 mg once daily

Pharmaceutical company
Otsuka America Inc. Rockville, MD.

Source
University of Pittsburgh Drug Information and Pharmacoepidemiology Center. Pittsburgh, PA.

 Vess chair

Description
adaptive seating device with ergonomic design and tilting flexibility; for modified barium swallow study, assures proper patient positioning; provides departments of imaging and speech-language pathology with proper posi-tioning of patient

Source
Vess Chairs Inc. product information. Wauwatosa, WI.

VestaBlate system balloon device

Description
conformable balloon with temperature-controlled electrodes for endometrial ablation; electrode balloon conforms to uterine cavity, obviating device manipulation; allows uterine tissue to be necrosed to a predictable depth

Source
Vesta Medical product information. Mountain View, CA.

Vestibulator positioning tumble forms

Description
creates vertical stimulation and direct flexion, linear acceleration, rotational experiences, head righting opportunities, and range of motion exercises; Vestibulator II with prone net swing and mat, platform swing, net swing with positioning, roll swing, flexidisk, rope with ascender

Source
J.A. Preston Corp. product information. Jackson, MI.

Vexol

Generic name
see rimexolone

V1 halo ring

Description
maintains traction during application without having to remove tongs; cervical spine application kit provides 29 pin sites concentrated in areas most frequently used; offers enhanced imaging compatibility with x-ray, MRI, and CT scans; compatible with 2-pin tong systems and all major vest systems

Source
Jerome Medical product information. Trenton, NJ.

VIA arterial blood gas and chemistry monitor

Description
near-continuous arterial blood gas and chemistry monitor

Source
VIA Medical Corp. product information. San Diego, CA.

Viagra

Generic name
see sildenafil

G5 Vibramatic massage/percussion unit

Description
continuously variable speed range of 20 to 50 cycles per second; 30-minute timer with automatic shut-off provides consistent, precise treatment intervals; directional-stroking motion adapter for machine assisted physical therapy procedures; manipulates soft tissues to produce desired effects on nervous and muscular systems; enhances local and general circulation of blood and lymphatic tissues

Source
General Physiotherapy Inc. product information. Earth City/St. Louis, MO.

 ## Vidas estradiol II assay kit

Synonyms
none

Use
this sixty-use kit determines total estradiol concentration in plasma or serum and is for use with the Vidas and mini Vidas automated immunoassay systems

Method
automated quantitative enzyme-linked fluorescent assay for estradiol

Specimen
serum or plasma

Normal range
not applicable

Comments
none

Source
bioMerieux Vitek product information. Hazelwood, MO.

 ## video-assisted thoracoscopic thymectomy

Description
video-assisted thoracoscopic surgery (VATS) provides new approach to traditional transsternal thymectomy for myasthenia gravis

Anatomy
intercostal spaces; pleural symphysis; mediastinum; pleura; endothoracic fascia; pericardium; thymic isthmus; thymic horn

Equipment
0-degree telescope; Endoshears; endoscopic scissors; standard endoscopic equipment

Source
Adapted from Kay R, Ho J. Video-assisted thoracoscopic thymectomy for myasthenia gravis. Chest 1995;105(5):1440-1443.

videostroboscopic diagnostic determination

Synonyms
videoendoscopy; strobovideolaryngoscopy

Indications
differentiation of true vocal fold cysts from polyps

Method
videostroboscopic examination evaluated according to stroboscopic established parameters for symmetry, amplitude, periodicity, mucosal wave, and closure

Normal findings
mucosal wave was diminished or absent in 100% of true vocal fold (TVF) cysts, and present or increased in 80% of TVF polyps (most important parameter)

Comments
stroboscopic evaluation of mucosal wave is helpful in preoperative differentiation of TVF cysts and polyps

Source
Adapted from Shohet JA, Courey MS, Scott MA, Ossoff RH. Value of videostroboscopic parameters in differentiating true vocal fold cysts from polyps. The Laryngoscope 1996;106:19-26.

 Viewing Wand

Description
neurosurgical device held by the surgeon; connected to CT or MRI scanner; CT or MRI image can be manipulated for image-guided surgery

Source
ISG Technologies Inc. product information. Ontario, Canada.

 vigabatrin

Brand name
Sabril

Use
treatment of refractory epilepsy

Usual dosage
oral: 2-3 g daily in 1 or 2 divided doses increasing up to 4 g daily as needed

Pharmaceutical company
Marion Merrell Dow. Kansas City, MO.

Source
University of Pittsburgh Drug Information and Pharmacoepidemiology Center. Pittsburgh, PA.

Villalta retractor

Description
ergonomically designed 4-bladed abdominal surgical retractor with auto-matic self-locking mechanism; increases surgical exposure, visibility, and instrument maneuverability; less potential for ecchymoses and/or femoral nerve damage

Source
Advanced Surgical Inc. product information. Princeton, NJ.

 Villasenor-Navarro fixation ring

Description
ophthalmic fixation ring and degree gauge surgical instrument for globe fix-ation and axial alignment of corneal incisions to correct astigmatism

Source
Accurate Surgical & Scientific Instruments Corp. product information. Westbury, NY.

 viloxazine

Brand Name
Catatrol

Use
bicyclic antidepressant for use in depression and sleep disorders

Usual Dosage
oral: 100 mg to 300 mg/day

Pharmaceutical company
Zeneca. Wilmington, DE.

Source
University of Pittsburgh Drug Information and Pharmacoepidemiology Center. Pittsburgh, PA.

 vinorelbine

Brand name
Navelbine

Use
single agent or in combination with cisplatin for the treatment of unre-sectable, advanced Stage III or IV non-small-cell lung cancer

Usual dosage:
intravenous: 25 to 30 mg/m^2 infused; dosage adjustment required in patients with hematologic toxicity or liver insufficiency

Pharmaceutical company
Bristol-Meyers Squibb Co. Princeton, NJ.

Source
University of Pittsburgh Drug Information and Pharmacoepidemiology Center. Pittsburgh, PA.

Viracept

Generic name
see nelfinavir

 viral neutralization assay for anti-HIV-1 antibody or antiserum

Synonyms
HIV-1 viral neutralization assay

Use
determination of anti-HIV-1 neutralizing activity of monoclonal antibodies and anti-HIV-1 immune sera

Method
HIV-1 viral load measured before and after treatment with anti-HIV-1 monoclonal antibodies or anti-HIV-1 immune sera, using HIV-1-infected peripheral blood mononuclear cells, p24 antigen ELISA, and HIV provirus synthesis PCR

Specimen
anti-HIV-1 monoclonal antibody or anti-HIV-1 immune serum

Normal range
not applicable

Comments
provides a functional measurement of anti-HIV-1 immune function for evaluation of infected patients and for vaccine development

Source
Adapted from Candotti D, Rosenheim M, Huraux JM, Agut H. Two PBMC-based neutralization assays depict low reactivity of both anti-V3 monoclonal antibodies and immune sera against HIV-1 primary isolates. Journal of Virological Methods 1997;64:81-93.

 Viramune

Generic name
see nevirapine

 Virazole

Generic Name
see ribavirin

 Visipaque

Generic name
see iodixanol

Visi-Tube catheter

Description
peritoneal dialysis catheter features a co-extruded radiopaque stripe for easy monitoring on x-rays; enables tracking of internal positioning; surface treated with Spi-Argent II; tapered intra-abdominal end for reduced irritation; adult and pediatric sizes

Source
Sil-Med Corporation product information. Taunton, MA.

 ## Vistide

Generic name
see cidofovir

 ## Visuflo wand

Description
surgical visualization instrument; fan-shaped tip delivers a light mist of humidified air which gently pushes blood away from surgical site

Source
Research Medical Inc. product information. Midvale, UT.

 ## vitamin D receptor (VDR or vdr) gene expression

Synonyms
none

Use
assessing the risk of osteoporosis in postmenopausal women and dialysis patients

Method
immunoassay detection and quantitation of VDR (or vdr) gene product

Specimen
blood

Normal range
not yet established

Comments
may have widespread utility in guiding pharmacotherapy for postmenopausal women

Source
Adapted from Ruggiero M, Pacini S. VDR (or vdr) gene study in assessing the genetic risk of osteoporosis: from experimental research on the dialysis patient to its routine use in the diagnosis, prognosis and therapy of postmenopausal osteoporosis. Epidemiologiae Prevenzione 1996;20:140-141.

Vitek automated susceptibility system for *Vibrio cholerae*

Synonyms
Vitek susceptibility testing

Use
determination of antibiotic susceptibility profiles for *Vibrio cholerae* isolates

Method
automated liquid-phase cell growth and metabolism measurement

Specimen
microbial culture specimen

Normal range
susceptible

Comments
emerging antibiotic-resistant strains of *Vibrio cholerae* necessitate susceptibility testing of all new isolates

Source
Adapted from Sciortino CV, Johnson JA, Hamad A. Vitek system antimicrobial susceptibility testing of O1, O139, and non-O1 *Vibrio cholerae*. Journal of Clinical Microbiology 1996;34:897-900.

 Vitinoin

Generic name
see retinoic acid

 Vitrasert

Generic name
see ganciclovir

 vitrectomy for proliferative retinopathy

Description
diabetic retinopathy with peripheral fibrovascular proliferation involving
equatorial and pre-equatorial fundus is an unusual syndrome; vitrectomy in
these cases differs from conventional approaches in that relief of retinal traction must be attained by scleral buckling and dissection of peripheral
fibrovascular disease; lensectomy and relaxing retinotomy may be required
in advanced cases; fibrovascular proliferation usually occurs in postequator-
ial fundus; in contrast, there have been cases of severe fibrovascular proliferation limited to equator or pre-equatorial fundus

Anatomy
anterior hyaloid body and ciliary body region; equatorial retina; equatorial
and pre-equatorial fundus; fundus; hyaloid membrane; macula; peripheral
fibrovascular tissue; retina; retrohyaloid membrane region; retrolenticular
body region; vitreous vitrectomy for proliferative retinopathy

Equipment
standard ophthalmic equipment; B-scan ultrasound; applanation tonometer; fluid-gas exchange: sulfur hexafluoride (SF6) 20% or perfluoropropane (C3F8) 10% to 20% in air; diode laser indirect ophthalmoscope; argon blue-green endolaser

Source
Adapted from Han DP, Pulido JS, Mieler WF, Johnson MW. Vitrectomy for proliferative diabetic retinopathy with severe equatorial fibrovascular proliferation. American Journal of Ophthalmology 1995;119:563-570.

 ## vitreous cells as indicator of retinal tears

Synonyms
none

Indications
for definition of relationship between vitreous cells and retinal tears in eyes without recent flashes or floaters

Method
after dilation, slit-lamp examination of the anterior to midvitreous was performed; density of vitreous cells graded; measurements taken using a 1 x 9-mm vertical slit-lamp beam to examine vitreous from immediately behind the lens to midvitreous

Normal findings
cell density ranged from 0 to 4+ with 0 indicating no cells; trace, occasional cells; 1, 1 to 9 cells per field; 2+, 10 to 30 cells; 3+, 31 to 100 (estimated) cells; 4+, innumerable cells

Comments
substantial number of vitreous cells is correlated with presence of retinal tear

Source
Adapted from Boldrey E. Vitreous cells as an indicator of retinal tears in asymptomatic or not recently symptomatic eyes. American Journal of Ophthalmology 1997;123:263-264.

 ## V-Lace digital video

Description
real-time digital video that offers light-to-dark contrasts, while preserving true color, for better visualization in all endoscopic procedures

Source
DigiVision Inc. product information. San Diego, CA.

Vmax series

Description
physiological tool kit of sensors and analyzers for pulmonary analysis, cardiopulmonary exercise testing, respiratory mechanics evaluation, and nutritional assessment; computer programs guide the user through testing and quality monitoring with a built-in tutorial

Source
SensorMedics Corp product information. Yorba Linda, CA.

 Volk Super Quad 160 pan-retinal lens

Description
diagnostic and therapeutic aspheric ocular lens allows 160 degree viewing inside the eye

Source
Volk Optical product information. Mentor, OH.

 Vortex Clear-Flow port

Description
rounded access port chamber with tangential outlet; fluid flows smoothly; the flow in turn cleans the chamber to prevent sludge

Source
Norfolk Medical product information. Skokie, IL.

 Vu-Max speculum

Description
vaginal surgical instrument that features an extremely wide rectangular yoke at speculum opening; eliminates chance of obstructing physician's view; blades size of standard speculum for comfort to patient

Source
Euro-Med division of CooperSurgical product information. Shelton, CT.

 Wagdy double-V osteotomy

Description
modifies Mitchell, Chevron, and Wilson oblique osteotomy treatment of flexible hallux valgus deformities; direct distal-V osteotomy and proximal-V osteotomy distally and laterally to join the first distal-V osteotomy at the junction between the medial one-third and lateral two-thirds of the transverse diameter of the metatarsal head; excise bone between the two osteotomies

Anatomy
metatarsal joints; foot; toes; proximal phalanx

Equipment
standard surgery equipment; tourniquet; osteotome; oscillating saw; hand pressure; below-knee nonweightbearing plaster cast

Source
Adapted from Wagdy S, El-Sheshtawy OE, Megahed A-HA. Evaluation of Wagdy technique for treatment of hallux valgus double-V osteotomy. Journal of Foot and Ankle Surgery 1995;34:65-73.

 Wallstent esophageal prosthesis

Description
flexible stent that expands after placement; makes palliation of malignant esophageal strictures less traumatic; consists of 2 layers with a silicone membrane in between to help prevent tumor ingrowth

Source
Schneider Inc. product information. Minneapolis, MN.

 Wave Web

Description
resistance glove used for therapeutic water aerobic rehabilitation exercises

Source
FlagHouse Rehab product information. Mt Vernon, NY.

 Wayfarer prosthesis

Description
modifiable foot prosthesis for wearing sandals and/or limited barefoot walking; available in 24 cm, 26 cm, and 28 cm sizes

Source
Kingsley product information. Costa Mesa, CA.

 Welch Allyn single fiber illumination headlight

Description
surgical headlight using fiberoptic cable and lightweight luminaire with 130 degree projection angle

Source
Welch Allyn product information. Syracuse, NY.

 West hand and foot nerve tester

Description
device detects and classifies peripheral neuropathy with increased grading accuracy; advanced version of Semmes-Weinstein test

Source
Sammons Inc. product information. Western Springs, IL.

Whitehall Glacier Pack

Description
cold therapy treatment; constructed with double-seamed 14-mil polyvinyl chloride (PVC) cover and flexible type filler that never freezes; pack conforms to area of treatment

Source
Whitehall Manufacturing Inc. product information. City of Industry, CA.

Whitney single use plastic curette

Description
curette used to remove excess cement; thumb notch allows user to tell orientation of tip even when it is hidden by implant

Source
Whitney Products Inc. product information. Glenview, IL.

Wichman retractor

Description
surgical instrument useful for exposure of acetabulum during hip replacement and acetabular reconstructive surgery; particularly helpful for exposure of posterior rim of acetabulum

Source
Innomed Inc. product information. Savannah, GA.

WIDEBAND urinary catheter

Description
soft silicon male external catheter with extra wide adhesive area for more secure fit

Source
Rochester Medical product information. Stewartville, MN.

Wiktor GX Hepamed coated coronary artery stent system

Description
heparin-coated stent to reduce incidence of clotting in coronary stenting procedures

Source
Medtronic Inc. product information. Minneapolis, MN.

Wilson-Cook esophageal Z-stent

Description
series of wire cylinders woven in a Z-configuration; sides covered with silicone membrane to prevent tumor ingrowth

Source
Wilson-Cook Medical Inc. product information. Winston-Salem, NC.

 ## WinRho SD

Generic Name
see rho (D) immune globuline intravenous (human)

 ## Woolley tibia punch

Description
orthopaedic surgical instrument designed to impact cancellous bone in subchondral weightbearing region of tibia; helps to improve mechanical interlock in cancellous bone/cement interface

Source
Innomed Inc. product information. Savannah, GA.

 ## Xalatan

Generic name
see latanoprost

 ## xamoterol

Brand name
not yet available

Use
positive inotrope used in the treatment of mild to moderate heart failure; may be useful in patients with angina complicating left ventricular dysfunction

Usual dosage
oral: 200 mg twice daily

Pharmaceutical company
Stuart. Rockville, MD.

Source
University of Pittsburgh Drug Information and Pharmacoepidemiology Center. Pittsburgh, PA.

Xelide

Generic name
see dofetilide

 Xeloda

Generic name
see capecitabine

 Xenical

Generic name
see orlistat

 Xosten

Generic name
see potassium bicarbonate

 XP peritympanic hearing instrument

Description
deep-canal hearing instrument with acoustical benefits; bony seal tip (BST) permits the hearing instrument tip to penetrate and make an active seal in the bony ear canal; seal is maintained with light pressure on the canal wall but remains active and comfortable when the patient is talking and/or chewing; BST comes with an integral wax guard and is easily removed for cleaning

Source
Philips Hearing Instruments product information. Mahwah, NJ.

 XTB knee extension device

Description
knee extension board for patients status post anterior cruciate ligament reconstruction, total knee replacement, below-the-knee amputation, and/or trauma

Source
Indiana Brace Co. product information. Indianapolis, IN.

X-Trel spinal cord stimulation system

Description
electronic device, implanted in a pocket in the skin for relief of residual pain; external transmitter worn as the power source

Source
Medtronic Inc. product information. Minneapolis, MN.

XXMEN-OE5

Generic Name
see edobacomab

Yashica Dental Eye II camera

Description
intraoral camera with a 100-mm macrolens and built-in ring flash

Source
PhotoMed International product information. Van Nuys, CA.

Youlten nasal inspiratory peak flow meter

Description
provides simple, rapid indication of nasal airway patency; suitable for assessment of response to provocation

Source
Clemens Clarke Inc. product information. Columbus, OH.

Yu-Holtgrewe malleable blade

Description
blade attaches to a standard surgical Balfour, Wexler, or Grieshaber self-retaining retractor; center groove allows the inflated Foley catheter to be trapped in place in the bladder while the bladder is retracted toward the patient's head; notched blade prevents the bladder from gradually slipping out of place; designed to enhance and maintain retropubic exposure during radical retropubic prostatectomy

Source
Rusch Inc. product information. Duluth, GA.

ZAAG (Zest Anchor Advanced Generation) guide and pin

Description
tools used by restorative dentists for measuring the degree of divergency from parallel for the placement of proper angle correction components; the angle measurement guide determines the angulation of the implant; the alignment pin is designed to be threaded into a divergent implant to extend the angle several millimeters above the tissue

Source
Zest Anchors Inc. product information. Escondido, CA.

 ZAAG (Zest Anchor Advanced Generation) implant anchor

Description
dental implant anchoring system with the choice of three female anchors allowing for the best placement regardless of tissue depth; the low intragingival design allows for more vertical height space for the prosthesis attachment in a close bite situation

Source
Zest Anchors Inc. product information. Escondido, CA.

 Zadaxin

Generic name
see thymosin alpha 1

 Zaditen

Generic name
see ketotifen

 zafirlukast

Brand Name
Accolate

Use
leukotriene antagonist used in the treatment of asthma

Usual Dosage
oral: 10, 20, or 40 mg twice daily was used in clinical trials metered-dose inhaler: 0.05 mg in four daily actuations or 0.2 mg in a single daily actuation was used in clinical trials

Pharmaceutical company
Zeneca. Wilmington, DE.

Source
University of Pittsburgh Drug Information and Pharmacoepidemiology Center. Pittsburgh, PA.

Zagam

Generic name
see sparfloxacin

 Zanaflex

Generic name
see tizanidine hydrochloride

 Zeldox

Generic name
see ziprasidone

 Zelicof orthopaedic awl

Description
cannulated awl designed to help in placement of guidewire for cannulated screws; awl helps hold bony fragments in position
Source
Innomed Inc. product information. Savannah, GA.

 Zemuron

Generic name
see rocuronium bromide

 Zenapax

Generic name
see daclizumab

 Z-epicanthoplasty

Description
double-lid procedure that enhances the aesthetic result by lengthening the palpebral fissure, producing the image of a larger, open eye; used extensively in Asian patients
Anatomy
supratarsal fold; eyelid; lacrimal lake; ocular globe; medial canthal fold; orbicularis oculi muscle

Equipment
fine felt-tip marker; scalpel

Source
Adapted from Park JI. Z-epicanthoplasty in Asian eyelids. Plastic and Reconstructive Surgery 1996;98:602-609.

 Zerit

Generic name
see stavudine

 ZEUS robotic system

Description
computer and voice-controlled robotic system that positions and maneuvers an endoscope and instruments for microsurgical procedures for cardiothoracic surgeries including endoscopic coronary artery bypass graft (E-CABG); allows for multiple occluded coronary arteries to be bypassed without thoracotomy or mini-thoracotomy currently used; expected to be commercially available in 1998 and will be distributed by Medtronic, Inc.

Source
Computer Motion product information. Goleta, CA.

 zileuton

Brand name
Leutrol

Use
agent with varying degrees of efficacy in the treatment of mild to moderate asthma, ulcerative colitis, and allergic rhinitis

Usual dosage
oral: 600 mg four times daily for the treatment of asthma; 800 mg twice daily in the treatment of ulcerative colitis

Pharmaceutical company
Abbott Laboratories. Abbott Park, IL.

Source
University of Pittsburgh Drug Information and Pharmacoepidemiology Center. Pittsburgh, PA.

 Zimmer Pulsavac wound debridement system

Description
fan spray tip for soft tissue and wound debridement, irrigation, and cancellous bone preparation; includes radial spray tip, aggressive femoral tip, single stream tip, adjustable tip, shower spray tip, and revision femoral tip

Source
Zimmer Patient Care Division product information. Dover, OH.

zinc acetate

Brand name
Galzin

Use
used after chelation therapy in the treatment of Wilson disease

Usual dosage
oral: 50 mg 3 times a day for adults or 25 mg 3 times a day for pregnant women and children over 10 years of age

Pharmaceutical company
Teva Pharmaceuticals. Sellersville, PA.

Source
Stadtlanders Managed Pharmacy Services. Pittsburgh, PA.

 ## zinc lozenges

Brand name
Cold-Eeze

Use
over-the-counter homeopathic lozenge for prevention and reduction of common cold symptoms

Usual dosage
oral: each lozenge contains 11.5 mg of zinc; during cold season, take 2 lozenges a day to prevent common cold symptoms; if the cold symptoms have already started, take one lozenge every 2 to 4 hours until the symptoms have ceased; also Cold-Eezer Plus with 14.5 mg zinc per lozenge

Pharmaceutical company
Quigley Corp. Doylestown, PA.

Source
Stadtlanders Managed Pharmacy Services. Pittsburgh, PA.

 ## Zinecard

Generic name
see dexrazoxane

 ## Zipper anti-disconnect device

Description
tracheostomy tie prevents accidental ventilator disconnection from tracheostomy tube site; one-piece neck-band with Velcro fasteners

Source
Zipper Medical product information. Kensington, MD.

ziprasidone

Brand name
Zeldox

Use
atypical antipsychotic agent with both dopaminergic and serotonergic receptor-blocking activities for the treatment of schizophrenia

Usual dosage
oral: 60 to 80 mg twice a day in clinical trials

Pharmaceutical company
Pfizer Pharmaceuticals Inc. New York, NY.

Source
Stadtlanders Managed Pharmacy Services. Pittsburgh, PA.

 ## Z-Med catheter

Description
peripheral, high-pressure balloon catheter; low deflation profile; rapid inflation/deflation time

Source
Braun Cardiovascular Division product information. Bethleham, PA.

 ## Zoladex implant

Description
goserelin acetate implant provides pain relief and reduction of lesions in treatment of endometriosis; monthly gonadotropin releasing hormone (GnRH) agonist administration in prefilled, ready-to-use syringes; also indicated as palliative treatment of advanced breast cancer in pre- and postmenopausal women

Source
Zeneca Pharmaceuticals product information. Wilmington, DE.

 ## zolmitriptan

Brand name
Zomig

Use
second generation selective serotonin receptor antagonist for the acute treatment of migraines

Usual dosage
oral: 10 mg dose was used in clinical trials

648

Pharmaceutical company
Zeneca Pharmaceuticals. Wilmington, DE.
Source
Stadtlanders Managed Pharmacy Services. Pittsburgh, PA.

 Zomig

Generic name
see zolmitriptan

 zonisamide

Brand name
Excegran

Use
benzisoxazole derivative used in the treatment of incurable epileptic convulsions

Usual dosage
oral: clinical trials have used doses of 100 to 600 mg daily in single dose or 2-3 divided doses

Pharmaceutical company
Warner Lambert. Morris Plains, NJ.
Source
University of Pittsburgh Drug Information and Pharmacoepidemiology Center. Pittsburgh, PA.

 zopolrestat

Brand name
Alond

Use
an aldose reductase inhibitor for use as an adjunct to diet to lower blood glucose in patients with non-insulin-dependent diabetes mellitus

Usual dosage
oral: clinical trials have used doses in the range of 50-1200 mg/day

Pharmaceutical company
Pfizer Laboratories Inc. New York, NY.
Source
Stadtlanders Managed Pharmacy Services. Pittsburgh, PA.

 Zorac

Generic name
see tazarotene

Zyban

Generic name
see bupropion hydrochloride

 zymosan

Brand name
Betafectin

Use
prevention of postoperative infection

Usual dosage
intravenous: 0.1-2mg/kg doses were investigated in early clinical trials

Pharmaceutical company
Alpha-Beta Technology Inc. Los Angeles, CA.

Source
Stadtlanders Managed Pharmacy Services. Pittsburgh, PA.

 Zyprexa

Generic Name
see olanzapine

 Zyrkamine

Generic name
see mitoguazone
▶ *As of June 23, 1997, the FDA Oncologic Drugs Advisory Committee found that there was not substantial evidence that Zyrkamine was effective for treatment.*

 Zyrtec

Generic name
see cetirizine

A

A to Z Index

A to Z Index

A to Z Index

A to Z Index

A to Z Index

A to Z Index

A to Z Index

A to Z Index

A to Z Index

A to Z Index

A to Z Index

A to Z Index

A to Z Index

A to Z Index

A to Z Index

A to Z Index

A to Z Index

692

A to Z Index

A to Z Index

A to Z Index

T

A to Z Index

A to Z Index

Cardiology

Dermatology

Specialty Index

Specialty Index

Emergency Medicine

Endocrinology

ENT, Plastic and Reconstructive Surgery, Oral Surgery, and Maxillofacial Surgery

Specialty Index

Gastroenterology

Specialty Index

Gynecology (*see* Obstetrics and Gynecology)

Hematology (*see* Oncology and Hematology)

Imaging (*see* Radiology and Imaging)

Infectious Disease

Maxillofacial Surgery (*see* ENT, Plastic and Reconstructive Surgery, Oral Surgery, and Maxillofacial Surgery)

Neurology and Neurosurgery

Specialty Index

Specialty Index

Neurosurgery (*see* Neurology and Neurosurgery)

Obstetrics and Gynecology

Specialty Index

Specialty Index

Occupational Therapy (*see* Orthopaedic and Rehabilitation Medicine)

Oncology and Hematology

Specialty Index

Specialty Index

Ophthalmology

Specialty Index

Oral Surgery (*see* ENT, Plastic and Reconstructive Surgery, Oral Surgery, and Maxillofacial Surgery)

Orthopaedic and Rehabilitation Medicine (including Sports Medicine, Chiro, Podiatry, OT, and PT)

Specialty Index

Specialty Index

Pediatrics

Specialty Index

Pharmacology (refer to Drugs in Topic Index)

Physical Therapy (see Orthopaedic and Rehabilitation Medicine)

Plastic and Reconstructive Surgery (see ENT, Plastic and Reconstructive Surgery,

Oral Surgery, and Maxillofacial Surgery)

Podiatry (see Orthopaedic and Rehabilitation Medicine)

Pulmonary and Respiratory

Specialty Index

Specialty Index

Radiology and Imaging

Rehabilitation Medicine (*see* Orthopaedic and Rehabilitation Medicine)

Respiratory (*see* Pulmonary and Respiratory)

Sports Medicine (*see* Orthopaedic and Rehabilitation Medicine)

Surgery

Specialty Index

Specialty Index

Specialty Index

Specialty Index

Specialty Index

Specialty Index

Specialty Index

Specialty Index

Specialty Index

Diagnostic Procedures

Topic Index

Drugs

Topic Index

Should future issues of Stedman's WordWatcher be available via the Internet?

YOU TELL US!

Now that you've seen the book, will you take just 2 minutes to tell us what you think about an ELECTRONIC version of Stedman's WordWatcher content delivered direct to you over the Internet?

When you're done, just pop this card in the mail. No postage needed. THANK YOU!

Here's how we see it...

Stedman's ELECTRONIC WordWatcher would be a WIN/WIN95-only product. The content would be organized and searchable along the same lines as the current print publication. You'd be able to look up data alphabetically, and by topic or specialty.

You'd get the complete program via download from the Stedman's Online website (www.stedmans. com) and be able to receive downloadable updates 3 times a year. Each update would include approximately 260 entries, each consisting of drugs, clinical trials, instruments/devices/equipment, surgical operations, lab tests, and diagnostic procedures.

The cost of the first issue and each update thereafter would be $19.95. You would decide how often you wanted to update and would owe no money until right before you actually download the update.

Now tell us what you think...

1. What is your initial impression of Stedman's ELECTRONIC WordWatcher as described?
   ☐ Very favorable   ☐ Favorable   ☐ Negative   ☐ Very negative
   Why? _____

2. Would three updates per year be adequate for your reference needs?
   ☐ yes. Why? _____
   ☐ no.   If not, how many updates per year would you prefer to see?   ☐ 1   ☐ 2   ☐ 4 or more

3. What do you think of the $19.95 price for each installment?
   ☐ Very reasonable   ☐ Reasonable   ☐ Unreasonable   ☐ Very unreasonable
   Why? _____

4. What do you think about receiving Stedman's ELECTRONIC WordWatcher via Internet downloads only? *(Circle the number that best describes your feelings.)*
   1—— 2 —— 3 —— 4 —— 5 —— 6 —— 7 —— 8 —— 9 —— 10
   hate it   no opinion   love it
   Why? _____

5. If you could sign-up for Stedman's ELECTRONIC WordWatcher right now as described — would you?
   ☐ Yes   ☐ No   ☐ Maybe
   Why? _____

ANY OTHER COMMENTS?
_____
_____

Thanks again for your assistance!

May one of our researchers contact you again? If so, please provide the following information. Otherwise, feel free to leave blank.

Name _____ Title _____

Firm _____

Address_____

City _____ State _____ Zip _____

Day Telephone (_____) _____ Ext. _____

Fax (_____) _____ E-Mail _____ @ _____

BUSINESS REPLY MAIL

FIRST CLASS   PERMIT NO. 724   BALTIMORE, MD

POSTAGE WILL BE PAID BY ADDRESSEE

ATTN: STEDMAN'S EDITORIAL
PROFESSIONAL LEARNING SYSTEMS
WILLIAMS & WILKINS
PO BOX 1496
BALTIMORE   MD   21298-9724

Topic Index

762

Topic Index

Topic Index

Topic Index

Topic Index

Topic Index

Topic Index

Topic Index

Instruments, Devices, Equipment, Implants

Topic Index

Topic Index

Topic Index

Topic Index

Topic Index

Topic Index

Topic Index

Topic Index

Topic Index

Topic Index

Topic Index

Topic Index

Topic Index

Laboratory Tests

Topic Index

Surgical Operations

Topic Index

Topic Index

Topic Index